TREATMENT OF NEUROSIS IN THE YOUNG: A PSYCHOANALYTIC PERSPECTIVE

Edited by

M. Hossein Etezady, M.D.

JASON ARONSON INC.
Northvale, New Jersey
London

The author gratefully acknowledges permission to quote the first eight lines of "The Beginning," from *The Crescent Moon*, by Rabindranath Tagore. Reprinted with permission of Macmillan Publishing Company from *Collected Poems and Plays of Rabindranath Tagore* (New York: Macmillan, 1937).

This book was set in 10 point Palacio by Lind Graphics of Upper Saddle River, New Jersey, and printed and bound by Haddon Craftsmen of Scranton, Pennsylvania.

Library of Congress Cataloging-in-Publication Data

Etezady, M. Hossein.
    Treatment of neurosis in the young : a psychoanalytic perspective /
    by M. Hossein Etezady.
        p.   cm.
    Includes bibliographical references and index.
    ISBN 0-87668-500-9 (pbk.)
    1. Neuroses in children—Treatment.   2. Neuroses in adolescence—
Treatment.   3. Child analysis.   4. Adolescent analysis.
5. Psychoanalytic Therapy—in adolescence.   I. Title.
    [DNLM: 1. Neurotic Disorders—in infancy & childhood.   2. Neurotic
Disorders—therapy.   3. Psychoanalytic Therapy—in infancy &
childhood.   WS 350.6 E83t   1993]
RJ506.N48E83   1993
618.92'85'20651—dc20
DNLM/DLC
for Library of Congress   93-231

Manufactured in the United States of America. Jason Aronson Inc. offers books and cassettes. For information and catalog write to Jason Aronson Inc., 230 Livingston Street, Northvale, New Jersey 07647.

CONTENTS

CONTRIBUTORS

Helen R. Beiser, M.D.

Training and Supervising Analyst (adult and child), Institute for Psychoanalysis, Chicago. Clinical Professor of Psychiatry, Emeritus, University of Illinois College of Medicine.

LeRoy J. Byerly, M.D.

Visiting Professor, Thomas Jefferson University, Philadelphia, Pennsylvania. Visiting Professor (Adolescent and Child Analysis), College of Physicians and Surgeons, Columbia University, New York. Supervising and Training Analyst (Child Analysis) and Instructor, Child Analysis, Philadelphia Psychoanalytic Institute. Assistant Clinical Professor, Medical College of Pennsylvania.

M. Hossein Etezady, M.D.

Board certified in adult and child psychiatry and trained in child and adult psychoanalysis. Active member of American Psychoanalytic Association, member of Association for Child Psychoanalysis, faculty member of Philadelphia Psychoanalytic Institute, assistant clinical professor at Medical College of Pennsylvania. In private practice. Former clinical director of the psychiatric services at Paoli Memorial Hospital, Paoli, Pennsylvania. Past president of the Regional Council of Child and Adolescent Psychiatry (Eastern Pennsylvania and Southern New Jersey).

Selma Kramer, M.D.

Training and Supervising Analyst, The Philadelphia Psychoanalytic Institute. Professor of Psychiatry, Jefferson Medical College. President, Margaret S. Mahler Psychiatric Research Foundation.

Robert C. Prall, M.D.

Life Fellow APA, AACAP, Life Member APsAnA, IPsAnA, Philadelphia PsAnSoc. Private practice of child, adolescent and adult psychoanalysis

v

and psychiatry in Austin, Texas. Visiting professor, Medical College of Pennsylvania, Philadelphia. Consulting child analyst, Austin State Hospital Children's and Adolescent Units and The Meridell Achievement Center.

Bertram A. Ruttenberg, M.D.

Graduate of the Institute of the Philadelphia Association for Psychoanalysis in adult and child psychoanalysis; also a trained and practicing adult, child, and infant psychiatrist and psychoanalyst. Emeritus Professor of Psychiatry and Human Behavior, Jefferson University College of Medicine, Medical Director of the Center for Autistic Children in Philadelphia.

Charles A. Sarnoff, M.D.

Lecturer, College of Physicians and Surgeons, Columbia University, Department of Psychiatry, Psychoanalytic Clinic for Training and Research, New York. Formerly Director of Child Psychiatry Fellowship Training; lecturer and supervisor in Child and Adolescent Psychiatry, Hillside Hospital, Glen Oaks, New York. Life Fellow, American Psychiatric Association; fellow, American Academy of Child Psychiatry.

G. Pirooz Sholevar, M.D.

Professor and Chairman, Department of Psychiatry, Cooper Hospital/ UMC, Robert Wood Johnson Medical School at Camden, University Medicine and Dentistry of New Jersey. President, Society of Professors of Child and Adolescent Psychiatry. Faculty, Philadelphia Association for Psychoanalysis.

Martin A. Silverman, M.D.

Clinical Professor of Psychiatry, Training and Supervising Analyst, and Chairman of the Child and Adolescent Analysis section at The Psychoanalytic Institute, New York University Medical Center.

PREFACE

Psychoanalytic treatment has traditionally been considered the treatment of choice for neurotic conditions. In fact, the history of psychoanalysis, from its very inception and throughout its later development, has been intertwined with the conceptual and clinical implications of this class of disorders. Even though many practitioners have made extensive use of other modes of treatment in dealing with neurotic symptoms, and while more severe disorders have been subjected to the widening scope of psychoanalysis, neurotic conditions continue to rank most prominently among the indications for psychoanalytic treatment.

Unique to analysis as a modality of treatment, in contrast to all others, is its emphasis on the pathogenic influence of unconscious conflicts. The therapeutic objective of this mode of treatment is the resolution of these unconscious intrapsychic conflicts which may lay the foundation for a multitude of symptomatic manifestations and behavioral disturbances. Since symptoms are merely the surface manifestation of deeper layers of unconscious conflict, addressing the outer crust of these deeply rooted disturbances would be of limited value. Psychoanalytic treatment uses symptoms and manifest behavior in order to reach the deeper elements that are involved in conflict and compromise formation. This modality of treatment may, therefore, be considered the most ambitious of all forms of treatment. Once this treatment has succeeded in adequate resolution of these conflicts, resources once invested in the perpetuation of these conflicts can be available to promote psychological growth and fulfillment of one's potential. Resolution of anxiety-producing conflicts results in enhancement of a sense of security and control, and the establishment of autonomy and inner equilibrium. The ability to realistically assess and appreciate one's own inner resources and values, as well as those of others, expands. One's relationship to others and the world of reality is strengthened. Mature mutuality and social adaptation become sources of joy and self-confirmation. Creativity, sublimation, and enthusiasm can be sustained and nurtured through the liberation of resources that were previously tied up in maintaining fragile defenses, archaic compromise formations, and burdensome fixations. New channels of adaptive expression can be forged, and forward movement may be resumed. Developmental arrest, delay, or deviation may become amenable to repair and correction.

For children and adolescents who are in the throes of rapidly evolving stages of their early development and whose potential and personality are in the process of being shaped and consolidated, this carries lifelong implications and consequences of immeasurable significance. Successful psychoanalytic treatment for the young can pave the way for resumption of normal development and may be an agent of profound change that could enrich the quality of life for the young patient in the present and lay the foundation for a fulfilling and rewarding future. Freedom from disabling anxiety, inhibition, regression, or fixation enables the young individual to meet challenges of development and, in time, to pursue the ambitions and responsibilities of adult life.

Compared with other methods, psychoanalytic treatment is time consuming and places great demands on patient and therapist alike. For the therapist, it requires extensive and highly specialized training only feasible for, and available to, selected individuals who have the acumen and the personal qualities essential to such an ambitious undertaking. It requires a special blend of devotion, sensitivity, empathy, emotional maturity, availability, and personal integrity. It requires self-awareness and mastery of one's own unconscious conflicts, which can be achieved only through the undertaking of one's own therapeutic analysis—for psychoanalysts, a basic training requirement. For the young patient and the family that supports it, psychoanalytic treatment involves expenditure of time as well as emotional and financial resources. It requires a capacity for tolerating substantial frustration. The process itself is slow, often perplexing, and in many ways runs counter to the native trends and the defensive mechanism of the psychological structure. Unconscious resistance against the repressed instinctual drives is ever-present, in both the patient and the therapist. In fact, the success of the treatment itself hinges upon the success with which such resistances are perceived, appreciated, and dealt with.

Resistances against the emergence of the repressed and defenses directed at intrusion of forbidden wishes are ubiquitous features of normal development in children. Mastery of the immature ego over the derivatives of the instinctual drives and the intrusive urgency of the primary process is tentative in young children and is in a state of precarious transition in young adolescents. For these reasons, the age-appropriate normative processes of development may militate against the aims of treatment, which tend to threaten the integrity of the repressive barrier that helps to maintain the dominance of secondary process and to hold in check unwelcome infringements from forbidden infantile impulses. Treating children therefore calls for special familiarity with and awareness of the phase-specific tasks and age-appropriate manifestations of each stage of development. These considerations in turn greatly influence the technique that organizes the approach to the therapeutic objectives.

The technique of treatment of the young differs in major aspects from that of adults. It was originally derived from the understanding gained from the work with adults and was gradually adapted to the treatment of children and adolescents. As our understanding of the analytic process became more refined and observations on early development produced fruit, the technique of treatment of the young also became more coherent and was enriched by ongoing research, observation, and clinical experience. Decades of clinical work and psychoanalytically informed research in early childhood increased our knowledge of the effects of internal as well as environmental factors on object relations, internalization, structure and identity formation, and pathology, as well as our knowledge of the influence of early experience on later development. These contributions not only expanded our grasp of normal and pathological development, they also established a firm theoretical and practical foundation for technique and clinical application. Coincidentally, the treatment of adults had also been strongly influenced by what was learned from our work with children. Although the psychoanalytic treatment of children was originally derived from its adult antecedent, in time it grew to become a guiding light and a major source of enlightenment for treatment of adults.

Both theory and technique of psychoanalytic treatment in children have evolved toward higher levels of complexity and sophistication and continue to be increasingly refined and further elaborated to reach new states of integration and clinical utility.

The present volume has been prepared and organized with the purpose of presenting a comprehensive account of the psychoanalytic treatment of neurosis in children and adolescents, and to present an in-depth update of this important modality of treatment in its present state. It is intended as a source of reference for clinicians of all persuasions who are concerned with the treatment of children and adolescents. For students of the field, as well as those who teach or train future clinicians, this reference offers an update on the current concepts as it clarifies questions of technique and areas of controversy. Presentations have been prepared by experienced clinicians whose contributions are grounded in their own work and bear the mark of their own individual style and unique approach to the topics under consideration. Rather than emphasizing uniformity and tightness of organization, the material presented here is characterized by variety of form and freedom in selection of content.

Topics under discussion consist of beginning treatment; formulating the dynamics; the working alliance and the real relationship; the conduct of the psychotherapeutic interview; transference; the use of dreams, play and fantasy; resistance; interpretation; countertransference; and termination.

At a time when the economic, social, and political realities of our environment militate against application of the more ambitious and long-term methods of treatment, intimate familiarity with this mode of intervention is needed to assure judicious case selection where the potential for success might be high and achievement of satisfactory results might be reasonably expected. To all those who are involved with treatment and mental health of the young, this familiarity can also be helpful in recognizing the need and to seek, recommend, or apply this ambitious modality when clinical indications so dictate. Otherwise, under the ever-increasing pressures and the restrictive influence of third-party providers, suitable candidates might be deprived of the first-choice, long-term treatment that their condition requires.

M. Hossein Etezady, M.D.

1

Child Analysis Today

Selma Kramer, M.D.

Historical Perspectives

Sigmund Freud discovered and explicated the relationship between the child's experiences within the context of his family and the development of neurotic problems in the adult. From its inception, the clinical application of psychoanalysis was limited to the treatment of adults; it was many years before the field of psychoanalysis could span the gap between this direct treatment of adults and the direct treatment of children. (Today, some of Freud's early cases, such as that of Dora [Freud 1905], would be considered to be adolescents.)

Kramer and Settlage (1962) reported that

> Direct work with children was not undertaken by Freud or other early analysts, for at that time they had neither the tools nor the inclination and time to learn the language of the child's communications. The well-known case of Little Hans was the first attempt by Freud to treat a neurotic problem in a child (1909). . . . While this treatment was of exceptional importance, for it had confirmed in the person of the child the truth of what Freud had already established as occurring in children from his experience with adults, this treatment was done not directly but through the child's father, with whom Freud worked and through whom he directed treatment. Subsequently, Ferenczi made one of the first attempts to treat a child directly (1913). He was not successful in adapting the technique used with adults to children, offering as the reason for his feelings that the child "did not cooperate because he wanted to play." [p. 512]

Victorian and post-Victorian men were not accustomed to interacting with children so as to provide the foundation for an analytic experience.

Furthermore, "they also did not fully understand the peculiarities of the child's psychic structure or the needs of the child's undeveloped ego to be helped withstand the onslaught of impulses" (p. 513). Those who could interact with children and understand the child's productions came, in the main, from two fields: teaching (A. Freud, Klein, Hug-Hellmuth, Aichhorn, and others) and pediatrics (Mahler and Winnicott).

As contributions to theory and technique of analysis of the adult burgeoned, the relationship between childhood experiences and later character structure as well as neurotic problems was delineated with increasing precision. However, psychoanalysis of children and adolescents continued to take a back seat to adult analysis. Mahler (June 1, 1962, personal communication) felt that this may have been so because most early child analysts were young women who discussed their work at what was called the "kinderseminar."

Child psychoanalysis slowly gained increasing respect in the late 1920s and 1930s. Wartime immigration of European-born child analysts strengthened the position of child analysis in the United States. However, this writer recalls shock and dismay upon hearing a beloved European-born adult analyst comment at a meeting of the American Psychoanalytic Association in the mid-1950s, "There can be no psychoanalysis of the child; his personality is not sufficiently formed."

Fortunately, this attitude no longer exists. Child analysis is well respected today. With few exceptions, most recent contributors to psychoanalytic theory and technique, especially those areas subsumed within "widening scope of indications for psychoanalysis" (Stone 1954), make excellent use of theoretical and technical contributions from child analysis.

RECENT TRENDS

As taught in the United States, the theory and technique of child analysis derives, for the most part, from concepts spelled out by Anna Freud and her early co-workers. Some parts of England, Europe, and South America reflect a strong Kleinian influence on child analysis. I focus on Anna Freud's child analysis theories because they are the basis for training in the United States. Just as Sigmund Freud's contributions were never static, so did Anna Freud's concepts change over the years, notably in her recognition that an introductory phase was no longer necessary and in her acceptance that some form of transference neurosis may take place in some child or adolescent analyses.

Child analysis no longer rides on the coattails of the psychoanalysis of adults. In fact, it is in the vanguard of psychoanalysis, especially in growing respect for the significance of observational research for understanding and treating the adult, and for the application of certain aspects of child analysis technique to the understanding and treatment of the adult patient. (As I will discuss later, because the child cannot verbally free-associate, the child analyst must be attuned to nonverbal cues, which include many kinetic clues.)

DEVELOPMENTAL PHASES

Theories of infant and child development, based on longitudinal observational research as well as on observation of the growing child, have emerged over the last 40 years. This is to the great advantage of adult as well as child psychoanalysis. These findings interdigitate with Freud's original developmental theories and add to them. Among the contributors are A. Freud (1965), Spitz (1959), Winnicott (1958), Mahler (1979), Greenspan (1979), and Emde (1981). Mahler's developmental theories have had a national and international impact on studies of the development of object relations, together with its applications to the analysis of the "normal neurotic" child and adult as well as to the analysis of patients with borderline or narcissistic pathology.

PREOEDIPAL AND OEDIPAL ISSUES

Mahler's formulation of the symbiosis–separation-individuation process provides ample evidence that conflicts arising in the rapprochement subphase of development may form the basis for, and provide the "shape" of, the infantile neuroses (Mahler 1975). During the rapprochement subphase, the child experiences conflicts between the desire for fusion with the mother and an opposite strong push towards separation-individuation and autonomy.

In this subphase, while development and maturation go apace, there are coexisting oral, anal, and early oedipal phase pressures and conflicts. Superego precursors, often very severe and distorted representations of parental prohibitions, may give rise to intrapsychic conflict when they interact with forbidden impulses and thus create a neurotic picture or a full-blown neurosis. Silverman (1978) referred to Anna Freud's (1965) comment that it is difficult to know "whether seemingly pathological phenomena represent serious disturbances for which therapeutic intervention is indicated, temporary difficulties which the child can be expected to overcome spontaneously in the course of further development, or reactions that are normal at certain developmental stages" (p. 110).

Observers know that in the course of development all children will develop transient evidences of intrapsychic conflict including separation problems, stuttering, tics, and obsessive-compulsive mannerisms, among others. The meaning and tenacity of these symptoms, the appearance of pathological defenses, and interference with normal development must be taken into account when evaluating whether psychoanalysis is indicated for a troubled child.

EVALUATION OF THE CHILD

It is very important to evaluate a child with great thoroughness in order to determine whether psychoanalysis is the treatment of choice. It is equally important to evaluate the family to determine whether they are capable of, and interested in supporting, analysis. Without parental support, analysis. Without parental support, analysis of a child is not possible.

My preference is to interview the parents together as well as separately even before seeing the child. During these interviews, while I obtain the child's developmental history, I attempt to assess the measure of parental health and pathology; to determine the meaning of the particular child and his symptoms to the parents; and to evaluate the strength of the marriage. I prepare them for bringing the child to visit me, hoping to establish that the parents do not present to the child the visit to the analyst as punishment. I also rehearse with the parent what to call me. (A "worry doctor" to the young child; a psychiatrist who wants to determine why the child is unhappy, with the older child.) I emphasize this because too often for my comfort, a parent who is reluctant to help the child face this particular bit of reality may tell the child that I am a friend of the mother, or someone who helps parents choose a better school for the child. When this occurs, even a very young child becomes alarmed at seeing diplomas designating me as a medical doctor. For the child feels that I must be a very frightening person if the parents cannot be truthful.

During an evaluation, I formulate the level of development the child has reached; his frustration tolerance, that is, his ability to delay gratification; the juxtaposition of ego strengths and weaknesses. If I know that my schedule will not permit me to take the child into my own practice, should treatment be necessary, I prepare the parents and the child for a referral to another child analyst during these early interviews. As much as I attempt not to hurt the child by a referral, not to make him feel rejected by me, all who know children will anticipate that this measure does not obviate the likelihood of hurt feelings in the child. But it should help.

In evaluating the milieu of a child of the '90s, it is important to determine whether either parent is a single parent who must work and rear the child. If in an intact family the mother works, as she must in so many two-career families, I ask about child care, its constancy and efficacy. I do not ignore the father as I estimate his role in the family.

That child-care practices in a family have a decided influence upon the transference was made clear to me in the analysis of an adolescent who was afraid to like or trust me. Her fear was that I would be fired, since her mother had fired every nanny the child felt close to. This mother could not spend much time with her children; however, she felt inordinately jealous of care-givers her children seemed to like.

INDICATIONS FOR CHILD ANALYSIS

Anna Freud (1945) stated that

> the decision as to whether a child needs therapeutic help or not can be based on the state of libido development. An infantile neurosis can be treated as a transitory disorder as long as the libidinal organization of the child remains fluid and shows progressive tendencies. Infantile neuroses disappear whenever the normal forward movement of the libido is strong enough to undo neurotic regression and fixation. *When the libido constellations become rigid, stabilized, and monotonous in their expressions the neurosis is in danger of remaining permanently. This means treatment is indicated.* [p. 141, italics mine]

Related to the increasing interest in problems of early development and its vicissitudes, speculation concerning whether the analytic process (not merely in its role in undoing regression and fixation) can constitute a developmental experience has been a subject of contention between some analysts. I think that all child analysts have had the experience in which the child's development appears to proceed, in part at least, from internalizations and identifications with the analyst, together with

concomitant loosening of pathological identifications with primary objects. Psychic structure formation, that is, development, may proceed
because it is facilitated by the analysis. This concept has been challenged
by some analysts. The conflict can perhaps be laid to rest by the
reporting of a sufficient number of child analyses, such as those that are
presented in this volume.

THE AIM AND TECHNIQUE OF CHILD ANALYSIS

This subject was presented in 1945 with a clarity that has not been
surpassed.

> Psychoanalytic technique aims at, in the adult as well as in the child,
> rendering unconscious psychic material conscious, no matter to what
> psychic institution the unconscious belongs. This is effected through
> *interpretation* of those pathological formations of the ego with which it
> wards off the instinctual impulse or its derivatives. By confronting the
> sound, mature portions of the ego through interpretations with those
> pathological formations, we gradually enable the ego to dispose of those
> defenses, so that the deeper unconscious conflict in its ramifications can be
> brought within the searchlight of the conscious. [Mahler 1945, p. 271]

While the aim is the same as that of adult analysis, the *method*
depends upon the physical maturity and emotional development of the
child. A child cannot be expected to be recumbent on the couch; he is
too motor-minded. He cannot be expected to verbally free-associate.
Much of what we expect of the adult patient (to follow the analytic rule)
cannot be expected of the child. The child analyst must be exquisitely
aware of variations in the affect of the child; he or she must translate the
child's kinetic clues and be aware of somatic responses to the evolving
unconscious content of his ideation. In short, the analyst must be
mindful of all kinds of nonverbal communication. These characteristics
of child analysis are becoming increasingly important to analysts of
adults.

I quote from Greenacre and McLaughlin to emphasize that child
analysis is no longer the second-class form of psychoanalysis. Indeed,
child analysis has come of age and is recognized to be in a position of
leadership in psychoanalysis. Tolerance for regression, sensitivity to
transference and countertransference issues, and translation by the
analyst of kinetic signs and somatic symptoms into meaningful analytic

content are among the many contributions from child analysis to adult analytic technique.

Phyllis Greenacre (1971), a most creative and sensitive adult analyst, said:

> I would be even more empathic now about the need to pay attention to nonverbal communication . . . than I have been in years past. The psychoanalytic situation stresses the importance of speech in contrast to action. The analysand's position on the couch, by subtle suggestion, limits the extent of active movement, and the suggestion is furthered by the direction to the analysand to speak whatever thoughts and feelings he becomes aware of during the hour. Yet the movements on the couch, postures, mannerisms, changes in tone and intensity of voice, flushing, sweating, and special states of body tension are all part of the expression of feeling and may represent explicit communications. [pp. 61–62]

A reference to the contributions of child analysis and child developmental studies to transference and countertransference in adult analysis was spelled out by McLaughlin (1981) as follows:

> New knowledge of the complexity and content of transference has come to adult analyses from the fields of child and adolescent analysis and child development . . . and from studies of narcissistic and borderline patients. While they have broken no theoretical ground for countertransference, they have provided opportunity and challenge to the work-ego of the adult analyst to integrate both cognitive and experiential understandings of the range of separation-individuation experiences and the vicissitudes of narcissism in the patient himself. [p. 650]

REFERENCES

Emde, R. N. (1981). Changing models of infancy and the nature of early development: remolding the foundations. *Journal of the American Psychoanalytic Association* 29:179–219.

Ferenczi, S. (1913). Stages in the development of the sense of reality. In *Sex in Psychoanalysis*. New York: Basic Books, 1950.

Freud, A. (1945). Indications for child analysis. *Psychoanalytic Study of the Child* 1:127–149. New York: International Universities Press.

—— (1965). *Normality and Pathology in Childhood*. New York: International Universities Press.

Freud, S. (1905). Fragment of an analysis of a case of hysteria. *Standard Edition* 7:7–122.

—— (1909). Analysis of a phobia in a five-year-old boy. *Standard Edition* 10:5–149.

Greenacre, P. (1971). Discussion of Eleanor Galenson's paper "A Consideration of the Nature of Thought in Childhood Play." In *Separation-Individuation—Essays in Honor of Margaret S. Mahler*, ed. J. McDevitt and C. F. Settlage, pp. 60–69. New York: International Universities Press.

Greenspan, S. (1979). Intelligence and adaptation: an integration of psychoanalytic and Piagetian developmental psychology. *Psychological Issues*, Monograph 47/48. New York: International Universities Press.

Kramer, S., and Settlage, C. F. (1962). Principles and technique of child analysis. *Journal of the Academy of Child Psychiatry* 1:509–535.

Mahler, M. S. (1945). Child analysis. In *Modern Trends in Child Psychiatry*, ed. N. Lewis and B. L. Pacella, pp. 265–290. New York: International Universities Press.

_____ (1962). Personal communication, June 1.

_____ (1975). On the current status of the infantile neurosis. In *Selected Papers of Margaret S. Mahler*, vol. 2, pp. 189–192. New York: Jason Aronson.

_____ (1979). *Selected Papers*. New York: Jason Aronson.

McLaughlin, J. (1981). Transference, psychic reality, and countertransference. *Psychoanalytic Quarterly* 50:639–664.

Silverman, M. A. (1978). The developmental profile. In *Child Analysis and Therapy*, ed. J. Glenn, pp. 109–127. New York: Jason Aronson.

Spitz, R. (1959). *A Genetic Field Theory of Ego Formation: Its Implications for Pathology*. New York: International Universities Press.

Stone, L. (1954). The widening scope of indications for psychoanalysis. *Journal of the American Psychoanalytic Association* 2:567–594.

Winnicott, D. W. (1958). *Collected Papers: Through Paediatrics to Psycho-Analysis*. New York: Basic Books.

2

Working with Parents at the Beginning of Treatment

Martin A. Silverman, M.D.

I have frequently heard from mental health professionals who work with children in intensive psychotherapy or psychoanalysis something like the following:

"Working with children is so great. It's exciting. It's fun. It's challenging. The only problem with seeing children is that they have parents. That's where all the problems come from. They don't cooperate. They make impossible demands. They do things that undo the very things you're trying to accomplish. They don't appreciate or value what you're doing for their children. They rank tutors and tennis lessons as more important than therapy. They repeatedly inconvenience you with requests for schedule changes. They take their children away on trips. They pull them out of treatment just when you're beginning to get somewhere. If only children didn't have parents!"

But children do have parents. In fact, most of the time, if it weren't for their parents, they wouldn't get into treatment in the first place. Very few children ask for treatment on their own; usually it is their parents who bring them for treatment. Even when they have been encouraged to do so by the school authorities or by the pediatrician or by friends or relatives, it is the parents who are concerned enough about their children's welfare to bring them for evaluation and to be willing to go to the trouble and the expense of placing them in treatment when that recommendation is made to them. And it is far from infrequent that we find ourselves relying on the parents to keep their children in treatment, especially at the outset, in opposition to the internal resistance being thrown up against us by the children's neurotic defense constellations.

9

So how can we understand the discrepancy between parents' role as the principal allies and supporters of treatment on the one hand, but also the source of so much difficulty on the other? It is not easy for parents to bring a child for treatment. Not only does it entail acknowledging that something is seriously enough wrong with the child to require professional assistance, but it also tends to imply that the parents have failed in their responsibility to foster healthy development. Parents tend to have painful feelings of shame and guilt, which, more often than not, are more latent or suppressed than they are apparent. Their child's public behavior exposes them as having failed in their quest to be perfect parents producing model children who will bring honor to them and, by narcissistic extension, will achieve and accomplish in exemplary ways that will enhance their own image and extend and enlarge upon their own accomplishments. Parents inevitably have a narcissistic investment in their children. They identify with them, feel responsible for them, feel proud of their successes, feel ashamed and embarrassed by their failures.

When parents bring a child for assessment and then for treatment, they feel conscious and unconscious guilt for having contributed to his or her problems, or at least for not having been wise and powerful enough to prevent them from having arisen. They expect to be blamed for the child's problems, an expectation to which the mental health community has intermittently contributed. When I was a resident in psychiatry, for example, the inpatient children's unit had a sign on the door that read: "Save a boy and you save a man. Save a girl and you save a family." I was pleased to see that this bit of mother-bashing was eliminated by the time I started my child psychiatry fellowship.

It is not easy for parents to transcend their narcissistic wounds, overcome the temptation to protect themselves by subscribing to the seductive notion that emotional problems are chemical in nature and therefore have nothing to do with family experience, and bring their child for psychotherapeutic assistance rather than for pills and nostrums. Their doing so does not mean, however, that they are free from hurt and pain or that they are unencumbered by shame and guilt. It should not really be surprising that they mobilize a host of defenses that then constitute a barrier to smooth and easy, trustful cooperation with the person to whom they are turning over their child for care. The very fact that they have to engage a professional to do for their child what they feel they *themselves* should be able to do tends to be experienced as a narcissistic wound.

The professional who evaluates their child tends not infrequently to be perceived unconsciously both as the bearer of extremely unwelcome, bad news about their child and as the outside judge who pronounces them responsible for the child's problems. Feelings of resentment and hostility, however unfounded, get in the way in such circumstances of cooperating with the very person to whom they have come for help. It is only when these interferences are recognized and dealt with effectively by the professional that an effective therapeutic alliance can be established with the parents that will enable treatment to proceed. Psychotherapy with adults can succeed only if a good working alliance, both on a real relationship level and on a transference relationship level, can be established and maintained between therapist and patient. With children the working alliance has to be established not only with the child but also with the parents. Winnicott observed that there is no such thing as a baby without a mother. In the treatment of children, at least at the outset, there is no such thing as a child without the parents. It is not only the child who has to be evaluated as to the genetics and dynamics of the illness, the pain the symptoms are causing, the motivation for change, the capacity to tolerate the impact of therapeutic regression and withstand the rigors of treatment, the transference potentials, the configuration of the defenses and the kinds of resistances that are likely to emerge, the life situation and the likelihood of its impinging positively and negatively upon the treatment that is being planned, and so on. The parents (and, where they play a significant role in relation to the treatment, grandparents and other significant individuals) also need to be evaluated with regard to these critical matters.

Parents bring a number of fears with them when they bring their children for assistance. They often are afraid that the treatment will not help. They may have known of children who have not been helped by various forms of treatment. They certainly are not encouraged in this regard by what they have been reading in the popular press. Care needs to be taken to dispel unwarranted pessimism, but it also is necessary to include the parents actively in the evaluation and planning process and to describe the kind of treatment that is being proposed and its likely outcome clearly, understandably, and in realistic terms, without undue pessimism but also without embellishment or overambitious promises.

Another fear that parents frequently harbor is that their child will become overly dependent upon the therapist; that is, that they will lose their status as the primary love objects upon whom the child relies for care, protection, nurturance, and love. They consciously or unconsciously worry that the child will develop a greater affection for and allegiance to the therapist than to them. This stems from their unconscious guilt for not having protected their child from developing emotional problems in the course of their development or even for having contributed to their emergence. Their unconscious fear is that in the course of treatment the child will come to blame the parents for his or her troubles and turn away from them. This is an outgrowth from, and exaggeration of, the difficulty parents have in general in coming to terms with their own limitations and human deficiencies. Children need to idealize their parents initially as omnipotent, omniscient, perfect, even exalted beings and to de-idealize them only gradually as they develop their own strengths, capacities, and ability to tolerate the imperfections of life and of the human species of which they are a part. Parents, in their participation in the child–parent interaction that takes place, not only try to live up to their idealization but tend to find the de-idealization process painful. This is so both because of the narcissistic blow that is entailed and because it connotes the passage of their own importance to their child and hence the ebbing of their own strength and vitality, the movement on in their life cycle toward eventual enfeeblement, superannuation, and death. Therapists need to be very sensitive to this latent set of anxieties in parents who bring their children for treatment, so that they can inculcate a sense of trust in the therapist as an ally who will not blame them, take over their role in the child's life, or strip them of their sense of primary strength, power, importance, and respect in their child's heart and mind.

It is also necessary when working with parents at the outset of evaluation and treatment of a child to be sensitive to the possible presence of secret (conscious) worries and of unconscious worries about their child's health derived from historical, familial factors, which they may not initially be able to share because of excessive shame, guilt, or fear. Parents may worry, for example, about having passed on to the child a serious genetic disturbance they believe might run in their family, or a genetic trait they secretly fear they may themselves harbor. There may be a history in themselves or in close family members of what they believe might be a link to manic-depressive illness or some other serious psychotic disorder. They may harbor the secret, painful belief that they may have passed on a learning disability, or they may worry about the possible implications of a past history of severe adolescent turmoil or a childhood behavior disorder. A family history in near relatives of psychopathic traits, alcoholism, suicide, homosexuality, neurologic disorders, or other conditions they may fear are genetically transmitted may be frightening them. If they are afraid of revealing such things or believe that it is best to let sleeping dogs lie and are afraid of therapy stirring up things that are better left untouched, there may be a serious impediment to possible treatment. Such latent concerns need to be gotten to and dealt with sensitively, patiently, and cautiously, while building up a good, trusting, working relationship with the parents. The same is true of any secret, guilt-ridden history of past episodes of loss of temper with the child on a parent's part, or of overly seductive or overly stimulating behavior that a parent is concerned may have played a part in generating the child's problems.

A particularly difficult issue to deal with is the presence, which more often than not is not readily apparent at the very beginning of treatment, of an unconscious reluctance on the part of one of the parents or at times both parents, namely, of unconscious reluctance to give up certain practices that are contributing to a child's neurotic disturbances. This may be so because the practices are gratifying to the parent or parents, or because they are necessary to sustain a particular family equilibrium that would be upset if those practices were to be given up. A parent may be reluctant, for example, to stop bathing with a child. Or there might be a family practice of walking about nude or scantily clad, rationalized as offering the children a "positive" attitude toward interest in the human body as something to be viewed as natural and free from guilt and shame. A parent may surreptitiously, and without conscious awareness of the ulterior motives involved, encourage a child to come into the parents' bed at night or insist that one of the parents sleep with the child because the parent wishes to be prevented from being able to engage in an intimate, sexual relationship with the marital partner. Parents may give one message to the child, usually verbally, while giving a very different, contradictory message via their actions and subtly communicated attitudes.

These kinds of active, unconsciously motivated and implemented contributions to the very problems for which the parents are bringing their child for help need to be approached and dealt with very differently in different instances. Sometimes it may be possible to ally oneself, patiently and progressively, with the parents' rational desire to help their child, with the result that the parents come to trust the therapist, reveal what is taking place, reflect on it with the therapist, and decide to make sacrifices necessary to facilitate the child's recovery through treatment. Sometimes they prove capable of carrying out their resolve. At other times, however, parents may ask directly, or accept a referral, for consultation with someone else that leads to the conscious decision to give up a gratifying practice that is not in their child's best interest, only to replace it with a more disguised form of the behavior involved. I once analyzed a youngster, for example, whose learning problems stemmed in part from the need to cloud his mind and be unable to grasp the import of what his senses perceived in response to his very attractive and seductive mother's habit of permitting him to periodically observe her nude or only partially dressed. She consulted another child analyst about it after I had expressed some reservation about what she was doing. When he recommended to her that she discontinue the practice, she dutifully complied. Some time later, however, I learned from her son that although she no longer openly exposed him to her unclad body, she periodically carried on a conversation with him while he stood in her room watching her towel herself after a shower, via the mirror that was mounted on the bathroom door that stood slightly ajar.

At times, it is necessary to guide one or another parent into treatment of his or her own in order to permit the treatment of a child to have any chance of succeeding. This was so with regard to the mother who could not stop herself from holding her son's interest in her by surreptitiously exposing herself to him despite her conscious awareness that it was necessary for her to discontinue it. At other times, it becomes evident that there is so much irremediable, neurotic acting out within the family or so much irreducible turmoil that although intensive psychotherapy or psychoanalysis clearly is indicated for a youngster brought for treatment, it has to be postponed until later on or replaced altogether by one form or another of family therapy.

A 7-year-old girl, for example, was brought for treatment because of phobic preoccupations and a behavioral disturbance that took the form of temper tantrums and of clinging, demanding, abusive behavior with her mother at night and in the morning. Although evaluation of the child clearly pointed in the direction of intensive psychotherapy for her largely oedipal, neurotic conflicts in the presence of favorable motivation and a strong, core ego organization, she insisted on her mother being present during all her sessions after the initial, evaluative ones. It soon became clear that her neurotic struggles were intricately interwoven with a dysfunctional family interaction in which an overwhelmingly powerful sadomasochistic interaction between her parents had become organized around disputes between the parents over their relationships with her. Her father was insisting that she be in treatment "to stop creating the distress and turmoil in the family" that actually stemmed primarily from what was going on between the parents. A complex family therapy approach, involving a shifting pattern of sessions with individual family members and various combinations of family members, emerged out of what turned out to be a protracted evaluation process. To have collaborated with her parents in forcing this little girl to undergo intensive psychotherapy for what was viewed as "her problems" without involving her parents (who would not accept referral to another therapist) would have been detrimental in that it would have given an authoritative stamp to a fictional attribution to her of responsibility for the family troubles.

The ways in which the individual, neurotic struggles of a child brought for treatment fit in with and interdigitate with the family dynamics always need to be elucidated at the beginning of treatment. The importance of the child's struggles, as reflected in the presenting symptoms and their underlying dynamics, in the overall patterns of interaction within the family is an essential ingredient of the initial evaluation. It is necessary to determine not only how the family dynamics are influencing the child's dynamics, but also how changes in the child's dynamics are likely to affect the family dynamics and therefore the ability of the parents to accept changes in the child without having to oppose or interfere with further change.

Two dramatic examples involve an 8-year-old girl who was brought by her parents for assistance because of incapacitating phobic and phobic-obsessive symptoms of which her parents wanted her cured, and a 17-year-old girl whose anorexia and school phobia caused her parents enormous grief. When the 8-year-old girl expressed powerful motivation to enter psychoanalysis, it quickly emerged that her parents had an enormous investment in her being ill to distract them from their intense hostility toward each other and to pull them together on her behalf instead of being so enraged at each other that they harbored terrifying, murderous feelings toward one another. As soon as she began to settle down, feeling more secure in the knowledge that help was on the way, one rationalization after another emanated from the parents to interfere with the beginning of the analysis, which, of course, never could get under way.

The 17-year-old girl was referred by someone who practiced at such a distance from the family home that it was impracticable to see her more than once or, at most, twice a week. We moved toward and then into a three-times-weekly psychotherapy in which the patient began to overcome her immaturities and summon up the courage to begin to pull away from her anxious clinging to her mother, to get a job, to begin to date young men, and to think about moving out of the parental home. Her mother, who, it then became clear, was extremely unhappy in her marriage to the patient's father, began to place one obstacle after another against the treatment, despite all the efforts expended by patient and therapist alike to work with her so as to save the treatment situation. The mother soon broke off the treatment, with the support of the patient's father, and brought her back to the initial therapist for twice-weekly treatment, rationalized by an argument he accepted. That treatment too was disrupted, predictably, 6 months later, with the rationalization that traveling that far for treatment interfered too much with activities that were necessary for the girl, who agreed with her mother at that point to quit her job, break off with the boyfriend of whom her mother disapproved, enter a local college, and live at home.

Even where there are no formidable resistances on the part of the parents against intensive treatment that leads to major change in the child and within the family dynamics, careful assessment of the family patterns and of what is going on psychologically within the parents is invaluable in pointing the way toward appropriate technical decisions during the opening phase of a psychoanalysis or intensive psychotherapy. This is illustrated by the contrast between the opening phase of the psychoanalytic treatment of a 5-year-old boy with a gender identity disorder and that of a 6-year-old girl with intense phobias, obsessions, and panicky temper tantrums. The boy's mother had bonded to him initially in a highly ambivalent manner that had interfered with his capacity to achieve a secure, safe sense of his own identity and intactness and had contributed to a burden of enormous guilt that aggravated her deep distrust of and ambivalence toward males in general. Following signs from both the boy and his mother that the opening phase had to include the two of them, who had not psychologically differentiated from one another but were ambivalently interlocked with one another, the analyst agreed to have the mother present during the psychoanalytic sessions, which were gradually increased in frequency, for 6 months before they were ready to shift to sessions for the child alone.

The little girl, in contrast, was brought for analysis after the mother had been advised by her own therapist to shift from twice-weekly psychotherapy to psychoanalysis four times a week, which her mother was very reluctant to do. It became evident during the evaluation that the mother, whose own mother had become irreversibly psychotic during the mother's childhood, had been terrified of the recommendation for psychoanalysis for herself because of the unconscious fear that she would respond to the regressive impact of psychoanalysis by becoming psychotic. She had unconsciously decided to bring her daughter to a psychoanalyst for evaluation and treatment instead of placing herself in analysis, to try it out on her, as it were. It became clear that psychoanalysis was indicated for the little girl, but the analyst was mindful of the circumstances in which the treatment had been initiated. When this patient, with subtle encouragement from her mother, sought to have the mother join her for the opening sessions of the analysis, the analyst did not agree to the request but made it clear that the treatment was for the little girl alone and that he would wait for her to become able

3

The Therapeutic Alliance

L. J. Byerly, M.D.

The concept of the *therapeutic alliance* (Greenson 1967, Kanzer 1975, Zetzel 1956), since its inception, has been considered as "ambiguous and controversial" (Moore and Fine 1990, p. 195). In this regard, the therapeutic alliance shares a fate similar to many other analytic terms and concepts. Anna Freud (1968 [1967]), commenting on the progression of the usage of most analytic concepts, makes the following observations: "Most of these concepts owe their origin to a particular era, or to a particular field of clinical application, or to a particular technical procedure (p. 96)." The tendency in psychoanalysis is then to carry these concepts forward unaltered and unresponsive to the changing clinical field, subjecting it to increasing ambiguities and controversies. The therapeutic alliance is just such a case in point, and A. Freud's remarks are relevant to our understanding of the conflict surrounding it.

The therapeutic alliance had its origin in the earliest beginning of psychoanalysis. It was conceived in its rudimentary form by Freud as a technical procedure that, in many ways, has proven to be its nemesis. In the interim,

> psychoanalytic theory has been a gradual shift from viewing objects as the repositories of drives (Freud 1905/1953), to objects as fantasy figures (Klein 1948, Fairbairn 1962), to objects as psychic representations of real people (Sandler and Rosenblatt 1962). Alongside of this shift has been a continuing debate about whether human social motivation is best conceived as motivated by the desire for sexual/sensual pleasure or the desire for human contact and relatedness. [Weston 1990, p. 27]

The last major reformulation of the treatment alliance occurred at a time when the entire analytic process was being examined from a fresh perceptive (Loewald 1960, Stone 1960).

It is characteristic of most analytic concepts, when they evoke controversy, to generate considerable emotional commitments to the various arguments and positions that follow. Perhaps no area of psychoanalysis is invested with more emotional intensity than the field of psychoanalytic technique. It has harbored some of the most fiercely fought battles in psychoanalysis (Greenson and Wexler 1969). One of the direct points of conflict around the therapeutic alliance deals with the technical aspects of transference. For many, analysis, psychoanalytic technique, and transference are inseparable terms. Child analysis, in developing its own technique, despite the fact that it incorporated the general principles and theories of adult analysis, had to ward off the same technique—transference biases (Kramer and Byerly 1978).

The nominal disagreement in defining and conceptualizing the therapeutic alliance does not do justice to the depth and extent of the conflict engendered. It is important, for example, to recognize that therapeutic alliance issues are not simply relegated to disputes over separating the treatment alliance from the transference. More fundamentally, therapeutic alliance issues disturb the very hearthstone of analytic technique—the rule of abstinence, analytic neutrality, and the blank-screen concept. It brings onto center stage the difficult problem of reformulating and dealing with the frustration–gratification problem inherent in the analytic process.

The therapeutic alliance (Zetzel 1956) and the working alliance (Greenson 1967) are "roughly equivalent terms" (Moore and Fine 1990, p. 175). The term *working alliance* is considered by some analysts to convey more concisely the concept of the collaborative, unified effort of both the patient and the analyst in their engagement of the therapeutic process (Greenson 1967, p. 192). The concept of the therapeutic alliance rests on two major premises:

The separation of the therapeutic alliance from the transference. The rational aspects and the nontransference elements of the analytic process are assigned to the therapeutic alliance, while the irrational aspects and the regressive elements are assigned to the transference.

The establishment of a real relationship within the analytic process. This implies "that the analyst can be perceived as and reacted to in part as a 'real person,' a dynamism free of transference conflict" (Moore and Fine 1990, p. 195).

HISTORICAL REVIEW

Freud's humanism and human reactions with certain patients are frequently cited as indicative of his acceptance of the concept of the

analytic process providing for a new experience (the analyst as a new object) as well as providing for the transference neurosis (the analyst as a transference object). The documented cases of the Rat Man (Freud 1909) and the Wolf Man (Freud 1918) are most frequently mentioned. In both cases, Freud utilized educational means, gratification, and empathetic responses along with interpretation in the therapeutic process. Both cases involved Freud acting outside the circle of abstinence and neutrality. It should also be noted, however, that these cases probably represented borderline pathology (Blum 1974, Glenn 1981) and that his principles of neutrality and abstinence were not well developed when he was engaged in these cases (Aronson 1986).

Even though Freud never explicitly described the concept of a therapeutic alliance, its existence is implied from the earliest stages of his writing to the end of his work. As early as 1895, Freud spoke of making the patient a collaborator in the treatment process, and as late as 1938, in his last work, he advanced the idea of a therapeutic pact between the patient and the analyst (Freud 1938, Sandler et al. 1973). There is ample evidence to indicate that Freud paid particular attention to establishing a treatment alliance with his patients to support the analytic work. As part of this rapport, Freud considered the analyst's primary role to be one of nonintervention and "sympathetic understanding" (Freud 1913, pp. 139–140). Freud divided the transference into a positive transference component and a negative transference component. The positive transference was further divided into warm and affectionate feelings directed toward the analyst, which were within the patient's conscious awareness; and unconscious return of repressed transference elements (Freud 1912). Statements are frequently made in the literature that for Freud the presence of a positive transference was sufficient to support the analysis, that the need for a separate therapeutic alliance was unnecessary. Sandler and colleagues (1973) correctly noted, however, that this is an "incorrect use of the term, 'the positive transference,' to designate the treatment alliance" (p. 25). As Sandler commented, warm and affectionate feelings toward the analyst do not constitute a treatment or therapeutic alliance. Such a definition of the therapeutic alliance would be deceptively simplistic. We need to keep in mind that the therapeutic alliance contains both conscious and unconscious elements (Sandler et al. 1973).

With the advent of the structural theory, Sterba (1934) was able to forcefully draw attention to the fate of the ego in the analysis. His paper on the identification with the analyst emphasized the importance of their mutual interaction and effect on the therapeutic process (Greenson 1967). The delineation of the observing ego and its separation from the experiencing ego became an essential part of understanding ego identification in the therapeutic alliance and the transference. By 1936, the debate around the nature of the therapeutic action was increasingly devisive. Sterba maintained the predominant view that although attachment was a preliminary factor in analysis, interpretation was the nature of analytic cure. At that time, however, psychoanalytic technique was predominantly controlled by Strachey's (1934) pivotal paper on the nature of the therapeutic action. Strachey's paper served to incorporate Freud's structural theory into clinical psychoanalysis. His formulations included the introjection (internalization) of analyst's superego by the patient. This set the transference interpretation (mutative interpretation) as the sine qua non for therapeutic intervention. All other forms of interpretations were regarded as inconsequential. Even as late as 1961, at the Edinburgh Conference, Gitelson had to reassure his audience that he believed in the primacy of the interpretive process in therapeutic action, as he defended the importance of a therapeutic alliance in the opening phase of analysis (Blatt and Behrends 1987).

It was not until Rapaport and Gill (1959) moved psychoanalysis into the era of the metapsychological points of view that the advances of ego psychology, defense analysis, and the general aspects of development impacted on the understanding of the analytic process (Sandler et al. 1973). The marked increase and interest in viewing the analytic process from different perspectives led to direct consideration of separating the rational from the irrational aspects of the transference. Fenichel (1941) was one of the first to describe a "rational transference," which he defined as an aim-inhibited positive transference that was necessary for analysis. Zetzel (1956) introduced the term *therapeutic alliance*, which has become the predominant analytic term to describe these concepts. Stone's (1960) work on the analytic situation led him to differentiate between a mature transference and the oppositional primordial transference. By 1965, Greenson had introduced the term *working alliance* and described the clinical manifestations of the treatment alliance.

Increasingly, the work of child analysis, infant observations, and the interest in preoedipal pathology precipitated the "widening scope of psychoanalysis" (Stone 1954, Valenstein 1980). This activity allowed the analytic process to be viewed from another and different perspective. Loewald's (1960) seminal paper on the therapeutic process was the keystone paper in this group. In it he explored the multitude of relationships that are encountered in the analytic situation. Gitelson (1962) contributed to the concept of an auxiliary ego as a component part of the treatment alliance. Greenacre (1968) used her vast experience with the analytic process to introduce and describe a basic transference.

THE IMPLICATIONS FOR CHILD ANALYSIS

Freud's emphasis on the absolute need to develop a positive transference before beginning the analysis had far-reaching implications for child analysis. The development of child analysis had two major and divergent sources of origin–Anna Freud and the Vienna School, and Melanie Klein and the Berlin School. Ultimately both of these groups became identified with the British Psycho-Analytic movement.

For Anna Freud, the imperative need for a positive relationship with the child led her to establish a mandatory, nonanalytic preparatory phase before initiating a child analysis. In attempting to duplicate (that is, to apply the technique of adult analysis to the child), she was faced with many impurities (A. Freud 1966). Among these impurities she listed the child's immaturity, his inability to free-associate, his incompletely developed and dependent superego, and finally his inability to withstand instinctual pressure. In addition to these developmental differences that separated the child from the adult, there remained the technical aspects of dealing with the child's strong defenses and resistances and the difficulty of interpreting the transference to the child. For these reasons, an introductory/preparatory phase was introduced by Anna Freud. Subsequently, both critics and advocates came to view this phase as one of gratifying the child and seducing the child into treatment. In brief, the gratification–frustration formulas implicit in the analytic process shifted considerably toward not frustrating the child, based on the rationale that the child's capacity for frustration was limited. His inability to tolerate abstinence permitted, indeed demanded, that the neutral position (neutrality) be abandoned.

Over time, Anna Freud changed much of her thinking and abandoned her position on the child's need for an introductory/preparatory phase (pre-analysis). Among the reasons for her change of attitude was Bornstein's ingenious use of defense interpretation, which, according to Anna Freud (1966), removed the difficulty of interpreting transference to the child and, importantly, "created a treatment alliance with the child" (p. 52). The correlation between interpretation and establishing a therapeutic alliance should be noted in Anna Freud's thinking.

Melanie Klein and her followers were less encumbered with differentiating the child from the adult as they developed their technique for dealing with child in analysis. They viewed the child as capable of using free association and did not encounter sparsity or difficulty in identifying a consolidated transference. In addition, they considered the child, in general, capable of withstanding moderate frustration in the analytic situation. Given these conditions, the Kleinians simply applied adult technique to the child analytic process, finding no appreciable need to modify technique. This included more or less maintaining the neutral position. Early symbolic interpretation from the beginning of the child's analysis became the hallmark of their technique. The shift among the Kleinians away from the phallic-oedipal phase of development to their predominant interest in the oral stage has provided considerable exploration of the preoedipal phases of development. In this regard, the oral phase in their theories has become the main source for the development of the superego and the formation of character, and has contributed materially to our understanding of the "widening scope of psychoanalysis" (A. Freud 1966, p. 52).

THE REAL RELATIONSHIP

Having considered and explored, to some degree, the therapeutic alliance from the vantage point of the transference, we need to consider another aspect of the alliance – the establishment of the real relationship within the analytic process. Zetzel (1956) described the therapeutic alliance as resulting in the formation of a new-ego identification, which was defined in terms of object relation. Both the new object and the transference object in the analytic process are variations of object relation, thus confirming the dominant role object relations play in the therapeutic alliance. A further consideration is important to note. The therapeutic alliance is an artifact, a functional construct of the analytic process. In contrast, the real relationship is "the realistic and genuine relationship between patient and analyst" (Greenson 1967, p. 217).

The importance of the real relationship for the analytic process, according to Greenson (1967), has primarily to do with reality testing. It provides a means of comparing what is real in the patient's relationship to the analyst against what is distorted (transference), and what is real in the analyst's relationship with the patient against what is distorted (countertransference). In outline form, we can then say:

In both the patient and the analyst, transference reactions are unrealistic and inappropriate, but they are genuine and truly felt.

In both, the working alliance is realistic and appropriate but it is an artifact of the treatment situation.

In both, the real relationship is genuine *and* real (Greenson 1967, p. 217).

These three modes of interrelating in the treatment situation form the matrix of therapeutic action. In addition, all three modes are not only interrelated structurally but condition and determine the function of each other. Kohut (1971) referred to the supportive elements in this interrelated state as the realistic bond, emphasizing the interplay between outer and inner reality.

Levine (1992) presented the proposition that there is an increasing polarization among analysts, reflected in their clinical approach in dealing with the real factors in analysis. He described the first of these two schematically opposite positions as consisting of those analysts who stress the real factors in the analytic relationship. They base their arguments on at least three major premises:

First, on *tradition*, in citing Freud's 1912 paper in transference in which he clearly distinguishes between non-objectable parts of the analytic relationship that do not need immediate interpretation and which foster the treatment alliance.

Second, arguments from *ego psychology*. The real elements in the analytic situation are considered as representative of the patient's ego functions (autonomous/conflict-free areas) and, as such, should be respected, since they lie outside of the transference area.

Third, *behavioral manifestations*. The patient's overt experiences have major therapeutic value that need to be directly and consciously managed.

In brief, those analysts who make a clear distinction between transference and nontransference elements in the analytic situation tend to accept more readily the existence of real factors in the analytic relationship. Such analysts lay increased emphasis on the analyst's characterological traits, such as empathy, honesty, fair-mindedness, dependability, reasonableness, and so on. These traits are regarded as indispensible in supporting the analytic situation and, by some analysts, as an important part of the therapeutic action. This group of analysts will also have more of a tendency to view the rule of abstinence in its strict application as a form of deprivation, and not as consistently helpful in the treatment situation.

The other polarized group of analysts will have a greater tendency to adhere to the classical model (Valenstein 1979) and will tend not to deviate from this model. The triad of premises that unite this group can be stated as

1. The primacy of interpretation in the therapeutic action

2. A relatively strict adherence to the rule of abstinence and maintaining neutrality
3. The tendency to treat the different factors in the patient–analyst relationship in the analytic situation as suspect of transference.

The psychoanalytic dialogue around the therapeutic alliance between these two groups is expressed in their respective tendency to view the alliance as either an enabler or a resistance (Hanly et al. 1991). Brenner (1979), as spokesperson for the latter group, has been critical of Zetzel, Stone, and Greenson, in particular, for their departure from the principles of abstinence and neutrality. Although Brenner argues against the necessity for and existence of a therapeutic alliance phase in analysis, his arguments are less than convincing. From a clinical point of view, it is easier to agree with Sandler and colleagues (1973) that the transference elements are extensive and are carried into the other modes of relationship (the therapeutic alliance and the real situation). The same arguments can also be made for the appearance of conflict elements in all three modes. That is, the concept of conflict-free, aim-inhibited states in the therapeutic alliance and the real relationship is a relative concept (Schowalter 1976). The transference is pervasive and can dominate the therapeutic relationship in certain circumstances (i.e., the eroticized transference). Also, there are certain personality disorders controlled by sadomasochistic attributes that need to defeat the analyst's therapeutic efforts—an antitherapeutic alliance (Sandler et al. 1973, quoting Sodre 1990).

Most of the criticism logged against the concept of the therapeutic alliance is based on concern and fear that the shift of emphasis from the transference to the real relationship will go too far toward the real relationship. Curtis (1979) elaborated the danger inherent in such a shift, not only in terms of a failure to deal with hidden transference manifestation but also from the vantage point of endangering other nuclear analytic concepts. He enumerates these nuclear analytic concepts as unconscious intrapsychic conflict; free association; and a failure of interpreting resistances. The perceived danger is that the therapeutic action will stop forming along transference lines and a substitute therapeutic alliance will provide a new and corrective object relationship that will become the goal of therapy (Sandler et al. 1973).

Disagreements and conflicts in the course of psychoanalytic development over manipulating and controlling real relationships as a therapeutic end in itself have been anathema for psychoanalysis. In the 1920s, Ferenzi and Rank's active technique caused an intense debate (Glover 1924, 1928). Alexander and French (1946) created a second major crisis when they proposed replacing the transference neurosis with the transference relationship, the corrective emotional experience (Rangell 1954).

OBJECT RELATIONS AND THE THERAPEUTIC ALLIANCE

Both the transference and the therapeutic alliance are composed of various features of object relations. The unfolding of object relations in an individual is based not only on ego psychology (defense, etc.) but on development itself (Byerly 1990, Meissner 1989, Pine 1985). Masterson (1992) is typical of many of the present analysts who, increasingly, are emphasizing viewing the therapeutic alliance from the theoretical approach of object relations. In addition to the advantage of providing for the utilization of the real object and reality testing as an instrument to measure and judge the analytic relationship, he also describes further advantages in correlating object relations with the therapeutic alliance:

> [The therapeutic alliance] provides an architecture of the patient's inner emotional life—self and object representations with their linking affects, ego defense mechanisms and functions—which allows the therapist to identify and understand the ebb and flow of the patient's emotions; it informs the therapist as to what emotional state must be dealt with and how to deal with it. [p. 179]

Masterson's work (1992) deals primarily with the borderline and narcissistic disorders. These personality disorders are characterized by a less consolidated transference and a weakened capacity to form a therapeutic alliance. Typically, individuals with these disorders do not relate to the analyst in a transference manner, but rather in a transference-acting out manner (behaviorally). This represents their style of relating as well as their style of defending against their anxiety and depression. The etiology of these disorders is generally considered to be developmental arrests during the narcissistic (preoedipal) phase of development. Clinically the child in analysis, particularly the preschool child and the regressed adolescent, will present the analyst with similar technical problems as those encountered in working with patients with narcissistic and borderline disorders. In both, the establishment and the maturing of the therapeutic alliance becomes the critical factor in establishing and maintaining the transference reaction. That is, in both the child and the patient with narcissistic disorder, the tendency toward transference of affect into action (self-activation) is controlled by the therapeutic alliance.

The literature contains two divergent views regarding the manner in which object relations are correlated with the therapeutic alliance. Anna Freud (1962 [1961]) does not feel that early developmental stages are carried forward, incorporated in any meaningful way, in the formation of the therapeutic alliance. Rather, she considers the oedipal phase as the major stage of object relations, the stage that contributes the most significant components to the formation of the therapeutic alliance. Among the developmental achievements of the oedipal period she cites, as major constituents of the therapeutic alliance: the observing aspect of the ego, the capacity for insight, and the give-and-take development of the ego. It is the establishment of object constancy that permits the ego differentiation necessary for this increased ego participation in the analytic process. In many ways, her position describes an advanced, more idealized state of structure development that also permits a correspondent increase in a consolidated transference reaction. Settlage (Van Dam 1966) maintains that structuralization during these developmental stages results in object constancy, ego autonomy (control and modulation of drive derivatives), and crystallization of the superego (incorporation of parental values). Accompanying functional features include increased capacity for self-concept differentiation, reality testing, and secondary process. Consistent with this finding, many child analysts hold that the latency period, in part because of these developmental achievements, represents the best time for analyzing a child (Fraiberg 1964).

The more acceptable view regarding the interrelationship between object relations and the therapeutic alliance holds that early object relations contribute significantly to the formation of the therapeutic alliance. The early mother–child dyadic relationship has become the central issue about which such understanding of the therapeutic alliance has been formulated (Greenson 1965, Loewald 1960, Modell 1976, Zetzel 1956). The major emphasis is the similarity and correlation between the mother–child matrix and the dyadic relationship in the therapeutic alliance (the basic transference). As Gitelson (1962) and Spitz (1956) have stated, in this view, the mother–child matrix in early development is the basic foundation for the therapeutic alliance in adult analysis.

Mahler's (1963, 1967, 1972) work and her work with colleagues (Mahler et al. 1975) in the area of mother–child interaction, and her skill in integrating her findings into the mainstream of psychoanalysis have been instrumental in permitting an ongoing reformulation of the therapeutic alliance. For example, Furer (1976) described the therapeutic alliance in terms of Mahler's separation-individuation theory. He called particular attention to the residual aspects of the practicing subphase and the rapprochement subphase of individuation in the therapeutic alliance. As a result of the multiple mutual interactions between the mother and child, a state of empathy is formed. In this regard, empathy becomes the functional extension of basic trust (Erikson 1950), which has developed over the first year of life. In the developing dyadic matrix gestures, somatic responses, signaling, and other preverbal responses between mother and child form the individuation process and are the genetic precursors, the determinants of the therapeutic alliance.

With the explosion of knowledge about infant development (Emde 1980, 1981, Lichtenberg 1983, Stern 1973, 1977, Tyson 1989), there is a growing awareness of the infant's subjective and affectual life, and of the likelihood that many functions and structures may occur earlier in development than we had previously recognized. The impact of our increasing knowledge of these early stages of development should lead to a clearer understanding of the concept of basic trust and early primary methods of identification. Both these concepts are important to the formation of the therapeutic alliance and transference.

An area of exploration that has implication for the therapeutic alliance is the infant's first subject experiences during an undifferentiated, preobject stage of development (symbiosis). The contention would be the infant's capacity in this stage to subjectively experience and identify with the maternal process, that is, with the process itself. Based on our understanding of this preobject related state, we could explore the analytic patient's identification, not with the analyst as a real or transference object but rather with the analytic (therapeutic) process itself. Such conceptualizations would lead us to reexamine the therapeutic alliance as having its precursors and origin in earlier preobject developmental stages and would allow for a primitive identification with a maternal process reconstructed in the therapeutic alliance. Within our clinical work, such identifications with the therapeutic process are more or less familiar and are separate from clear identification with the analyst. For example, we ascribe importance to the patient's wish and desire to be well, attributing such motivational force to his mature ego organization, which can then be enlisted in the working alliance.

Based on these motivational forces, the patient accepts (identifies) with the analyst as a therapeutic agent. The same positive desires are equally instrumental in aiding the patient to accept (identify with) the limitations and contingencies of the analytic (therapeutic) process. In a true therapeutic alliance, both the patient and analyst are subject to the impositions of that process. Even in children and adolescents, where the motivation to change or to be well is not always primary, it remains an important component awaiting expression in the therapeutic alliance. One of the fascinating aspects of child analysis is observing the child struggle with the analytic process in the initial stages of his analysis. The identification of the child with the analytic process is recognized with the passing of his naiveté and openness, with his increasing awareness. At such times he may grudgingly admit or demonstrate that he knows what is going on. Only then, when the child has gained sufficient familiarity with and understanding of the analytic process, will his own insights begin to contribute to the analytic work. It is at this point that we can say "now the child is *in* analysis" (Kramer and Byerly 1992, p. 220).

Bollas's (1987) work has provided us with a possible explanation of the patient's capacity to identify with the therapeutic process in the working alliance. He has postulated a transformational object as a predecessor to the transitional object in development. He reminds us that there is no clear delineation of the object-self in the undifferentiating phases. Within the symbiotic matrix the mother, in the dyadic relationship, is first associated with a process of transformation or an agency of change. According to Bollas, this process of transformation is identified with the "cumulative internal and external transformation" (p. 13) that are the infant's first subjective experiences. By repeated interaction with the mother, the infant experiences changes in his world that are attributable to a process that alters his sense of physical and emotional well-being. The mother literally transforms the infant's internal and external world, not only in terms of libidinal gratification but also in terms of functional ego activities (Bollas quoting E. Jacobson 1965). Consequently, these preobject representations will be retained not as an object relation that emerges from desire but from a perceptual identification of the object with its function: the object as an environmental somatic transformer of the subject (p. 14). If we accept Bollas's premises, then the residual and regressive components of the symbiotic phase of development can be expressed not only in terms of the search for fusion and merger (that is, possession of the object) but also in terms of a search for an object (place, thing, etc.) that alters and changes the self.

Mahler (1967) and Bollas (1987) are in agreement that the holding or facilitating environment (Winnicott 1965) is the organizer of the symbiotic phase. Many analysts would also regard a similar holding or facilitating pattern as the organizer of the therapeutic alliance. They would view the therapeutic alliance not only in terms of a supporting structure to facilitate and maintain the transference but also as a structure that permits and facilitates identification with the analytic process and the real object of the therapeutic alliance. For Mahler, the transformational activity during the symbiotic phase consists of mutual reflections, mirroring functions, and mirroring frames of reference. These primary methods of identification determine the stability or disturbances of the infant's primitive self-feelings. They will lead increasingly to the delineation of the self and beginning of individuation. We will again see these same patterns of mutual interactions between the mother and child when locomotion induces a second major cathartic shift, in the practicing subphase (Mahler 1972). Both the differentiating phase and the practicing subphase are critical in the infant's developing sense of reality and his capacity to integrate. The infant utilizes the mother as an auxiliary ego (Spitz 1956), importantly as a point of reference to whom he looks to make sense out of (integrate) his explorations into his transitional world (inner/outer reality). It is from this primordial sharing position (Werner and Kaplan 1963) that mutual cueing and signal function will lead to symbol formation, a major tool in the developing sense of reality and integration. When the toddler reaches the practicing subphase in individuation, the primitive identification and subjective experiences of the child during the first year of life lead to an increased shared-perceived reality and affectual organization at a higher structural level. The increased capacity of the child to share his "romance with the world" with his mother, and the capacity to share limited intimate separation (Stone 1960), are essential features of the practicing subphase. It is from these shared experiences that the capacity for empathy (Furer 1976) develops in this object relation stage: "A path leads from identification by way of imitation to empathy, to the comprehension of the mechanisms by means of which we are enabled to take up any attitude at all towards another's mental life" (Freud 1921, p. 110).

In summary, we have been considering the possible prototype behavior from the early object relations stage (before the oedipal phase) that could contribute to the functional aspects of the therapeutic alliance. We have identified an analytic holding environment (Modell 1976, Winnicott 1960) that serves at different levels of organization as the organizer of both the symbiotic phase and the therapeutic alliance. We have been following Bollas and have speculated on the contribution of an earlier (preobject relation) stage to the therapeutic alliance. Early identifications with a transformational object would lead to a re-identification with the analytic process itself (i.e., the desire to be well, correlated with the self's desire to be changed).

In addition, we have also placed emphasis on the prototypical functions of the therapeutic alliance found in early object relations states. These included the capacity from a shared position (mother–

child) for the infant/toddler to check reality against one's experience, using another (the maternal object; auxiliary ego) as a point of reference, and using another to make sense out of one's experience (reality testing and integration). In this regard, particularly in treatment with children, the therapist will, at times, need to function in the role of an auxiliary ego (Gitelson 1962). It is important to make a distinction from the original auxiliary ego status of the maternal object and the therapist functioning as an auxiliary ego (Spitz 1956). And, finally, following Freud's direction, we have traced primitive identifications to the formation of empathy in an early object relation stage. Child therapists might, in general, lay more stress on the importance of empathy than would therapists working with adults. There is general agreement that empathy is a facilitator of interpretations and serves an important and useful function in this regard. In addition, however, many child analysts would consider empathy an essential ingredient not only in establishing the therapeutic alliance but also in reestablishing empathic attunement after transference disturbance. Few, if any, child therapists would regard empathy as a mutative factor in and of itself. (For an excellent review of empathy and the analytic process, see Basch 1983.)

Even as the symbiotic and practicing phases may hold special implication for the formation of the therapeutic alliance, it should be noted in passing that the transitional phenomenon (differentiating subphase) may have special implication for the formation of the transference (Byerly 1990). In general, two shared aspects of the transitional phenomenon and the transference neurosis are:

1. the loosening or poorly defined boundaries between inner and outer reality, aspects of a continuing differentiation,
2. a particular form of internalization–externalization aspects of a continuing integration.

In the origin of the transitional phenomenon, the transactional field (mother–child matrix) is frequently described in terms of potential space (Winnicott 1965). A similar phenomenon is considered operative in the transference where boundaries are once more not clearly defined and serve as an explanation of the illusionary quality of the transference neurosis. The point being emphasized is the genetic determinants of the transference process. Each developmental phase contributes its own unique properties to later developmental stages and to the therapeutic alliance and the transference process. However, it is the rapprochement subphase of separation-individuation, as a recapitulation of the separation-individuation process, that leaves its indelible imprint on the transference process and defines more clearly the common characteristics of the transference process.

The disturbances in reality testing characteristic of the transference neurosis have their early determinants in the major shift in the ego's developing function from a dominant defensive stance to a predominant integrative stance in the rapprochement subphase. This major cognitive development results in the toddler being capable of creating his own reality (Lester 1983), that is, distorting reality as a means of integrating his interactional world (representational world). As Sandler and Sandler (1987) have noted, the transference neurosis is not only a distortion of the reality involving the analyst but also involves the recreation of a distorted reality that is representative of a disguised repetition of an earlier experience, a relationship.

A second important common characteristic of the transference neurosis is found in the mutative qualities (therapeutic action) ascribed to the resolution of the transference. Following Stone's (1960) concept of deprivation in intimacy, Blatt and Behrends (1987) concluded that the mutative power in the analytic situation derives from the ongoing tension between closeness and distance in the analyst–analysand matrix. This mechanism (oscillation) is regulated by the transference. It can also be described as the oscillation between gratification and deprivation (the gratification–deprivation formula central to the analytic process previously discussed). The basic model in normal development of deprivation in intimacy, the oscillation between closeness and distance, is found in the toddler's rapprochement struggle between oneness (merger) and separateness (independence). The resolution of this conflict (individuation) is achieved through the process of internalization. It is Blatt and Behrends's (1987) contention that internalization is the basic process through which all psychological development occurs including therapeutic change in analysis. In this regard, they quote Tolpin (1971) in her discussion of the transitional object (transitional phenomenon) that links each step in the separation-individuation process with internalization.

Early transitional stage elements contributing to the transference can be briefly followed through Bollas's (1987) description of the transitional phenomenon. He regards the fate of transformational object as displaced from the "mother-environment (where it originated) to countless subject-objects" (p. 15). The importance of this development is twofold:

1. The infant now has the ability to play with an illusion of his own omnipotence.

2. The movement from his first subjective experiences to his first creative act, which is a cardinal feature of the transitional phenomenon as expressed in the formation of the transitional object.

According to Bollas (1987), the transitional phenomenon takes the infant's experiencing the process and shifts it to articulation of the experience. That is, what was process is displaced into symbol formation. This important aspect of internalization and its relationship to the transitional phenomenon may hold far-reaching implications for understanding transference distortion and resolution. This interrelationship between the transitional phenomenon and the transference is particularly significant if we are in agreement with Blatt and Behrends's (1985) view that assumes "the mechanism of internalization to be the same at all levels [of development], but to involve gradations of self and object differentiation" (Moore and Fine 1990, p. 102).

As stressed previously, object relations theory allows for the integration of development with the tenets of ego psychology. Not only do object relations from all stages of development contribute to the therapeutic alliance and the transference, but their integration leads to the multiple and varied types of therapeutic alliances and transferences we encounter in the analytic process.

CLINICAL CONSIDERATIONS

For Greenson (1967), the "reliable core of the working alliance is formed by the patient's motivation to overcome his illness, his sense of helplessness, his conscious and rational willingness for cooperation, and his ability to follow the instructions and insights of the analyst" (p. 192). Unfortunately, children and adolescents rarely are able to qualify for such a level of motivation. Appropriately, Greenson recognizes that technique needs to be modified to deal with children and certain areas of pathology. It remains that one of the fundamental tasks of the therapeutic alliance is to bring out the child's desire to be well and to change. Unfortunately, children and adolescents suffer more than is generally perceived.

Novick (1990), writing on the therapeutic alliance in children, indulges in a fantasy. In his fantasy, Freud's original patients were all children and the analytic process was derived exclusively from the treatment of children. In this scenario, Novick comments that the therapeutic alliance would not have been taken for granted nor would its core be the desire to get well. Rather, in his judgment, the analytic task would be to create a therapeutic alliance, and its constant maintenance would be the task of the analyst and patient. The central position of the therapeutic alliance is one of the more important subtle differences between child and adult analysis. Child therapists customarily need to, and do, pay more attention to the therapeutic alliance. This is particularly evident in the distinctions the child therapist needs to make between establishing a working alliance and maintaining it. For the child therapist, establishing the therapeutic alliance may involve developing the informative alliance with the parents, and in some cases this may be critical in maintaining the working alliance with the patient (Harley 1974). Invariably, even in dealing with adolescents, the opening phase should include contact with the parents. Depending on the situation, the adolescent's wishes, the nature of the crisis, or a subjective feeling regarding the adolescent's need for independency (to tell his story first), the therapist may elect to see him before seeing the parents, with their consent.

Built into the therapeutic alliance is the structure of treatment. In this opening phase the parents, not the child or adolescent, will be responsible for fees, maintaining regular appointments, missed appointments, and vacations. It is around this integral structuring of fees and appointments that the therapeutic alliance is frequently most vulnerable. The parents' absolute control of time and money—two major aspects of reality for the developing child—may increase the child's feelings of helplessness. They may also serve as a growing resistance for developing transference. A case may illustrate some of these points:

Sarah, 6 years of age, the oldest of three sisters born to two active professionals, came to treatment because of her uncontrolled outbursts of aggression at school. The parents had made an informed and diligent search for a therapist. They belonged to a prepaid health plan to which the therapist did not belong. There was a manipulative and coercive quality to the father's attempt to pressure the therapist to join this group for the financial advantage to the parents. When his efforts failed, he decided to proceed with his daughter's therapy anyway, with the stipulation that the therapist would cooperate with his plan.

During the initial stage of treatment, Sarah on one occasion literally assaulted the therapist, smashing her in the face with a closed deck of cards. When she threatened the therapist again and was restrained lightly, she "tapped" the therapist, threw the cards all over the room, knocking down articles. She ran from the room and told her father the therapist had touched her. During her aggressive outbursts, Sarah screamed at the therapist, "You don't care about me. All you care about is money. I don't want to be here anyway." Even though the father took control of the situation and is supporting treatment, it raises the

question of his unconscious commitment to treatment by which Sarah, acting
out the parents' unconscious, expresses their ambivalent feelings. In a diffuse
manner, transference elements around Sarah's self-concept and self-worth have
invaded the therapeutic alliance. From her history, we can speculate that
transference distortions and displacement from her mother to the therapist will
involve her mother leaving her for work, caring for money more than her, and
her anger over being sent to another "mother" to care for her as she had been
relegated to her father with the birth of her siblings.

Establishing a therapeutic alliance with Sarah will be difficult. It will
depend on the success of finding a means to separate out and isolate the
disruptive transference and displacement elements from the early stages
of treatment until they can be dealt with later in treatment. In equally
broad terms, the therapist, in establishing limits, will facilitate a
"holding position." The major task will be to establish a dialogue
between Sarah and the therapist. Even as it is important to separate out
the irrational from the rational features in her behavior, it will be
important to help her separate her observing ego from her experiencing
ego—by increasingly giving her behavior meaning (interpretations). Her
capacity to identify with the analytic process will be critical to drawing
Sarah into treatment.

Sarah's case illustrates two other major components of the informative alliance—the parents' commitment to treatment and the way
parents prepare the child for treatment. At some point, Sarah's parents
may need to be confronted regarding their unconscious attitude toward
money and the meaning Sarah has for them. Often such issues fade into
transference issues, and confrontations are best dealt with when there is
ample material in the therapeutic setting.

Carlos, a pre-latency-aged child, had been in treatment for over a year. His
parents were inconsistent in supporting therapy and required constant efforts
on my part to support therapy. This included frequent change of appointments,
canceled appointments, and irregular payments. Despite this, Carlos did well in
treatment, bed wetting stopped, and he became a much more alert, interested
child. One day he brought me $500 in play money from his sister's Monopoly
game to pay his bill. I understood that Carlos was telling me that the therapeutic
alliance was in danger and needed my immediate attention. A conference with
the parents established that a long-overdue bill had caused open parental
conflict, which Carlos had overheard. A compromise on payment was reached,
and treatment continued. The transference and displacement issue, as you
might suspect, consolidated as we dealt in the transference with his pseudoma-
ture defenses (his need and tendency to take charge coincided with his longing
and regressive needs to be cared for).

Many children and adolescents are not very well prepared for treatment. Unless parents are particularly careful in the preliminary stages of considering treatment for the child, symptoms, including behavioral problems, can be concretized into being bad; that is, unacceptable or undesirable. The child may then assume, despite parental reassurance to the contrary, that he is bad, and thus treatment is frequently seen as punishment. The parents themselves may see treatment as punishment, judgment against their failed efforts in raising the child. Not only may this interplay of guilt directly set the mood in the informative alliance, but if perceived by the child, it may set the tone for the therapeutic relationship. (Sarah's case may contain some of these factors.) Because the child's entry into treatment cannot be adequately controlled, the meaning treatment has for the child needs to be worked out in the therapeutic alliance and converted or sustained as a mutual effort to effect change in the patient. It is especially important that the therapist maintain a nonjudgmental attitude, despite the child's attempts to align him with the negative aspects of being in treatment. It is around such issues that the character of the therapist becomes a dominant and critical factor in the working alliance. From the therapist's being fair, nonpunitive, reasonable, and understanding, the organization of a new object will form in the therapeutic alliance. It is here, as a bridge from the therapeutic alliance mode to the new object mode, that emphatic attunement serves another one of its ancillary functions. The therapist's conception of the child and his feelings, conscious and unconscious, about the child will not only be evident to the child but will control much of his behavior toward the child. One of the major areas of problems in working with children centers around this topic, which we can only touch on briefly here. Because children live so close to their affects, and because the secondary process is not as well stabilized in children as in adults, the child therapist repeatedly faces dealing with affectual and regressive issues in himself to a greater degree than does an adult therapist. When one adds to this the tendency of the child to transfer affects into action (self-activation), maintaining a positive attitude toward the child is difficult and not always possible. It is only through repeated attempts at understanding the child that the therapist can maintain a therapeutic distance. In this sense *understanding* is to the child therapist what *interpretation* is to the child patient.

After the beginning of treatment, the purpose of the informative alliance is to maintain the treatment (Harley 1974). Frequently, as treatment progresses, the growing involvement of the therapist and child may cause considerable competitive feelings in the parents. Parents deal differently with the child's growing closeness to the therapist and often his accompanying acting out or assertiveness at home. The interplay of guilt we mentioned previously can also result in parents feeling left out, and their guilt over not being able to help their child themselves can also result in narcissistic injury. Resistances generated in the informative alliance can be formidable but, in general, are not the major source of resistance in treating the child.

Two major areas for concern are to be noted in this regard. It is essential to remember that it is *the child* who is in treatment. Information from the informative alliance should always be regarded as secondary to the primacy of the child's material. The child's material should be regarded as adequate for the treatment process. That is to say, the material from parents should follow the treatment process and not lead it. This is equally true in dealing with resistances suspected of coming from the informative alliance. The therapist should first reexamine the possibility of the resistance coming from the child. For example, a missed appointment, despite the parent's responsibility for keeping appointments, may have more to do with the child than the parents. Second, in a related manner, it is not unusual for the parents to deal with some of their resistances to the child's treatment by drawing the therapist into a treatment situation with them. Being involved in such a relationship may be subtle and outside the therapist's area of awareness (unconscious). Such situations are to be avoided. This does not mean that questions regarding the child cannot be answered, or that joint therapeutic goals and plans for the child cannot be worked on together. It is often a judgment call when to refer a parent for treatment, but a cardinal rule would be to do so when their interference with the child's treatment threatens that treatment.

Maintaining the therapeutic alliance can be an arduous task in child and adolescent treatment. It becomes increasingly more difficult as parental influences are disengaged and the developmental thrust is toward independence (individuation). Adolescents by far comprise the group that most frequently discontinues treatment prematurely. Novick (1990), drawing attention to this fact, considers this to be based on the development aspects stated above. There may well be another important factor involved. Sandler and colleagues (1973) comment that with the disappearance of symptoms, the major motivation for treatment also disappears. The motivation for treatment now needs to shift emphasis to the desire to know oneself and understand one's inner world. Generally, with adults in treatment, this is achieved with a smoother transition than it is in the child and adolescent. The child's disruptive manner of dealing with this shift is seen more characteristically with adults in crisis. Once the crisis has passed, one has to "start all over again getting the individual back into treatment." With younger children, the parents' sincere efforts to understand the child can be conveyed to the child and will support a shift in emphasis in treatment. In adolescence, often self-activation, externalization of the adolescent's conflicts and the involvement with the process of experiencing holds more promise of understanding than does the treatment situation. This need not be regarded as a therapeutic failure. If we have achieved the best possible position for the child's ego, and development is progressing, then we may need to interrupt treatment to let the child go (Mahler 1974). Both Mahler and Maenchen favor reentry into treatment, where the child reenters treatment at a later developmental stage (the revolving-door concept of treatment). They consider prolonged treatment in the child and adolescent as possibly interfering with the synthetic (integrative) functions of the ego.

The first and foremost principle in establishing a therapeutic alliance with the child and adolescent is based on his or her need to feel safe, held and understood (Novick 1990). Novick felt that if Freud worked only with children, this would have been the fundamental rule of psychoanalysis. In a schematic, arbitrary manner, we might say that the need to feel safe and to be held will engage more directly the emphatic and realistic aspects of the therapeutic alliance; moreover, understanding will predominantly be the province of interpretation. It is essential that the child therapist act as an auxiliary ego for the immature child whose development and functional capacities are limited. Empathy is fundamentally used in such incidents in an ancillary manner. For example, children may have difficulty verbalizing their feelings, and the analyst's role as a verbalizer may be imperative to forming a working alliance. The manner in which an interpretation is conveyed will also be an ancillary function of empathy. For example, the child and adolescent are particularly susceptible to narcissistic injury (narcissistically vulnerable). Empathy will serve to control the danger of narcissistically injuring the child. Narcissistic elements in the child are important in establishing the therapeutic alliance. It is one of the major ways the child invests in and becomes a participant in the working alliance. Feeling safe represents a reinvestment in basic trust; to be held represents his reinvestment in a *holding position* that will grow into a shared, *mutual sharing position*, and his need to be understood will facilitate the process of interpretation (integration). To summarize, it is essential the child feel it is *his* treatment, *his* time, and that you are *his* therapist.

Many of these characteristic features of the working alliance, as we have argued, have their genetic origin in early stages of object relations. Frequently, in the treatment of the child or adolescent you can see the residual elements of the transitional phenomena as the stage is set for the recreation of past experiences. The child or adolescent will often use the treatment setting itself (i.e., the office, the analyst's possessions) to aid in establishing a transitional phenomena (Byerly 1992). It is the purpose of the therapeutic alliance as a construct of the treatment process to move the therapeutic alliance closer to the transference and to create a new object relationship. That is to say, the therapeutic alliance will contain the seeds of both the transference or displacement elements and the nature of the new object relationship.

David, a mid-adolescent who had many borderline features, repeatedly "forgot the time for his appointments" and always appeared an hour or so early in the beginning of treatment. He would bring his homework and settle in. He told me it was quiet in the waiting room and he didn't mind waiting. He felt comfortable there. David's home was not a happy place. He was essentially an only child who was left at night with his mother, who was an alcoholic. His father stayed out most nights and was rarely at home. David was frequently in a panic state at home, feeling responsible for the home and his mother. Our brief encounters between patients served to reassure him of my acceptance of him. The fact that I did not throw him out, reject him as his parents did, formed the pathway through the therapeutic alliance to a situation where David could engage me as a new object. His being in the office was later analyzed as serving to check up on me and determine if I were having an affair, as his unconscious recognized his father was having, but which he couldn't accept.

Mary was a pre-latency-aged child whose case was in supervision. Her therapist shared an office with another therapist. This other therapist had contributed a large tree to the office furnishings. Mary became "attached" to the tree, using it as a safety base, playing contentedly under the mother tree, as she designated it. Over one weekend the other therapist moved precipitously and took the tree with her. Mary was unreconcilable at the loss of the tree. Allowing her to effectively mourn the loss of the tree became an integral part of establishing the therapeutic alliance. It also heralded the future transference elements of depression and loss.

As Anna Freud has indicated, the therapeutic alliance is established through interpretation. It is by interpretation that the analyst conveys his understanding to the child. Interpretation of the defenses, not the transference, establishes the working alliance. A brief review of defense analysis would contain the following: Defense analysis is well suited to children because children live closer to their instinctual wishes than do adults (Mahler 1945). In children, affects are more transparent, and analysis of affects leads directly to unconscious instinctual conflicts (fantasies). The closer proximity of affects and defenses to the ego and the ego's relative distance from impulses, which remain more frequently closer to the id, make defense analysis possible (Bornstein 1951).

As Hartman (1956) reminds us, interpretations and insight create a sharper differentiation between the ego and the id, result in a more flexible relationship to the external world, and alienate the id more effectively from reality. Hartman emphasizes, in treatment, the importance of new information and personal understanding that facilitates reality testing, which in turn leads to better control over affects and enhances adaptation (Blatt and Behrends 1987). Before the child can deal with interpretations, however, he must be prepared to hear the interpretation.

The workaday "dialogue" of treatment is the process by which the child engages the treatment process and is prepared for treatment. Kramer and Settlage (1962) have commented extensively on technique in child analysis. Kramer and Byerly (1978) have outlined the "dialogue" in child therapy as consisting of *running comments, confrontations*, and *interpretations*.

Running Comments. Running comments by the therapist allow his active participation with the child in the treatment situation. It creates a relatively neutral position of not interfering with the child's production but rather monitoring them. This in turn acts to facilitate the presence of an observing ego in the person of the therapist. The child and his productions serve as the complementary part to the observing ego—the experiencing ego. By repetition of this mutually complementary behavior, the child gradually learns that his actions, productions, and so forth have meaning and make sense. He learns the treatment method as he increasingly attaches more meaning, significance, and importance to his own productions. With time, the child becomes more identified with the treatment process. This leads to the reinforcement of his own observing ego or, in part, helps him to develop some aspect of an observing ego. Finally, through a more complete understanding of the treatment process and by his identification with the function of the analyst, the child, through articulating (verbalizing) his experiences, develops the capacity for insight. Working together in such a complementary manner fosters the holding position, where the singular purpose of understanding the child holds other variables at a minimum. The therapist does not become the child's playmate, nor does he compete with the child for center stage; rather, he continually invites the child to join him in the search to understand himself.

It is interesting to note the close correlation between the development of the observing ego and organizing capacity of the oedipal complex.

The search for understanding in treatment can be seen as a journey that two people take together (Loewald 1990). Invariably, the child and adolescent conceptualize the treatment process in some type of metaphorical terms. In the child, both conscious and unconscious elements contribute to this concept formation. If the child "sees" the treatment experience as a journey toward understanding himself, oedipal characteristics will, in different developmental stages, influence (color) his conceptualization of treatment as a journey. For example, the oedipal- and latency-aged child frequently, in conceptualizing the treatment as a journey, an adventure of two companions, will emphasize the oedipal aspects of discoveries and fighting the force of the unconscious; the pre-adolescent will lay more stress on the oedipal aspect of solving mysteries and finding out what and how things happened; the adolescent will emphasize the oedipal aspects of a true quest where the search for and possession of abstractions (love, beauty, truth) become the goals. The point to be made is that the oedipal organization can give to the treatment process an interesting, vital, and shared experience quality with a common goal.

Confrontations. As Kramer (Kramer and Byerly 1992) has noted, confrontations are closely related to running comments. Here not only are present observations commented on, but past observations are tied into recurrent patterns. This establishes integration as part of the treatment process. The therapist uses his own ego functions to a much greater extent than previously. He may show surprise, puzzlement, or frank confusion over the child's inconsistent, irrational, or illogical behavior and productions. In a way, he establishes a point of reference for reality testing. By separating out the irrational, placing the emphasis on reality allows reality testing and the formation of new (real) objects to come into play. It is by making use of reality that the therapist makes the child aware that a defense is being used. The use of past observation is one way the child becomes acquainted with his unconscious (present unconscious). In order to form patterns and configurations about his behavior and productions, the child often has to dig deep into his past unconscious to come to conclusions. It is important to recognize that defenses rarely exist in isolation and generally appear in clusters. Being able to identify a defense is a major step forward for the child. This prepares the child to explore with the therapist what is being defended against (prepares the child for an interpretation).

Interpretations. By the time an interpretation is made, the child should have the means (tools) to discover defenses and should be familiar with defenses. That is, he will know that his productions have more than one meaning and that defenses occur in clusters and form patterns. The more repetitious defenses are, the more we can assume they are characterological. The child is then ready to proceed to the next step — to know the purposes of the defense; namely, what is being defended against. The timing and manner of interpreting will be accomplished through the use of the ancillary function of empathy. It is important to make an interpretation based on the affectual content of the child's material, not on the overt content of the material. By understanding the defended-against material, the child is in a better position to give up a defense that is no longer needed. In such an experience, the ego is enhanced in terms of reality testing and integration.

John was a mid-adolescent who came into therapy willingly. He was a self-reliant, self-sufficient boy who prided himself in not needing anyone. In treatment, when his parents could not bring him, he literally walked several miles or rode his bike. His parents supported his self-sufficiency to the degree that he was out of control, and he recognized it. His parents were aware of his night wandering and suspected his use of drugs (marijuana), but were not aware of his delinquent acts such as breaking into cars and stealing money. John had two younger brothers whom he mocked and teased unmercifully, repeatedly challenging their masculinity. He regarded his father as a weakling, controlled and dominated by his mother. He blamed his mother for most of his and the family's difficulty and for her self-interest in taking care of herself, not caring for him. That is, his mother was a "health and exercise freak," who physically maintained herself well and made this her main priority.

Running comments established, among other things, that when he was particularly angry with his mother, he would act out. Despite his tendency not to ask anyone for anything, he was able, with help, to approach his mother and ask her for protein supplementary food to help him gain weight. This soon became a conflict area where his mother would forget to keep him supplied and argued with him, claiming it cost too much money. Her inattention to his need made him furious and enhanced his sense of impotency (on an oedipal level) and feelings of helplessness (on a preoedipal level). It was on such occasions that he and his friend would break into and "search" cars for anything they could find. In the therapeutic alliance he was eventually confronted with his behavior, his reaction to his anger, and disappointment with his mother's inattention to him. On one occasion, a phone call I chose to take drew my attention from him for what he felt was a significant time. He was furious, enraged, and acted out in the familiar pattern as he did when angry with his mother. Following his anger at me, it was possible for me to admit my inattention to him, an action uncommon with his parents. Based on his now familiar and recognized affectual response (anger, belligerence), I was able to interpret the conflict surrounding his generalized attitude of self-sufficiency and feelings of rejection—his fears of being insignificant (helpless, impotent, and unmasculine) with his need to take risks in the belief that he was proving his masculinity.

The other side of the conflict was pointed out in terms of his strong desire to identify with his mother, particularly her ambivalent caretaking qualities. As he worked through these thoughts, both the stealing and use of marijuana stopped. They became "childish and stupid" activities. He made a strong identification with the therapist's caretaking attributes and began talking his friends out of using drugs and breaking into cars, despite his fears of being isolated by them. Second, he found and brought home a stray cat, a loner and survivor like himself. He assumed full responsibility for the care of the cat, fascinated by the cat's nocturnal wanderings and always on edge wondering if the cat would return home. The therapeutic alliance developed in two directions—his identification with the analyst as a "new object" along the lines of a concerned caretaker and along the lines of allowing the transference elements around his mother to progress and develop. In later work the transference implications of the "searching" of cars and wandering behavior had multiple oedipal and preoedipal determinants.

In the above interpretation of defense, we have been following A. Freud's (1936) "proposed differentiation of transference phenomena, in which former defense measures against the drives are repeated" (Sandler et al. 1973, p. 42). This is in contrast to transference of libidinal impulses, in which instinctual wishes attached to infantile objects break through toward the analyst. The concept of the transference is in transition: the historical view versus the modernist view (see Cooper 1987). The multiple controversies surrounding the transference (neurosis), externalization, and developmental relationship to transference are unresolved. In children and adolescents the concept of past transference and present transference (Kanzer 1953) is clinically practical. That is to say that not all transferences are regressive (Schafer 1977) but, in children, may also involve present-day parental object interactions with the child that are carried into the treatment situation. Regardless of the classification as transference or displacement, such material needs to be dealt with in the same careful and discernible manner as one would deal with transference proper material.

John's case raises two interesting points that we have been following. The first deals with the principle of abstinence or the gratification–frustration equation. John's early preoedipal pathology and his adolescent strivings for independence placed particular stress on self-gratification (control issues) in the treatment situation. In such cases, Winnicott's admonition to gratify the patient's ego needs but not his id wishes becomes critical in maintaining the therapeutic alliance (Kingston and

Cohen 1986). The gratification of ego needs may address such issues as early trauma and developmental arrests. The analyst must be constantly aware of the level of frustration the child or adolescent can tolerate. John's polarization of his identity, the nature of his identity crisis in adolescence, reflected an earlier and more fundamental split in his identification with his mother. This was primarily reflected in his need to take care of himself and belief that others could not or would not meet his needs. The therapeutic alliance and the transference paralleled this basic conflict.

An equally important area that dominated John's case is acting out. Again, we can only briefly comment on this area and its implications for treatment in children and adolescents. Action language or the tendency to self-activation is synonymous with children and adolescents who are in treatment. Generally, it is not regarded as pathological until after latency development (A. Freud 1968). The determinants of acting out are multiple (Byerly 1990) and surround such pressing issues as enactment versus acting out, externalization, and projective identification. John's initial acting-out behavior was not confined to the treatment situation, although later in treatment he did act out in therapy. The general concept behind his acting out was based on his tendency to externalize his conflicts when they, and later the transference itself, intensified to an uncontainable degree.

The intensification of John's conflict was dependent on factors both outside and within the treatment situation. In the treatment situation the shifts in modes of functioning between the therapeutic alliance mode, the real object mode and the transference mode were correlated with such disruptions in the treatment relationship as acting out. This is consistent with Blatt and Behrends's (1987) description of disruptions in the treatment which they describe as experienced incompatibility, defined as

> [occurring] either unconsciously or consciously, presymbolic or symboli-cally . . . [it] comes about for a variety of reasons including the possibility that the other person either no longer wants to or is no longer able to gratify one's need. Incompatibility may occur when one of the individuals, in his or her own right, feels ready to move the relationship to a more mature or less mature level. If the disruption in the relationship is premature, the individual may not be prepared to internalize aspects of the relationship and thus will be forced to resort to less successful means of adaptation. [p.285]

Blatt and Behrends (1987) experienced incompatibility concept can be understood to include disruption in the interrelated therapeutic modes (i.e., the real object and alliance object level of relationship) as well as the familiar disruptions in the transference. The role interpretation serves, not only in maintaining the therapeutic process at one level of object-relations, but also its function in causing shifts (disruption) to other levels of object-relations deserves further consideration. The therapeutic process may be most susceptible to gratification failures (experienced incompatibilities) at the interfacing of these different object-levels of the therapeutic process. The risk of internalization failure at such points, and the resultant transference of affect leading to acting out, may be increased by the shift from one functional mode to another. If we follow this line of reasoning, then the oscillations between the real mode, the alliance mode, and the translation may result in the gratification–deprivation cycle important to the core of the therapeutic process.

In conclusion, our technique, particularly therapy with children, is an ongoing process. There is an increasing tendency to incorporate developmental and object relations theories into the understanding of the therapeutic process.

Technique is also faced with a growing understanding that the most serious psychopathology is not necessarily id-ego conflicts but failure to negotiate successfully the developmental issues around the separation-individuation process (Eagle 1984). Many of our future advances in technique with children may well be determined by a more complete exploration and understanding of the interrelationship of the separation-individuation process in development, the different modes of functioning in the therapeutic setting, and the mutative regulating aspect of therapeutic core.

REFERENCES

Alexander, F., and French, T. (1946). *Psychoanalytic Therapy*. New York: Ronald.

Aronson, M. (1986). Transference and countertransference in treatment of difficult character disorders. In *Between Patient and Analyst*, ed. H. Meyers, pp. 13–29. Hillsdale, NJ: Analytic Press.

Basch, M. (1983). Empathic understanding: a review of the concept and some theoretical considerations. *Journal of the American Psychoanalytic Association* 31:101–126.

Behrends, R., and Blatt, S. (1985). Internalization and psychological development throughout the life cycle. *PSOC* 40:11–39.

Blatt, H., and Behrends, R. (1985). International and psychological development throughout the life cycle. *PSOC* 40:11–39.

———— (1987). Internalization: separation-individuation and the nature of the therapeutic action. *International Journal of Psycho-Analysis* 68: 279–296.

Blum, H. (1974). The borderline childhood of the Wolf Man. *Journal of the American Psychoanalytic Association* 22:721–742.

Bollas, C. (1987). *The Shadow of the Object: Psychoanalysis of the Unthought Known*. New York: Columbia University Press.

Bornstein, B. (1951). On latency. *Psychoanalytic Study of the Child* 6:279–285. New York: International Universities Press.

Brenner, C. (1979). Working alliance, therapeutic alliance and transference. *Journal of the American Psychoanalytic Association* 27:137–157.

Byerly, L. (1990). Neurosis and object relations. In *The Neurotic Child*, ed. H. Etezady, pp. 159–195. Northvale, NJ: Jason Aronson.

_____ (1992). Unresolved separation, masochism and difficulty with compliance. In *When the Body Speaks: Psychological Meanings or Kinetic Clues*, ed. S. Kramer and S. Akhtar, pp. 114–130. Northvale, NJ: Jason Aronson.

Cooper, A. (1987). The transference neurosis: a concept ready for retirement. *Psychoanalytic Inquiry* 7:569–585.

Curtis, H. (1979). The concept of the therapeutic alliance: implications for the "widening scope." *Journal of the American Medical Association* 27:159–192.

Eagle, M. (1984). *Recent Developments in Psychoanalysis. A Critical Evaluation*. New York: McGraw-Hill.

Emde, R. (1980). Towards a psychoanalytic theory of affects. Part I. The organizational model and its propositions. In *The Course of Life: Infancy and Early Childhood*, Vol. I, ed. S. Greenspan and G. Pollock, pp. 63–83. Publication No. (ADM) 80–786. Washington, DC: National Institute of Mental Health.

_____ (1981). Changing models of infancy and the nature of early development: remodeling the foundations. *Journal of the American Psychoanalytic Association* 29:179–219.

Erikson, E. (1950). *Childhood and Society*. New York: W. W. Norton

Fairbairn, W. (1962). *Psychoanalytic Studies of the Personality*. London: Routledge and Kegan Paul.

Fenichel, O. (1941). *Problems of Psychoanalytic Technique*. Albany, NY: Psychoanalytic Quarterly Press.

Fraiberg, S. (1964). Panel discussion: child analysis at different stages. (Reporter, G. Abbate.) *Journal of the American Psychoanalytic Association* 12:135–150.

Freud, A. (1962 [1961]). The theory of the parent–infant relationship. Contribution to the discussion. In *The Writings of Anna Freud, vol. V, Research at the Hampstead Clinic and Other Papers*, pp. 187–193. New York: International Universities Press, 1969.

_____ (1966). A short history of child analysis. In *The Writings of Anna Freud, vol. VII, Problems of Psychoanalytic Training, Diagnosis and the Technique of Therapy*, pp. 48–58. New York: International Universities Press, 1961.

_____ (1968 [1967]). Acting out. In *The Writings of Anna Freud, vol. VII, Problems of Psychoanalytic Training, Diagnosis and the Technique of Therapy*, pp. 94–109. New York: International Universities Press, 1971.

Freud, S. (1895). Studies on hysteria. *Standard Edition* 2.

_____ (1905). Three essays on the theory of sexuality. *Standard Edition* 7:125–245.

_____ (1909). Notes upon a case of obsessional neurosis. *Standard Edition* 10:153–318.

_____ (1912). The dynamics of transference. *Standard Edition* 12:97–108.

_____ (1913). On the beginning of treatment. (Further recommendations on the technique of Psychoanalysis.) *Standard Edition* 12:121–144.

_____ (1918). From the history of an infantile neurosis. *Standard Edition* 17:1–123.

_____ (1921). Group psychology and the analysis of the ego. *Standard Edition* 18:110.

_____ (1938). An Outline of Psycho-Analysis. *Standard Edition* 23:141–207.

Furer, M. (1976). Panel discussion: current concepts of the psychoanalytic process. (Reporter, M. Morganstein.) *Journal of the American Psycho-Analytic Association* 24:184–188.

Gitelson, M. (1962). The curative factors in psychoanalysis. *International Journal of Psycho-Analysis* 43:194–205.

Glenn, J. (January, 1981). *The Ratman: Historical and contemporary views of Freud's psychotherapeutic approaches.* Paper presented at the Joint Meeting of the Long Island Psychoanalytic Association and the Nassau Psychiatric Association.

Glover, E. (1924). Active therapy and psychoanalysis. *International Journal of Psycho-Analysis* 5:269–311.

_____ (1928). Lectures on technique in psychoanalysis. *International Journal of Psycho-Analysis* 9:7–46; 181–218.

Greenacre, P. (1968). The psychoanalytic process on transference and acting out. In *Emotional Growth, vol. 2, Psychoanalytic Therapy and Training*, pp. 762–775. New York: International Universities Press, 1971.

Greenson, R. (1965). The working alliance and the transference neurosis. *Psychoanalytic Quarterly Press* 34:155–181.

_____ (1967). The working alliance; the real relationship. In *The Technique and Practice of Psychoanalysis, vol. I*, pp. 190–216; 216–224. New York: International Universities Press.

Greenson, R., and Wexler, M. (1969). The non-transference relationship in the psychoanalytic situation. *International Journal of Psycho-Analysis* 50:27–29.

Hanly, C., Rangell, L., and Schachter, J. (1991). *Psychoanalytic Dialogue: Therapeutic Alliance: Resistance and/or Enabler.* Audiotape, APSA–162. Recorded 12/91.

Harley, M. (1974). Panel discussion: a comparison between adult and child analysis. (Reporter, C. Fiegelson.) *Journal of the American Psycho-analytic Association* 22:603–611.

Hartman, H. (1956). Notes on the reality principles. In *Essays on Ego Psychology*, pp. 241–267. New York: International Universities Press, 1964.

Jacobson, E. (1965). *The Self and Object.* London: Hogarth.

Kanzer, M. (1953). Past and present transference. *Journal of the American Psychoanalytic Association* 1:144–154.

_____ (1975). The therapist and the working alliance. *International Journal of Psycho-Analysis* 4:48–73.

Kingston, W., and Cohen, J. (1986). Primal repression: clinical and theoretical aspects. *International Journal of Psycho-Analysis* 67:337–355.

Klein, M. (1948). *Contributions to Psychoanalysis, 1921–1945.* London: Hogarth.

Kohut, H. (1971). *The Analysis of the Self.* New York: International Universities Press.

Kramer, S., and Byerly, L. (1992). Technique of psychoanalysis of the latency child. In *Child Analysis and Therapy*, ed. J. Glenn, pp. 205–236. Northvale, NJ: Jason Aronson.

Kramer, S., and Settlage, C. (1962). On the concept and technique of child analysis. *Journal of the American Academy of Child Psychiatry* 4:509–535.

Lester, E. (1983). Separation and cognition. *Journal of the American Psychoanalytic Association* 31:127–156.

Levine, F. (1992). *Unconscious fantasies and theories of technique.* Paper presented at a joint meeting of the Philadelphia Psychoanalytic Association and Society. Accepted for publication, *Psychoanalytic Inquiry*, January.

Lichtenberg, J. (1983). *Psychoanalysis and Infant Research.* Hillsdale, NJ: Lawrence Erlbaum.

Loewald, H. (1960). On the therapeutic action of psychoanalysis. In *Papers on Psychoanalysis*, pp. 221–256. New Haven, CT: Yale University Press.

Mahler, M. (1945). Child analysis. In *Modern Trends in Child Psychiatry*, ed. N. Lewis and B. Pacella, pp. 265–289. New York: International Universities Press.

_____ (1963). Thoughts about development and individuation. *Psychoanalytic Study of the Child* 18:307–374. New York: International Universities Press.

_____ (1967). On human symbiosis and the vicissitudes of individuation. *Journal of the American Psychoanalytic Association* 15:740–763.

_____ (1972). On the first three subphases of the separation-individuation. *Journal of the American Psychoanalytic Association* 53:333–358.

_____ (1974). Panel discussion: a comparison between adult and child analysis. (Reporter, C. Fiegelson). *Journal of the American Psychoanalytic Association* 22:603–611.

Mahler, M., Pine, F., and Bergman, A. (1975). *The Psychological Birth of the Human Infant*. New York: Basic Books.

Masterson, J. (1992). Psychotherapy and the borderline and narcissistic disorders in the adolescent: establishing a therapeutic approach. *International Annual Adolescent Psychiatry* 2:179–191.

Meissner, W. (1989). The viewpoint of a devil's advocate. In *Significance of Infant Observational Research for Clinical Work with Children, Adolescents and Adults*, ed. S. Dowling and A. Rothstein, pp. 175–194. Madison, CT: International Universities Press.

Modell, A. (1976). "The holding environment" and the therapeutic action in psychoanalysis. *Journal of the American Psychoanalytic Association* 24:185–307.

Moore, B., and Fine, B. (1990). *Psychoanalytic Terms and Concepts*, pp. 195–196. New Haven, CT: The American Psychoanalytic Association and Yale University Press.

Novick, J. (1990). The significance of adolescent analysis for clinical work with adults. In *Child and Adolescent Analysis: Its Significance for Clinical Work with Adults*, ed. S. Dowling, pp. 81–94. New York: The American Psychoanalytic Press.

Pine, F. (1985). *Developmental Theory and Clinical Process*. New Haven, CT: Yale University Press.

Rangell, L. (1954). Similarities and differences between psychoanalysis and psychotherapy. *Journal of the American Psychoanalytic Association* 2:734–744.

Rapaport, D., and Gill, M. (1959). The points of view and assumptions of metapsychology. *International Journal of Psycho-Analysis* 40:153–162.

Sandler, J. (1978). *Projection, Identification, Projective Identification*. Madison, CT: International Universities Press.

Sandler, J., Dare, C., and Holder, A. (1973). The treatment alliance. In *The Patient and the Analyst*, ed. J. Sandler and U. Dreher, pp. 23–36. Madison, CT: International Universities Press, 1992.

Sandler, J., and Rosenblatt, B. (1962). The concept of the representational world. *Psychoanalytic Study of the Child* 17:128–145. New York: International Universities Press.

Sandler, J., and Sandler, M. (1987). The past unconscious and the present vicissitudes of guilt. *International Journal of Psycho-Analysis* 68:331–340.

Schafer, R. (1977). The interpretation of transference and the conditions for loving. *Journal of the American Psychoanalytic Association* 25:335–362.

Schowalter, J. (1976). Therapeutic alliance and the role of speech in child analysis. *Psychoanalytic Study of the Child* 31:415–436. New Haven, CT: Yale University Press.

Sodre, J. (1990). *Treatment alliances: therapeutic and anti-therapeutic*. Paper presented to a Weekend Conference for English-speaking Members of European Societies. London.

Spitz, R. (1956). Transference: the analytic setting and its prototype. *International Journal of Psycho-Analysis* 37:380–385.

Sterba, R. (1934). The fate of the ego in analytic therapy. *International Journal of Psycho-Analysis* 15:117–126.

Stern, D. (1973). *The Interpersonal World of the Infant*. New York: Basic Books.

_____ (1977). *The First Relationship: Infant and Mother*. Cambridge, MA: Harvard University Press.

Stone, L. (1954). The widening scope of indicators for psychoanalysis. *Journal of the American Psychoanalytic Association* 2:567–594.

_____ (1960). *The Psychoanalytic Situation: An Examination of its Development and Essential Nature*. New York: International Universities Press.

Strachey, J. (1934). The nature and therapeutic action of psychoanalysis. *International Journal of Psycho-Analysis* 15:127–159.

Tolpin, M. (1971). On the beginning of a cohesive self: an application of the concept of transmuting internalization to the study of the transitional object and signal anxiety. *Psychoanalytic Study of the Child* 26:316–352. New Haven, CT: International Universities Press.

Tyson, P. (1989). Two approaches to infant research: a review and integration. In *The Significance of Infant Observational Research for Clinical Work with Children, Adolescents and Adults*, ed. S. Dowling and A. Rothstein, pp. 3–21. Madison, CT: International Universities Press.

Valenstein, A. (1979). The concept of "classical" psychoanalysis. *Journal of the American Psychoanalytic Association* 27:113–136.

_____ (1980). Preoedipal reconstruction in psychoanalysis. *International Journal of Psycho-Analysis* 70:433–442.

Van Dam, H. (1966). Panel discussion: problems of transference in child analysis. *Journal of the American Psychoanalytic Association* 14:528–537.

Werner, H., and Kaplan, B. (1963). *Symbol Formation. An Organismic-Developmental Approach to Language and the Expression of Thought*. New York: John Wiley and Sons.

Weston, D. (1990). Psychoanalytic approaches to personality. In *Handbook of Personality Theory and Research*, ed. L. Pervin, p. 27. New York: Guilford.

Winnicott, D. (1960). Countertransference. *British Journal of Medical Psychology* 33:17–21.

_____ (1965). *The Maturational Process and the Facilitating Environment*. London: Hogarth.

Zetzel, E. (1956). Current concepts of transference. *International Journal of Psycho-Analysis* 37:369–376.

4

The Conduct of the Psychotherapeutic Interview

Helen R. Beiser, M.D.

Literature

Although there is a massive literature about psychotherapy with children, most deals with how to treat specific conditions or how to use specific techniques. It is hard to put oneself into many treatment situations and prepare one's own setting to actually do psychotherapy. I (Beiser 1962) went through this problem when I was assigned my first administrative position in a state child guidance clinic, which was to purchase toys for the common playrooms shared by all therapists. At that time, I surveyed the literature and found Melanie Klein (1932) describing her room as containing a low table with wooden human and animal figures, houses, bricks, various toy modes of transportation, paper, pencils, and scissors. From about the same time period, Anna Freud (1946) did not mention any specific materials but talked about making herself useful to the usually resistant child patient by crocheting doll clothes, tying knots, and so on.

The first child analysis, Freud's (1909) famous "Little Hans," was conducted through the boy's father, and Freud saw the boy only once. Another pioneer, Hug-Hellmuth (1921), performed analysis in the homes of her child patients, so that their natural surroundings were used as the therapeutic environment. Frederick Allen (1942), one of the early child guidance psychiatrists, says only that the child should choose from a variety of play materials rather than those preselected by the therapist to deal with a specific symptom. Winnicott (1958) apparently also subscribes to this point of view, describing a miscellaneous mass of toys, including teddy bears. He also includes a diagram of his office, which has a split space, so that adult therapy is conducted in an area separate from the play space. A different philosophy is exemplified by Gardner (1975), who has a specific game with which to conduct his mutual storytelling technique. Winnicott (1958) also introduced a specific technique, "the squiggle game," which required only paper and pencil, with therapist and patient alternately completing and describing a "squiggle" of lines started by the other. Although a number of special setups have been described by various workers in the field, such as David Levy's (1939) release therapy using amputation dolls, and Margaret Lowenfeld's (1935) "world," these are more likely to be used in the diagnostic process or for research purposes than for psychotherapy. Toy companies, however, have advertised a number of special toys over the years, with more or less success. It is easy for children to ignore these, which is why I (Beiser 1979) learned long ago that latency children prefer board games, and if these are not provided, will bring their own. Of course, for most adolescents these play materials are not appropriate, and Sarnoff (1987) describes the stages of early and late adolescence, when the shift to verbalization takes place.

Other techniques may or may not require special materials. These include nondirective therapy, as described by Axline (1947), group therapy, as exemplified by Ginott (1961), and family therapy by Minuchin (1974). There are a number of general books on psychotherapy that describe a variety of techniques as well as the authors' personal philosophy, such as those by Mishne (1983), Haworth (1964), and others. Erikson (1977) has written extensively on the meaning of play and toys.

GOALS OF TREATMENT

The goals of treatment for the neurotic child must be kept clearly in mind when conducting the psychotherapeutic interview. Sometimes these may be lost sight of in trying to prove the efficacy of a given theory or technique. Relief from the neurotic conflict, allowing normal development to proceed, should be the stated goal. If regression is encouraged, it is for the purpose of helping the child to come to a healthier resolution of those conflicts. Educational techniques can have the same goal. There is no intrinsic virtue in great frequency or length of treatment, or the opposite, very brief contact, unless these accomplish the stated goal. Different goals and techniques are necessary when psychosis is the problem, as well as for character disorders. The need to free the superego in the neurotic child may be irrelevant in the autistic child and may actually harm the child with a character disorder who has an inadequate superego. Conflict with persons in the environment is not usually a major problem for neurotic children, but this might develop if regression occurs during the treatment process. Eventually, a more comfortable relationship with such persons should be part of the goal of treatment of the neurotic child. This is quite different from helping a psychotic child to be able to remain in society, and the character-disordered child to develop a less conflicted relationship with persons in his or her environment.

PHYSICAL SETTING

The physical setting in which psychotherapy can take place may be quite varied. As previously mentioned, if it occurs in a group clinic setting, it may have to be shared with other therapists. Also to be taken into consideration is what other work the space is to be used for. If special rooms are set aside for play therapy, then some regulations need to be made as how they are to be assigned to therapists, which cuts down on flexibility in the use of time. Also, housekeeping habits of different therapists may cause tension. Those therapists who promote regression through messiness may cause trouble with those whose patients are going through a progression phase. Similarly, if toys must be shared, the problems due to carelessness in handling materials, loss of game pieces, breakage, and so on with patients who are loosening their superego may cause trouble with patients in either earlier or later phases of treatment. Therapists must be held responsible for leaving materials and space in the condition in which they were found. I recall bringing a child who had already passed through a destructive phase into a playroom full of broken toys and wet plaster. She was upset, saying, "Who did this? I know it wasn't one of your children, because you would have cleaned it up." Another problem with sharing is that a toy that was being used may disappear, and a child may have difficulty continuing with the process of working out a problem. Even in my private office I had several figures disappear, apparently stolen by cleaning personnel. The disappearance of the girl member of the doll family was particularly distressing to a girl patient who had fears of being kidnapped.

A different problem may arise if the room is used as an office and contains records, papers, dictating machines, and the like. As these are objects of curiosity to a child, they must either be kept out of sight, become a part of the play equipment, or become the objects of a struggle over limits with the child patient. I learned early to file all papers and keep certain objects up high and out of the reach of little explorers. This situation can be a real stimulus to neatness for therapists. As well as the problems of seeing children in a setting built for adults, there is also the problem of seeing adults in a setting prepared for children. The conflicts of adults over the regression stimulated by a play-oriented setting can be disturbing. This can be handled by having separate but connected rooms, or by keeping play material in a closet or box out of sight of adults but easily available to a child. A sink may be useful for both adults and children, but if it is unavailable, water for children can be brought in by container. I have not found sand worth the mess and inconvenience. Each therapist needs to make a decision about smoking while seeing a child in psychotherapy. Children may not only be stimulated to smoke by example, but also be stimulated by the fire used in the lighting of cigarettes.

The decision as to what play materials to provide is an individual matter related to the theoretical leanings of the therapist. Perhaps the most important thing to keep in mind is that no material should be included that the therapist does not want the child to use. I recall a therapist I was supervising who, knowing I liked using formal games, had a number of them in his play setup. When it became apparent that the therapist became very annoyed playing games, I recommended that the games be removed. If the therapist believes it is best for a child patient to freely choose the materials for play, the toys can be either simple and few, or more extensive, but rarely complex. Usually this includes toys that stimulate or allow children to express their fantasies, which symbolically represent their conflicts. The most frequently used are human figures, such as doll families, but other figures such as cowboys, Indians, farmers, policemen, or soldiers may be helpful. In the early '60s I found a set of toy astronauts very useful in working out the separation problems of a boy with school phobia. Other toys may also be used to represent humans, such as Melanie Klein's famous trucks and other transportation toys, as well as animal figures. These do not always stimulate what the therapist expects. I once bought a toy alligator for the expression of oral hostility, which, as it turned out, no child ever used. I started out my practice with a baby doll but learned that little girls never played with it, because a baby doll has to belong to them personally. Some boys used it as a way of exploring sexual differences in the process of changing diapers. Therapists may wish to try out a number of ideas before coming to a decision about what toys they wish to provide. Perhaps it is most important to eventually standardize the toys so that a given child may be compared with himself or others in his or her play activity over time.

Other pretty standard materials are paper, pencils, crayons, scissors, and paste. Whether to provide paints depends on how much messing can be tolerated, as well as the availability of water. I found oil paints too much of a problem because of the time needed for drying, but watercolors and colored pencils are quite satisfactory. Clay is another material whose use depends on the therapist's tolerance. Some clays are less messy than others but may pose the problem of quick hardening. Here, as with models, rules are required as to what the child may take home. My first psychoanalytic supervisor thought *nothing should ever be removed* from the therapy room. My rule had been that nothing should be removed that can be used again, and constructions should not be taken home until they are finished properly. This avoids resentment about the cost of sloppily used materials. Drawings are dated and retained until the termination phase, to be reviewed and distributed at that time.

Therapy can be conducted quite adequately with the above materials. In fact, at the state clinic, in order to ensure some stability in the play materials for each child in therapy, individual boxes were designed to contain a doll family, two trucks, paper, pencil, crayons, scissors, watercolors, and clay. Other small toys could be added at the discretion of the therapist, and drawings could be stored in the box until termination. Such a small box could also be used when traveling to a clinic in another town.

Other toys that may be made available in a free-choice therapy situation may be a sandbox, a dollhouse, a soft ball, and a variety of games. The latter should be those that are well known to the therapist, span a variety of developmental phases, and incorporate a variety of principles, such as chance, physical skill, mental skill, strategy, and various combinations of these. It is better to choose according to categories rather than specific games, as toy manufacturers change their stock often. Some standards I find useful are dominoes, checkers, and Chinese checkers. I do not supply ordinary playing cards because it is too difficult to know if children are playing by correct rules. I found by experience that if games are not supplied by the therapist, latency children will bring their own, which might not be familiar to the therapist. Another principle to keep in mind with games is that it should be possible to complete them during the therapy hour. This eliminates otherwise valuable games such as Monopoly and chess. Except for a windup car with four forward gears and a reverse, which demonstrated the relationship of speed to power and control, I have not found mechanical toys useful. A toy hard to categorize, but which I found very useful, is the Nok-out Bench, which can release energy through pounding, teach colors, challenge the child to figure out its inner structure, act as a model of the gastrointestinal tract, and even be used as a missile launcher. The specially structured toys may also be used in the free choice situation but are not generally available through the usual sources. At one time David Levy's amputation dolls were quite popular but also frightened a number of children. Richard Gardner's mutual storytelling games are more likely to be used at present, and of course no special equipment is required to play Winnicott's squiggle game. Other useful toys may be found during explorations of toy stores and catalogues.

FREQUENCY AND REGULARITY

Wide variations are encountered in establishing the frequency of therapy sessions. Most classical psychoanalysis involves seeing a child four or five times a week. On the other hand, Winnicott (1978) writes that he analyzed a 2-year-old girl over a 2-year period for a total of seventeen sessions, "on demand." Most psychotherapy sessions are held once or twice a week, regardless of the profession of the therapist. Regularity has been generally thought to be an important aspect of therapy, but Winnicott's experience may call into question the universality of that. Greater frequency is designed to intensify the child's relationship to the therapist. More important is that a therapeutic process is established, which some children may be able to develop without being seen so often. Regularity has much the same function but can be more important in the treatment of some children than of others. With very resistant children it may be necessary to increase the frequency and allow irregularity on their part before a firm therapeutic alliance can be formed. It may also be necessary to vary frequency and regularity according to the resistance or realistic requirements of parents. Winnicott's patient lived in another town, and frequent and regular appointments were not possible. I once treated a child from another state whose mother had moved to the city for the summer so I could start treatment at three times a week. After school started, they flew in for Saturday morning sessions. In another family, who went out of town every weekend, I would have lost the case if I had insisted on seeing the child on Saturday. Establishing a therapeutic relationship is more important than following the optimal rules of a specific theoretical viewpoint.

COLLATERAL CONTACTS

Another controversial issue concerns who besides the child can be seen, and under what circumstances, when a child is being treated for a neurotic problem. I find it preferable to make a therapeutic alliance with both parents, if they are available, but essential to see whoever the child is living with. It is important to have the consent and cooperation of whoever is going to pay for the treatment, including insurance companies. Although the need for confidentiality is often used as justification for refusing contact with all collaterals, most neurotic children expect the adults in their lives to communicate about them. If the welfare of the child is kept in mind, no problems need occur. There is usually a countertransference problem in the therapist who cannot communicate with important others in the child's life.

The frequency of divorce has complicated the problem of relating to both parents, and it is important to remain neutral in the area of marital controversy. I have seen mothers who used therapy as a way of punishing the divorced father, whose relationship to the child may be worsened by his resentment over paying the bill. If a neutral person like a therapist can talk with the noncustodial parent, he or she is more likely to support treatment, both financially and psychologically. I even had one warring couple decide on remarriage to one another during the therapy of their daughter.

If the school has been the initiator of treatment, it is essential that some form of communication be arranged. This is particularly important if the child needs to be excused from school to come to therapy. Sometimes a teacher can be helped to be either more or less sympathetic with a child in therapy, as the situation demands. A similar attitude can be desirable for whoever referred the family in the first place. Many physicians consider psychiatrists lacking in courtesy when their referrals are not acknowledged, and unless at least some information is conveyed as to the problem and progress of the child. With neurotic children, courts usually are not involved but certainly need to be included in lines of communication if they are.

Rules for communication with collaterals may be somewhat different when the patient is an adolescent. It is still necessary to establish a relationship with whoever is to pay the bill, as well as with whoever is responsible for the adolescent. It is not advisable to promise the adolescent complete confidentiality, as he or she will find some way to get the therapist to recant for the patient's protection. I only promise that I will inform the adolescent of what, in general, I will say to whom.

MEANS OF COMMUNICATION

The type of communication with children in therapy depends a great deal on the age or stage of development, as well as on the problem for which therapy is being undertaken. Direct discussion of problems for any length of time, as in the treatment of adults, is not to be expected until mid- or late adolescence. Some obsessive-compulsive children may intellectualize, and seem to communicate like adults, but this is a defense, and very little change results from it therapeutically. Desirable communication is age and stage appropriate. Very young children tend to use a lot of fantasy and will use toys that express that fantasy. With various human or other figures provided, they may act out their conflicts. The therapist may translate what he or she sees into words, or join in the play. Too direct an interpretation of the meaning of the play may simply stop it, and the child may shift to a different activity. The ability to comment on fantasy play in a way to help the child come to some better resolution of a conflict is a skill that may take years of experience and/or supervision to develop.

Fantasy play with doll figures is almost too easy to understand. Drawings may not be as easy, especially in younger children whose visual motor skills are not well developed. It is important that poor skills not be given a psychological meaning. Drawings as communication can be the most meaningful with children who have some skill at drawing and want to portray their conflicts in this mode. This can be important with some relatively nonverbal but artistically gifted adolescents. Dreams are another form of communication, valued by therapists but likely to be avoided by many children. When produced, they can give valuable insights. The dreams of very young children are usually quite transparent and easy to understand, but the therapist's interpretations and responses are again a matter for training and experience.

The use of structured situations may be more controversial. I have a preference for formal board games with clearly written rules. In this situation children exhibit their attitudes toward winning and losing, toward the therapist's winning and losing, and toward the unseen writer of the rules. At the same time, playing something they enjoy may allow them enough relaxation to talk about problems and listen to the therapist's comments. The rules are especially important for latency-aged children, who are including persons and institutions beyond the home into their lives, and whose rights and attitudes must be respected. It is necessary for a therapist to teach children how to play some games, as well as helping them to win or lose gracefully, so that they can enjoy playing with peers.

Starting with preadolescence, there may be a transition to talking about sports or other outside activities, especially with boys. Here the seemingly omnipotent fantasies must be compared with the patient's realistic abilities. Can a short boy become a basketball star? I treated a very bright boy who fantasied he would rule the world by first being elected president of the United States. After dealing with his cheating and hostile impulses, I realized that with his abilities and his family's social status, the goal of at least running for some high elective office was a realistic possibility.

Although not as common with neurotic children as with psychotic or conduct-disordered children, much communication, at least in some phases of treatment, takes place around the need to set the limits of behavior during the therapy hour. Some therapists have an ideal of permissiveness, but there are certain conditions that require the therapist to control a child's behavior. The boundaries may vary with the tolerance of the therapist, but everyone's limits are reached at some point. One of the most common problems is the manipulation of the times at which the sessions start and stop. Of course, the penalty for lateness is loss of therapy time, which may not seem to concern some children, but which can be used to point out that they might lose out in some more enjoyable situation. Prolonging the end of the hour may be accomplished by dawdling, or not clearing toys away. The above boy who would be president went through such a stage and actually enjoyed it when I physically ejected him. I finally told him that his time was like a bank account, which he had been overdrawing. I would subtract the time he stayed over from his next hour. A very smart boy, he asked what would happen if he had *no time left*. After I said he would always have 10 minutes, and time would be deducted from subsequent hours, he stopped manipulating the ending of the sessions.

Other limits may also need to be set. One relates to personal attacks on the therapist. These are not frequent and may be a response to an attempt to limit some other form of behavior. For example, when a phobic boy started to leave the office before the end of the hour, and I stood in his way, he kicked me in the shin. Even though he was wearing rubber-soled boat shoes, it hurt. One day I took his shoes off and put them up high. The kicking then hurt his toes, and he stopped. Later in his treatment, when he had resolved his need to be in control, he mentioned the incident a number of times, appreciative of my ability to take control. Attacks on property can be stopped with an interpretation or diversion to symbolic behavior. For example, a 7-year-old girl was in treatment because she saw a witch in the shadows cast on her bedroom wall by a street light shining through the leaves of a tree. When she was gleefully annoying me by trying to invade the boxes in which other children kept their drawings, I asked her who that witch in her bedroom really was, and she shamefacedly admitted it was herself. The boy with the boat shoes once deliberately broke a wooden toy mannequin and also splashed me with red paint. I suggested we put these toys away, and he never played with them again, probably out of a guilt reaction. Preventive arrangements in the office are probably the best way of limiting fire and water damage.

A difficult mode of communication in preadolescence or early adolescence is total silence as well as refusal to use toys. If this occurs after a good therapeutic process has been going on, it can be explored and interpreted so that treatment can continue. If it persists, it may be necessary to terminate or interrupt treatment. Adolescents more usually communicate negative feelings through canceling or failing appointments. Unlike with adults, this cannot be handled by charging for missed appointments. It is unethical to charge an insurance company, and if parents are so charged, they may become so angry with the adolescent that the problem becomes worse.

It may be controversial for a therapist to give actual suggestions or educate the patient in some way. Much information may be obtained from whether the patient ignores, refuses, or agrees in an overly compliant way with suggestions. Somewhat related is when the child asks direct questions of the therapist, often regarding the personal life of the therapist. Responses may vary widely, from "Why do you ask?" to giving detailed personal information in an effort to provide the child with a role model. I have found giving a very brief, factual answer followed by the question, "Why do you ask?" the best way to explore the fantasy of the child about the therapist.

Similarly, I think an educational response to real, or not so real, ignorance in the child can promote communication. Many children fake competence in playing games. It is a mistake to accept the grandiosity of such a fake. I prefer to beat the child at the game, demonstrating my superior power, and then teach him or her how to win without faking.

That leads to a real increase in self-esteem. There is also something to be learned in observing how children respond to education. For example, after teaching a child the basic rules of Chinese checkers, and playing a few games at which I am likely to win, I offer to teach the child how to accomplish the longest possible move in the game, if he or she will let me go first and will mirror my every move. Any child who will not accept this offer is probably not treatable. Of course, after learning the move, the child will try his or her own way for a long time before asking me to demonstrate the winning move again. Some education needs to be at a much more primitive level, and I have taught some children how to blow their nose, take a pill, or draw anatomically correct details and proper perspective.

THE THERAPEUTIC RELATIONSHIP

A good therapeutic relationship is the ultimate basis for the treatment of the neurotic child. All other aspects are only supportive of that. The relationship depends on the personality, training, and experience of the therapist. The therapist must have the goals of treatment in mind, and work to get the child to participate in achieving these goals. Because few children initiate treatment, it may take some time to persuade the child to this participation. For this reason, the early techniques of Anna Freud may still be necessary, and a certain amount of seduction may be used. Actually, some therapists see the provision of toys as a seduction and a resistance to the therapeutic process. A more direct seduction may be the provision of food. I have not found this useful, and in fact, after treating the son of a dentist, found it a hindrance. The boy, already in trouble with his father, knew he was not supposed to eat candy and felt the therapist was wrong to provide it. Education may also be seen as a seduction if the therapist subscribes to a pure psychoanalytic philosophy in which abstinence requires the patient to work out problems almost solely on his or her own.

It is a matter of personal philosophy whether the therapist allows free choice of activities and materials or provides a structured situation to which the child responds. Of course, it is best not to offer a child patient any more freedom than the therapist is actually willing to grant. I have known therapists who have introduced a child to an office or playroom with the statement, "You can do anything you want to here." That either frightens an inhibited child with too much of an opportunity to express unacceptable impulses, or invites a less inhibited child to test out whether the therapist really means it. Going back on a promise does not promote a good therapeutic relationship. On the other hand, if the situation is too strictly structured, the child might not feel free to express himself in ways not designated by the materials or the expectations of the therapist. For example, I recall a case where the therapist had strong feelings that no outside situations should intrude on the therapeutic process. He could not understand his patient's depression, because nothing had happened in the treatment to explain it, and was astonished to learn eventually that the child's father had died. Flexibility is desirable in the treatment situation and in contact with collaterals.

With neurotic children, the therapeutic relationship is designed to help the child understand the basis for his or her neurotic conflict and come to a healthier or more phase-appropriate solution. Although interpretation is the psychoanalytic technique of choice, it may not always be the most therapeutic. Children often see, or feel, an interpretation as an attack or criticism, and become resistant, or regress. My first analytic patient was a 7-year-old girl who had the fantasy of growing thick blades of grass by watering a sand box. When I interpreted this as her wish for a penis, she moved toward an open window in an attempt to jump out. The interpretation was confirmed later when surgery was planned to correct inguinal hernias, and she expected the surgeon to supply her with a penis. She was angry with me when this did not occur, a severe strain on the therapeutic relationship.

There are other means of conveying meaning to children without direct interpretation. One common method is to enter into the child's fantasy play and suggest alternate solutions to the conflict portrayed. For example, if the child sets up a doll play situation in which the parent dolls are fighting, the child doll's dilemma can be discussed. Alternatives are encouraged, and positive ones supported. When boys play war games with soldiers, a peace conference can be suggested, with an exploration of what led to the conflict, as well as what might lead to a peaceful settlement. If the child does not go along with this suggestion, setting up a hospital for the care of the wounded might be tried.

A similar approach can be tried while playing board games. The question of cheating is hard to deal with without becoming angry and moralistic. It is necessary to help a child play fairly so that winning can be a realistic boost to the self-esteem, not a false one. It can be hard to know just what the origin of the cheating behavior is, although it is often from a misguided attempt of a parent to boost self-esteem by letting the child win. In the therapy situation I have simply explained to the child that cheating interferes with peer relationships, and I cannot play games with them if they cheat. It is then possible to offer to help them learn the game better in order to win. Some children need to be helped to play at a more appropriate level for their age and ability, rather than the therapist supporting a desire to excel at a more advanced level. It is doubtful if a 6-year-old should be encouraged to be a chess expert. I recall the treatment of a very bright 10-year-old only child whose father complained that she beat him at checkers. I said that was rather odd, because she could not beat me at dominoes, a much simpler game. By means of therapy, child and family are encouraged to support age and phase-appropriate behavior. Of course, as part of the training of a child therapist, it is important to learn what *is* age-appropriate behavior.

In the past, many therapists deliberately encouraged regressive behavior, on the theory that children could relive earlier stages of development in a healthier way and then be able to resume progress. Baby bottles were provided for a more satisfactory oral experience, and clay and finger paints to enjoy the messing of the anal period. The doll figures were to help the child deal with oedipal conflicts. In my experience, the theory has not been borne out, and the child sees the therapist as enjoying only regressive behavior, making it difficult to move on to more age-appropriate behavior. I prefer to allow the child to regress as this occurs during the therapeutic process, but then support the more age-appropriate behavior that usually follows. Again, knowledge of behavior suitable to various development stages is necessary. For example, a latency-aged child is likely, after losing a game, to move to fantasy, or compulsively making designs with the game pieces. Dominoes make pretty good blocks, which can be built up and knocked down. When ready, the child will move on to a renewed interest in playing the game according to rules, and the therapist can help the child be more successful at it. There are various levels of skill necessary for different games. When children attempt games beyond their abilities, they are likely to fail and regress or cheat. It is preferable to suggest an easier game, and when that is mastered, to go on to a somewhat more difficult one.

Adolescents may not be able to maintain a conversation related to their problems and may regress by shifting to some seemingly unrelated topic, or even wish to play a game. This sequence is more usually found in children who started therapy in the preadolescent years, and have a well-established therapeutic relationship. Again, a tolerant attitude on the part of the therapist usually allows the young person to return to discussing problems. When therapy is started in early adolescence, the patient is rarely able to regress to play, considering it too "babyish." At that age, silence is the most common regression and can be very difficult to overcome.

if possible, it is important to determine what stimulates regressive behavior. For example, I was treating a boy whose father was dying. His mother had visited his school to inform the principal, who said to the boy, "My boy, you will have to be a man before your time." He not only wet his pants immediately thereafter, but during his next therapy hour, he froze and wet his pants at the point in a game where a single move would allow him to win. Therapy not only helped him with his anxiety over losing his father but also relieved him of the fear that growing up had caused his father's illness and death. His strong wish to beat me twice consecutively at dominoes revealed a magical fantasy that it would change his very bad luck in losing his father, having a very sick mother, and needing two operations of his own. In general, the therapeutic relationship is used to help the child understand the nature of his conflicts, tolerate any regression that occurs, and promote moving on to a more age-appropriate solution, usually measured by more age-appropriate behavior.

SUMMARY

The details of conducting a psychotherapeutic interview, including the physical setting, the frequency and regularity of sessions, modes of communication, and contacts with collateral adults can vary greatly. Variations depend on the age and sex of the child, the condition for which he or she is being treated, and the situation and preferences of the therapist. The most important consideration is to promote a therapeutic relationship between child and therapist in order to achieve the goals of therapy.

REFERENCES

Allen, F. H. (1942). *Psychotherapy with Children*. New York: W. W. Norton.

Axline, V. M. (1947). *Play Therapy*. New York: Ballentine.

Beiser, H. R. (1962). Psychiatric diagnostic interviews with children. *Journal of the American Academy of Child Psychiatry* 1:656–670.

_____ (1979). Formal games in diagnosis and therapy. *Journal of the American Academy of Child Psychiatry* 18:480–491.

Erikson, E. H. (1977). *Toys and Reason*. New York: W. W. Norton.

Freud, A. (1946). *The Psycho-Analytical Treatment of Children*. London: Imago.

Freud, S. (1909). The analysis of a phobia in a 5-year-old boy. In *Collected Papers*, vol. 3. London: Basic Books.

Gardner, R. A. (1975). *Psychotherapeutic Approaches to the Resistant Child*. New York: Jason Aronson.

Ginott, H. G. (1961). *Group Psychotherapy with Children*. New York: McGraw-Hill.

Haworth, M. (1964). *Child Psychotherapy*. New York: Basic Books.

Hug-Hellmuth, H. N. (1921). On the technique of child analysis. *International Journal of Psycho-Analysis* 2:287–305.

Klein, M. (1932). *The Psycho-Analysis of Children*. London: Hogarth.

Levy, D. (1939). Release therapy. *American Journal of Orthopsychiatry* 9:713–736.

Lowenfeld, M. (1935). *Play in Childhood*. London: Camelot.

Minuchin, S. (1974). *Families and Family Therapy*. Cambridge, MA: Harvard University Press.

Mishne, J. (1983). *Clinical Work with Children*. New York: The Free Press.

Sarnoff, C. A. (1987). *Psychotherapeutic Strategies in Late Latency through Early Adolescence*. Northvale, NJ: Jason Aronson.

Winnicott, D. W. (1958). *Collected Papers*. London: Tavistock.

―――― (1978). *The Piggle*. London: Hogarth.

5

Transference

Charles A. Sarnoff, M.D.

Is transference possible in the psychotherapy of toddlers, latency-age children, and adolescents? This is a question that has often been asked by those who seek to understand the limits and potentials of psychotherapy. The question is tantamount to asking if dynamic therapy is possible for the young. After all, it is widely held in theory that therapeutic gain is achieved primarily when transference is worked through.

This challenge is well taken if one considers the fact that youngsters are involved in intense relationships with parental primary objects and that drive energies are absorbed into these relationships. This should drain force from the contribution of the child's drives to the therapeutic relationship. Such strong parent–child ties could in theory undermine sustained transference.

In spite of such persistent family ties, sustained transferences do occur. To understand this, one must take into account the circumstances that underlie the occasional appearances of transferences in child therapy. These occur where finding a new object (i.e., the therapist) toward whom to direct the drives helps in the process of individuation, in overcoming of passivity in relation to the parents, and in the protection of the parent–child relationship from the effect of incestuous and aggressive wishes, through the displacement of drives from parent to therapist. This chapter is devoted to a demonstration of the occurence and nature of transference in childhood and adolescence through the presentation of clinical case material and related theoretical concepts.

TYPES OF TRANSFERENCE

Characterological Behavior (Clichés of Character)

Characteristic patterns of behavior that mark the daily life of patients, when repeated in the psychotherapeutic situation, are often called *transference*. Freud (1912b) saw such "anticipating ideas" (p. 100) as inherent templates that contribute consistent and characteristic form to behavior. Words used to translate this concept are "stereotype plate" (Freud 1912b p. 100) and "cliché or stereotype" (Freud 1912a, p.313). Recognition of these clichés are useful in identifying personality problems in therapy. Freud (1914) noted that "the transference is itself only a piece of repetition, and . . . the repetition is a transference of the forgotten past not only onto the Doctor, but also onto all the other aspects of the current situation . . . [and] every other activity and relationship which may occupy his life at the time" (p. 151). They are not all that is transference. The patient may be aware of their existence.

Freud's description of transference has inherent in it two related phenomena. A group of generalized repeated patterns, often known to the patient before he started treatment, here called characterological behavior, should be set off from patterns that occur only in the therapy situation and are expressions of repressed infantile sexual wishes, here called transference proper. (This differentiation was early elaborated by Dr. Max Stern in an unpublished paper.) Most characterological behavior and symptoms are derived from the defensive structures that lead to the repression. Demonstration of the existence of these repressed wishes and their relationship to the character defenses and symptoms that maintain the repression is achieved through (Freud 1916–1917) "lifting the repressions, [to] . . . remove the preconditions for the formation of symptoms. . . ."

Freud's character "clichés" are manifestations of behavior shaped by defenses against unconscious fantasy rather than the direct manifestations of unconscious wish fantasies. Such "clichés of character" are surface phenomena. They are accessible even to the unschooled. As such they tend to draw attention away from transference proper (see below). The search to understand them long preceded the discovery of psychoanalysis. Indeed, unavoidable fates that repeat the manifest contents of one's dreams have awakened the attention and curiosity of many, including the wise men and ancient poets who preceded modern-day therapists.

The development of patterns of behavior reaches a point (usually by the age of 16) when responses become so predictable that it becomes possible to identify the reliability of response of a person and to give a diagnostic name to the pattern of behavior. Prior to this, character patterns are not sufficiently consistent to support a characterological diagnosis.

Character develops in the following way. Infantile wishes become masked by the appearance of defenses, especially repressions reinforced with symbols. Such symbols become linked and are organized into core fantasies, which in turn inform the interpretation of the behavior of others. These fantasies give rise to responses and behavior that may owe more of their content to the past and its patterns than they do to the inputs of current reality. These core fantasies become conduits for the transmission of preformed intrusions from the past that underlie repetitive behavior, fate neuroses, and clichés of character. The ability to detect and interpret these repeated patterns has become an important part of the technique of the psychotherapies.

There has been a growing tendency to see characterological behavior as it is manifested in the psychotherapeutic situation as the predominant manifestation of transference. This attitude is enhanced by the ubiquitousness of such behavior; the ease of its generation, detection, and interpretation; and the fact that such emphasis aids in the decathexis of energy theory concepts.

Early childhood and latency psychotherapies are not devoid of characterological influences. Budding character patterns in statu nascendi are quite fluid and changeable. Psychotherapy can shape and guide the outcomes during this period of metamorphosis. Characterological transference interpretation, identifications with the character of the therapist, and recruitment of behavior patterns with resulting metamorphoses are characteristic aspects of the psychotherapeutic approach to this age group.

Characterological transference becomes important in the therapies of adolescents, where much energy is expended in the recruitment of peers to play out the roles of characters in the fantasies, at the expense of symbols and symptoms.

There has been a tendency to use the word *transference* generically to describe characterological behavior. This has resulted in a loss of emphasis on other categories of transference, such as transference proper, primary transference, and primal transference. These must be clearly defined if transference as it is manifested in children is to be understood.

Transference Proper

Transference proper is defined as an unique situation created by the mind of the patient, which involves the analyst in a relationship whose content is derived from a repressed infantile wish. Defenses against these wishes have resulted in their repression. The defenses themselves contribute to the nature of characterological behavior.

This is the form of transference that underlies transference neuroses. It is rarely manifested in true form and strength in children. The closest I have seen that resembles transference proper in prelatency children occurs when a cryptic manifest symbol for the object of the infantile wish takes the form of the analyst.

Primary Transference

Primary transference is defined as the need for nurture and care from a well-regarded object (e.g., the therapist). The situation in which the loving parent puts a Band-Aid on the small child's hurt knee provides the paradigm for the child's expectations in the therapeutic situation. In child and adolescent therapy, primary transference is strong and, if encouraged, would dominate the child's relationship to the therapist. It can aid in the early establishment of the therapist as helper. In this form, it is called positive transference. It turns into negative transference when needs exceed the available responses of the therapist, as a result of either therapeutic needs or personal limitations. Primary transference is a derivative of immature oral dependent needs. The older the child, the less acceptable is it as an universal attitude. Its pervasive presence in the characterological behavior of a patient requires that it be attended to psychotherapeutically. In such cases, the resolution of primary transference is a developmental task that dominates the living-through and abreaction experiences of the child in treatment.

Primal Transference

Primal transference is defined as the emergence for the first time anywhere of infantile sexual and aggressive wishes during an ongoing therapy with a young child in the process of negotiating age-appropriate stages of infantile psychosexual development. (This concept was introduced en passant by Peter Neubauer, M.D. [1962] during a training seminar.) The presence of an accepting analyst in the course of a therapy encourages the first manifestations of both instinctual and cognitive maturational achievements in behavior symptoms and attitudes that involve the therapist. This phenomenon results in the bringing of unalloyed and scarcely altered elements of drive energy into the sessions. The ready appearance of primal transference is enhanced by the fact that in the prelatency years repression is weak (Piaget 1945). Weak repression encourages primary and primal transference. The energy and attention that could have gone into transference proper is dissipated. The need for and development of organizations of defenses is reduced. As a result, potentially adaptive characterological behavior, superego, and inhibitions fail to develop. Primal transference occurs predominantly in the prelatency years.

EGO ASPECTS OF TRANSFERENCE

On the level of ego function, the underpinnings of transference are not present at birth. They are the products of development. Transference is produced by the fantasy-forming function of the ego and is therefore intrinsically part of the group of psychological phenomena that includes fantasy, delusion, dreams, and creativity involving narrative elements. Transference differs from these in that the object of the drive in the fantasy is the therapist and the venue of the experience is a session within a psychotherapeutic situation. Drive intensity varies in transference as it does in these other, related phenomena. Primal transference is a continuation of the object seeking that makes up the establishment of early object relations. Primary transference in the early stages of life is derived from a positive aspect of transference proper. Theoretically, transference proper and the beginnings of characterological behavior can be present at the earliest only after the maturation of two functions: first, the ability to represent an object in the latent content through the use of a displacement-mediated substitute, and second, the ability to obliterate self-awareness of the relationship between what represents and what is represented in the displacement. The obliteration is syncretic with repression. The first of these functions is called primary creativity; the second is called symbol formation. At the earliest these functions are in place and working together by 26 months (Sarnoff 1970).

PRIMARY CREATIVITY

The capacity for transference at its most primitive level begins with the development of "primary creativity," a concept introduced by Winnicott (1953). Primary creativity was seen as an ability developed in the first year of life that made possible the transitional object, and which can be understood to be a precursor of creative sublimative fantasy and symbols as well as transference. Winnicott placed primary creativity at 4 to 12 months of age. He postulated an intermediate area of experiencing (1958), which exists somewhere between the observing self and reality. In this zone the child begins to create phantom beings suited to satisfy inner needs. Winnicott (1953) postulated that "at some theoretical point early in the development of every human individual, an infant . . . is capable of conceiving of the idea of something which would meet the growing need that rises out of instinctual tension" (p. 239). Through primary creativity, drives can seek gratification from a zone of experience that is neither self nor world. A very primitive form of transference can be mediated as a result. Through it a therapist or other real figure can be interpreted to be the fantasied object. In essence the identity of the gratifying object is displaced from a phantom in the intermediate zone of experiencing and onto a person who exists on the world-side edge of that zone.

A problem in child therapy is that these primitive forms of characterological transference are mediated primarily through immature cognitive structures such as behavior that demands, crying, and whimpering. Such expressed needs change only in response to corrective object relations and not to interpretations. Their presentation has to be modified so that the infantile psychosexual fantasies that they mediate can be brought into the zone of effective psychotherapeutic intervention using verbal interpretation. This requires that the therapist encourage the development of the child's ability to present needs through the acquisition of verbal concept formation. In addition, the ability to displace wishes and representations of potentially gratifying objects onto objects in the world must be developed to ensure that their estranged nature will hide the true meaning of the wished-for fantasy, which, if too close to the original, may be forbidden or threatening. In this way, the therapist gains control of the speed and intensity of interpretation and therapeutic work.

The functions that mediate the presentation to consciousness of the instinctual wish in the form of a symbol are two. These are repression and the function it primarily subserves in the third year of life, psychoanalytic symbol formation. These functions create an intermediate signifier (the psychoanalytic symbol) for the instinctual wish. This intermediate signifier serves as a conduit for drive gratification, which produces lessening of drive need tensions. In addition, the psychoanalytic symbol lends itself to being worked into a verbal therapy. The secrets of the psychoanalytic symbol (the substitute object in the world) can be read by a skilled therapist who conveys their meanings by the creation of a verbal pathway that strengthens the patient's feelings and wish expressions to the point that they are experienced intensely and the reality of their existence supported. Such calling of attention to obscure motivations intensifies self-reflective awareness and leads to insight.

SYMBOL FORMATION

In all forms of transference, the therapist serves as the substitute or intermediate signifier. Ergo, in all forms of transference, the therapist serves as a symbol. This is so even in primal transference, where the therapist as primal object serves in displaced form for a protosymbol (see below). Therefore the nature and course of the transference during the early childhood, latency, and adolescent psychotherapies can be seen as a development-linked process with parallels to the developmental vicissitudes of symbol formation.

There is an expansion of consciousness at the dawn of the mind. This is made possible by the appearance of mechanisms that enable delay of response to the awareness of sensation and affect that is shared by all creatures. In humans, this delay in response becomes long enough to permit time for reflection to occur. This can result in the introduction of deferral or alteration of response, including deferrals based upon the active alteration of perception. The latter process underlies neurosis. Such modified perceptions are the product of the symbolizing function.

PROTOSYMBOLS

Protosymbol is a term used to represent the process by which the apparatus of awareness responds to bodily sensations displaced from their original organs of origin to a different organ within the body boundary (Sarnoff 1989). Such phenomena as painful anospasm in place of sexual arousal, tearing of the eyes representing an affect of sadness, or encopresis as defiance are examples. The sensation is displaced to an organ that has an unrelated function. These sensations can be worked into drive discharge fantasies, creating fantasies whose total manifestations can be expressed in a mind awareness arena limited to the space within the boundaries of the self. Abraham (1924) described partial object relationships in which objects in reality are related to as though they were body parts or products of the subject. For example, the therapist could find himself related to by a child whose need to control has been expressed through anal function, as though the therapist were the child's bowel content. Should the misperceived object be a parent, the process is called a primary object relationship. If the therapist is the first to experience this relationship, the process is called primal transference.

When the cognitive capacities of the mind expand to appreciate sensations as originating in the world beyond the boundary of the self, reality perceptions are added to the sensory inputs that lead to response. This occurs first at about 8 months. There is little to produce reflection of meaning of these inputs in terms of past and future implications. Recognition for response and later naming is the initial step in this expansion of function. At that point playthings are concrete representations conveying no meaning but themselves. At 15 months, "play symbols" (Woodward 1965) appear. These may be used for the conscious representation of something known or hoped for. Primary transference, the seeking of the therapist to serve as a kindly healer like the parent, can occur and is a manifestation of this early level of development of the symbolizing function. At this time, emphasis on words to represent concepts apart from the concrete manifestation of that which the word describes becomes a part of the parental training of the child. Storage of these abstractions becomes a part of the child's working memory. The increased emphasis on verbal conceptual memory produces a rich word web of awarenesses about percepts that can be related to one another and enhance meaning and interpretation of sensations. Extended consciousness is crystallized around these verbal codifications of abstract relationships, which makes possible abstract interpretation of perceptions (e.g., concrete operational thinking of Piaget [1945], also see Woodward 1965) in terms of past experience and implications for future planning. Not all perceptions or affect-charged contents of memory are so encoded. Many remain outside the arena of verbally organized memory. One may justifiably say that they are unconscious but not repressed. Verbally conscious elements are at times so rich in uncomfortable affects that it is necessary to avoid thinking about them or being reminded of them. This exclusion from consciousness is achieved through denial, which is supported by a number of different mechanisms of defense. Foremost of these is displacement. Displacement alone produces paranoia.

PSYCHOANALYTIC SYMBOLS

Displacement accompanied by the countercathectic effects of symbol formation produces an exclusion from consciousness, which is called repression. The symbols so formed are called psychoanalytic symbols (see Jones 1916, also secondary Symbols of Piaget 1945).

One of the aspects of the psychoanalytic symbol is the use of visual puns in the selection of substitute representations of words. This type of symbol formation is the basis for oneiric (dream) symbols. Repression is produced by introducing perceptions whose verbal associations are on the surface removed from any percept or concept that could convey that which is being excluded from consciousness. Such a redirection of conscious attention is called countercathexis. In child therapy the role of substitute is played by toys used in play (called ludic symbols).

Repression becomes strong enough to become clinically effective in producing symbols by 24 to 26 months. The use of the therapist as such a symbol is part of the process of transference proper, as defined earlier. As will be discussed in a case to be presented below, such a transference contributed to the therapy of a 4-year-old boy with delayed symbol formation. However, as a general rule, transference proper is not common in therapies of early childhood.

The capacity for symbol formation is not necessarily accompanied by the appearance of transference proper. Another vicissitude in the development of psychoanalytic symbols is involved in this. That is the gradual shift of the symbol from the evocative to the communicative pole, which is a characteristic of much more mature ego function than can be expected to be strong before late latency–early adolescence. Symbols that serve drive discharge alone, without being part of a social structure that encompasses objects and discharge within a context, are commonly seen early on. These symbols are said to be operating in the evocative mode (Sarnoff 1987b). As in the cryptic symbols seen in dreams, these symbols have little communicative value. They dominate the play of latency-age children. In psychotherapy, fantasy play involving evocative ludic symbols diverts drive energies from the energies available for transference proper. Gradually, as children move through late latency into early adolescence, the symbols become more involved in communicating to objects and thus more easily interpreted. Often observers are actively told what the symbols mean. Such use of symbols places them in the zone of communication. These are called communicative symbols. The more toward the communicative pole a symbol leans, the more is the symbol apt to choose as its representation the therapist rather than a toy. As a result of the shift to the communicative mode, symbol formation is apt to use a relationship with the therapist as a manifest symbol and become accessible as a transference.

Toys and other play symbols tend to provide discharge through the evocative symbol pole. They distract attention from the core problems of instinctual discharge and reality problems to be solved. This further diminishes the impetus toward object seeking in the child who plays in therapy. As such, play symbols sap the strength from the processes that produce transference. Play (ludic) symbols lose their capacity to function in this way at the time (late latency–early adolescence) of ludic demise (Sarnoff 1987a). At ludic demise, maturation makes toys no longer attractive to young teenagers. It is then that the drive energies turn toward dream symbols and into the search for objects in reality to serve as symbols for the core fantasies. The available reality objects fall into three groups. These are parents, therapists and teachers, and peers. The off-putting aspects of a closer tie to the parent that is generated by incest fears, the heightening rage involved in the search for independence from parental authority, and the concomitant sense of passivity that pervades the psychic life of early adolescence, diminish the parental potential to serve as an object of fantasy. The therapist is found to be a relatively benign substitute object (symbol). In such turnings in the way of therapy, the therapist can play two roles. He can be the source of insight through interpretation of transference (both proper and behavioral) as well as a model for identification.

Early adolescent transferences are neither stable nor dependable. The drive-manifesting fantasies that had been removed from parents and play and brought into the therapy continue in their browsing search for an object that can offer a gratification more concrete and immediate than the frustration of drive that is inherent in the psychoanalytic therapeutic approach to transference. The transference situation may serve as only a way station on the route to object love, and removal of the instincts from play discharge to fantasy discharge in the form of transference proper continues to enlist objects to play out roles in their fantasies in the teenage world. As a result of this process, love relationships with peers drains energy from transference and may lead to the abrupt termination of treatment (Katan 1937).

Parallel to this process is a transition in the march of persecutory objects used as symbols in the developmental march of symbols. The earliest such symbols as objects of fear are plants and animals. With the onset of latency, amorphous figures who might break into the home are feared. At about 8½ years of age, creatures with human forms are feared, a process that foreshadows the giving up of toys in favor of people that occurs with ludic demise. With the step over the threshold into adolescence, real people are recruited to play out the fantasies. Evocation gives way to communication. Fantasy gives way to object love. The further toward these mature polarities of instinctual expression a child grows, the greater is the chance that the child will manifest his forbidden wishes in a transference manifestation. Conversely, as real objects become more in evidence in drive discharge phenomena, the real objects more and more vie for the instinctual energies and undermine the transference, much in the way that the presence of parents contributes to the vitiation of the transference during the latency years. Character is established when fixed patterns of drive discharge fantasy become involved with real objects. When these fixed patterns are acted on during psychotherapy, characterological patterns of behavior, often called transference, can be identified and interpreted.

Accompanying the loosening of inhibitions and the increased use of reality objects, neuroses (see Laughlin 1967, p. 566) become less in evidence in early adolescence. They return in early adulthood. At that time (by 28 years), an increase in inhibitions in the use of objects in reality and social wants reshape and strengthen the organization of defenses. The resulting limitation in alloplastic drive discharge results in the recathexis of unconscious fantasy life. This phenomenon is associated with an intensification of the use of the therapist as object (if a therapist is made available to encourage the focusing of energies on him or her as an object).

LIMITATIONS TO TRANSFERENCE MANIFESTATIONS IN PREADULT PERSONALITY ORGANIZATIONS

Economic and emotional dependence on parents who are still actively involved in parenting is a characteristic of the life of children and adolescents. The presence of such primary and permanent objects absorbs drive energies to such an extent that there is little energy left to be used to cathect a sustained transference to a therapist. Transference phenomena that do occur in prelatency children with toddler-appropriate ego function are dominated by immature types of transference, with emphasis on primal and primary transferences and bursts of characterological behavior based upon unmitigated demands for care, power, and supremacy. Adult ego states reflecting fixations and regressions to these levels of immaturity produce transference reactions akin to these.

The encouragement of a transference to the analyst with gain from abreaction holds less promise for latency-age therapy than for the psychoanalysis of adults. Because of the nature of their immature ego, which includes the intensity of their sense of reality (fantasy feels real) and the poor quality of their reality testing, abreaction and resolution of conflicts involving early infantile wishes can be achieved through fantasy play which is generated by the ego structure of latency. This diverts energy from fantasy involving the analyst.

During the latency years transference proper can and does occur. However, throughout latency and adolescence, transference is diminished by the diversion from it of drive energies. These energies discharge through fantasy; play; dreams; and the presence, especially in adolescence, of real objects articulated with maturation of those ego functions that mediate the capacity to fall in love, coupled with the increased drive energies of puberty.

TRANSFERENCE IN THE TODDLER

We now turn to a clinical illustration of the case of a child whose delayed cognitive development resulted in the manifestation of his conflicts in a primitive form of symbol (a protosymbol) and defiant characterological behavior. Therapy aimed at a mature symbolizing function made it possible for him to make his transference available to interpretation. In essence, the following material illustrates, in statu nascendi, the ontogenesis of transference.

The primary symptom was encopresis, defined as stool retention with leakage. Roy K., 4 years old when he was brought for therapy, had never been fully trained. He held back his stools. He stained when he could no longer restrain himself. He had temper tantrums that disorganized him and the family. He could tolerate no frustration.

When he was 33 months of age, there had been some progress in toilet training. Then there was a change in his personality, and progress in bowel control showed a regression. He became obstinate, overcontrolling, and highly personalized in his selection of the where and when of defecation. At that time, a sibling sister had been born. From the day that she was brought home, he became active, running from room to room (*Note*: This is one of the outlets of a child with impaired or limited use of the symbolizing function.) For 3 months he was persistently hyperactive. At 36 months he was sent to nursery school, where his pattern of overcontrol and retention of stool with leakage made him a somewhat odoriferous but "apparently toilet trained" 3-year-old boy. Retention in school evaded detection by his teachers. At home, his soiled clothes told of episodes of loss of control. He could be put on the toilet without product only to lose control when his clothes were rearranged. There was no question that he could sense bowel fullness. At $3\frac{1}{2}$ years of age he had fecal impaction, which was relieved by enema. This brought his problem to medical attention. Megacolon,

Hirschsprung's disease, disorders of colonic innervation, and absence of anal wink (sic) were ruled out and psychotherapy recommended.

Roy was weaned at 18 months. He sucked his thumb constantly; he had a distinct thumb-sucker's bump proximal to the first right carpophalangeal joint. He carried a security blanket with him continually when he was at home.

His mother is a tense, self-centered, money-occupied woman who tends to overweight, which she keeps under good control. After discovering that my time for parent visits were subject to a charge, she shifted to frequent telephone calls.

She could cooperate in changes in patterns of parenting required for the therapy, such as limitation of severe punishments, disengagement from stimulating fecal cleansing activities, neutralizing of parental rage, reinforcement of symbolizing function (e.g., through reading fantasy material, inquiring about dreams, and discussions of enhanced cultural experiences such as movies and plays for children and encouragement of play with passively conceived ludic symbols). She performed by rote, with little grasp of the dynamic balance of psychological ecologies, mutual influences and balances that characterize early child development and that inform therapeutic endeavors undertaken for people of that tender age.

Roy was a handsome, sturdy, very cooperative, verbal $4\frac{1}{2}$ year-old boy. Mental status was within normal limits except for deficiencies in the fantasy-forming functions. When asked about sleeping habits, he responded, "Sometimes I can't sleep—I think of having ice cream." He reports that he has never had a scary dream and doesn't make up stories.

When I began to make something with clay, he saw it as a snake but could not put it into a story context or elaborate on the snake form. I concluded that he was capable of symbolic play, first seen in the 15-month-old (Piaget 1945), but not of producing true ludic psychoanalytic play symbols. There seemed to be a limit on his ability to create fantasy symbols and fantasies, which would have provided him with a more socially acceptable displaced outlet through which he could have resolved conflicts.

We now digress to discuss the evaluation of the symbolizing function in the 4-year-old. Note that immediately above I said *a limit*. I did not say that the symbolizing function was totally absent in Roy. When it comes to the evaluation of the viability of the symbolizing function in the service of fantasy in children, one must conceptualize the process within a context of an evolving complementary series, remnants of each part of which may still be manifest after later stages have developed.

Relative health is determined by identifying the number and maturity of the symbolic forms available as well as the quality of the specific symbolic form that is utilized primarily in the production of manifest fantasy and behavior. If the reaction of the child aimed at adjustment to stress utilizes a manifest symbol selected from within the body boundary (Sarnoff 1989), we deal with a symbolic form expressing reaction utilizing a body organ or product (a protosymbol). This is a precursor of what will in later life be called a psychosomatic symptom, which is a truly evocative symbol with little in the way of a communicative pole. Were a child able to express his reaction through an external ludic (play object) symbol whose meaning is hidden from the therapist, we would say that we are dealing with a manifest symbol whose evocative pole is being emphasized (external and evoking, but not in the service of communication). At the more mature end of the complementary series is the psychoanalytic symbol used in the communicative mode. Here fantasy play contexts consist of symbol groupings that contain enough meaning detectable to the observer for the underlying (unconscious) meaning of the fantasy to be detected. With such symbols, conscious discussion, interpretation, and working through of the roots of represented problems can be introduced.

In the case of Roy, it became clear that the symbolic forms available to him were limited to simple verbalizations, non distortion dreaming and the use of body functions for a regressed, evocative-fantasy-level resolution of affect and conflict. Once this clarification had been established, that a developmental cognitive impairment (immature symbol formation) gave rise to his specific manifestation of anal-phase problems (fecal retention), it was possible to plan the treatment approach needed. First the symbolizing function of the ego had to be improved so that the interaction between therapist and patient could be conducted in the zone that would permit communication and interaction between the two, and open the way for a manifestation of transference. Then the conflict and misunderstandings underlying the transference could be interpreted, identified, and worked through, as illustrated in the following description of Roy's treatment.

Roy's initial way of solving problems in sessions gave the impression of superior intelligence. He was neat and asked questions about the objects in the playroom. As he became more comfortable, however, he began disorganized messing. Little was planned. There was also little in the way of organized fantasy. Attempts at painting, which dominated his activities, always resulted in mixed colors put on the paper in such large amounts that the table bore almost as much pigment as the paper. Early attempts at work with clay produced pizza, snakes without fantasy contexts, "duty," and a lot of clay on the floor and on our shoes. If he dropped something, he asked or ordered me to pick it up (a manifestation of characterological behavior). He ordered me to pick it up so often that we resolved his demands by drawing a line on the floor. Things that fell on my side, I picked up. Things that fell on his side, he picked up, sometimes.

There was poorly developed symbolizing function. His defensive resources were dominated by drive expression using primitive protosymbolic forms such as body parts and products. This shaped his behavior. When called upon in situations of stress, these primitive defenses produced ego dissolution, increased messing, anxiety, and loss of control instead of the comfort to be derived from age-appropriate fantasy formation. Mastery and discharge through the use of fantasy that employs symbols sufficiently removed from the latent content to obscure its meaning and its associated affects were not available to him. Because of this, I had recommended that the mother introduce the passive use of symbols through reading and storytelling. In addition, I introduced activities during the sessions that were aimed at enhancement of cognition and symbolizing function. The clay-molding technique described in my book *Latency* (Sarnoff 1976) was introduced. I molded small clay figures of amorphous form, asking him to guess what I was making. Whatever he guessed, I made. Once completed, these figures of his own creation were permitted to dry. Once dried, the figures could be used to introduce the employment of ludic symbols in fantasy. I asked questions that required the use of the figures in a story. I introduced use of his own symbols in fantasy stories.

In the 12th month of treatment, I went out to welcome Roy in the waiting room. He rose from his seat slowly and, having the sense that he had left something behind, turned back for an instant, further slowing his progress toward the door of my office and playroom. His mother jumped up from her seat and shoved him forward, pushing the base of his neck with such force that his head whiplashed backward. As she pushed him, she said, "Go faster, you're wasting money." Two elements were added to the therapy as a result of her action. In a trice, one could see an identification with mother's harsh controlling demands as one source of his characterological choice of bossiness. In addition, this situation provided an important inroad therapeutically. His mother's rejecting behavior turned his dependency needs toward a substitute object (the therapist). Removal of the primary object encouraged primary transference. Roy was so overwhelmed by feelings that he could not maintain his cold distance from me.

Tears streaming from his eyes, he cried to me, "Do you see that? Did you see what she did? She does that all the time." I had become his confidant. In turning to me, Roy had begun to live through or abreact the primary transference wish to be nurtured and cared for. In response to his mother's failure in this instance to give comfort, he turned to the analyst as a substitute object. In this way he overcame some of his resistances and defense against relating dependently and began to undo the stilted nature of his object relations. This corrective object-relationship experience apparently was followed by the mobilization of the communicative pole in the formation of symbols.

He marched from my consulting room into the playroom. Tears gave way to anger. The anger too resolved as he began the first of a series of fantasies played out in the playroom. He took small gummed labels and began to paste them on every toy in the room. On each he marked a value. He declared himself the owner of a store, and he invited me to come in and buy. The play was awkward without a medium of exchange. After a few sessions, this lack was responded to by the introduction of an industrial process that required my help because of its complexity. He organized the manufacture of coins to be used in his store. This included cardboard coins, gold foil-covered coins, and even Olympic commemorative coins. A final stage in this play, which lasted for months, was the production of gold credit cards.

While working on the credit cards, he dropped a piece of gold foil paper on his side of the line. He looked at me briefly and then curtly ordered me to pick up the scrap of paper. I pointed out its location. He cocked back his head, looked down his nose, and while pointing with haughty demeanor, commanded me to pick up the paper.

I looked straight back at him, while he continued his demands and bid me coolly to obey again and again. In this way, he focused his characterological behavior in the therapy. He drove toward converting me as an object external to his body boundaries into a symbol of the stool he controlled at will.

Then I said, "Who do you think you are?"

"I am a king," said he.

I was a little surprised. I realized at that moment that he had used a word that we could share to describe the sense of self that he demanded be recognized in his desperate need to undo the inferiority and narcissistic vulnerability that formed the core of his self-image. This demand aimed at me was a form of transference. Such transference is an example of the act of remembering through the utilization of styles of recall that exist before the development of speech informed by propositional thought (see below). Finding a name (*king*) could make it possible for us to share, look at, discuss, come back to, and make this barely conscious concept that had been used as defense available to the system consciousness. McCrone (1991) has described how "naming something makes it stand out more clearly from the surrounding background" (p. 110). Luria (1968) speaks of "the forms of reflection which are realized through speech" (pp. 120–123). And Sacks (1989) speaks of "the acquisition of conceptualizing and systematizing power with language" (p. 43). In a person who is fearful of harm from loved ones, some concepts have too much affect to be spelled out in words. In these cases symbolic substitutes are produced that are sufficiently removed from the original to hide meaning. The more fearful or autistic the child, the less are these symbols used in a communicative mode. Interpretation is needed to bring their true meaning into consciousness.

Insight and the possibility of working through occurred when we shared the aftermath of the reality situation in the waiting room. At that point Roy was able to represent drives through symbols that, although masking, had a communicative aspect that could be used for interpretation and expansion of consciousness to include explanations of previously inexplicable transference behavior.

In response to his declaration, my thoughts dwelled on the possibility of approaching insight through the symbol he had introduced (a king). He needed to be a king, I thought, because he felt so unimportant. I suspected that pursuit of the king symbol could provide knowledge with enough distance to be psychotherapeutically workable. However, it soon became clear that such working through would have to wait for another day, for he began to cut a long strip of cardboard creating a sawtoothed edge. He glued gold paper to the cardboard and then pasted on brightly colored clay "jewels." He twisted the strip into a loop large enough to circle his head and then, placing it on his brow, marked the end of the session by marching proudly from the room wearing a symbol of the king, a Golden Crown.

In subsequent sessions, we pursued his idea that he was a king. Logically he could not be a king, because a king's father is always a king. He had got the concept of king from the fairy tale books his parents had read to him, and in his experience, kings were the sons of kings. He was easily able to put aside naming himself a king. The underlying concept needed more attention. I pointed out the linkage of his kingship to his encopresis. I said, "When you thought you were a king, you could make a duty any place you want to." "And anytime I want to," said he. From that session forth his encopretic withholding came under control.

This insight was not enough to modify his character traits. There was left to be worked through the reason that he needed to feel he was something special, with special rules, like a king. We were embarked on an investigation of his sense of humiliation when scolded by his mother and his feeling that money was more important to her than he was. He also had feelings of envy toward his sibling, who was seen to be held in more value than he. The working through of these important areas was averted when his mother, encouraged by the subsidence of the encopresis and with a lack of psychological mindedness that caused her to see treatment results as the product of a sort of magic, withdrew the child from treatment.

Verbal Representation and Mental Content in the Toddler

Roy's anal-sadistic drives were expressed through body organ–based protosymbols when he came to treatment and so were not available at first to understanding that could be productive of verbal interpretation and influence.

A transition from affecto-motor memory to verbal concept memory, which Roy had only partially completed before he came for therapy, left much that was encoded in the affecto-motor memory system and unavailable to the awareness system to which psychotherapy is geared. That awareness system detects verbalizations primarily. Not every event or experience in the child's world finds a word. Roy was slow in this area, especially when it came to the cushioning effect of the symbolizing function, which makes representation possible, albeit in masked form.

When he started therapy, Roy had no words for what his anger expressed or meant to him. This is a form of repression that works by exclusion through an absence of a conduit to verbally organized consciousness (unconscious, but not a part of the system consciousness) (Schachtel 1949). Cognitive structures for use in producing symbolic or verbal communication were not yet adequately mature for utilization. Rather than through the use of symbols and fantasies, compensatory narcissism—generated in response to his mother's ease to anger and the birth of a sib—was manifested in messing; bowel withholding; and demanding, controlling behavior (transference) in the therapy. Therapeutic goals included verbalized insight. This required techniques to encourage more mature symbolic forms. This goal was achieved through the introduction of psychoanalytic symbols using words and concepts derived from the zone of experience beyond the boundary of the self. This raised the level of instinctual expression to the point at which communication and interpretation became possible. The verbalization and identification of an age-available form of transference were then realized.

Developmentally, the capacity to utilize psychoanalytic symbols in a communicative mode is a turning point with many implications. The development of latency, with its importance for civilization, begins. The introduction of communicative symbols and words to interpret them enhances verbalized insight and aids in the resolution of conflict.

When early infantile wishes or the memory residua of trauma can be symbolized communicatively, speech can be used in resolving transference. This entails the working through and disenabling of the contents of the core and masturbation fantasies that are the precursors of adult transferences, characterology, fate neuroses, and neurotic symptoms. Communicative discharge and confrontation are enabled by the development of speech and the evolving of decipherable cryptic symbols. These permit the organization and expression of fantasy-informed infantile sexual wishes on increasingly more mature, socially acceptable, and sublimated levels.

Organ protosymbols sidetrack this trend. The symbols are too primitive and evocative. The adjustment is interfered with, as in the case of Roy, whose use of control of his stools expressed his anger and control needs. Psychoanalytic symbols in the communicative mode serve compromise formation and permit discharge under more socialized conditions. Through the interpretation of such symbols, otherwise irretrievable transferences based on early infantile wishes or the memory residua of trauma can be converted from that which is only acted or felt to that which can be expressed in symbols that can be interpreted into verbal concepts that can then be worked through or associated to, confronted or challenged.

In Roy's case, a developmental step in symbol usage was introduced to the therapy so that interpretation of transference behavior could bring unconscious motivation into consciousness.

Verbalization in children enhances the working through of and disenabling of contents that are destined to underlie transference wishes in adults. Communicative discharge and confrontation followed upon the development of speech and the evolving of decipherable cryptic symbols. This permits the organization and expression of infantile sexual wish-informed fantasy, which can be interpreted in child therapy. This results in controlled reparative mastery, working through, and the confrontation of the sense of reality with reality testing.

The effective interpretation of transference results in a self-reflective awareness. This awareness places the content of past events and future effects, attitudes, and behavior within reach during the therapy session. The patient expands his consciousness, creating a lucid image by expanding the view he has of himself to include what had formerly been repressed or left unconscious. In this way, the person becomes aware of behavior and motivation, and can recognize what makes the behavior inappropriate. This brings into focus, with the therapist's help, reasons for stopping the behavior.

The evolution of consciousness is the evolution of self-reflexive verbal thought. This should be differentiated from other awarenesses such as awareness of reflex signals and the responses and awareness that accompany semifacultative automatic responses that have been learned or have become second nature, as in dancing or athletics.

A major transition in a child's awareness occurs when words representing abstractions become associated with percepts and affects and other experiences of the moment that previously had only called for reflex responses. Words that represent abstractions can be recalled and remembered. Such recall of abstractions opens the way to past and future, and expands awareness to encompass a view of life that adds insight and a sustained longitudinal history of meaning to experience. The role of interpretation is to expand this memory resonance.

TRANSFERENCE IN THE LATENCY-AGE CHILD FROM 6 YEARS OF AGE TO LUDIC DEMISE

There is no sharp division between the transferences of the toddler and the transferences of the child in early latency. Parents as primary objects continue to draw instinctual drive energies to themselves. In therapy sessions either fantasy play, athletic pursuits, or structured games hold the attention of the child, keeping the inquiring therapist at bay. Peers share the play experience in a socialized collusion that helps to keep the thin repression of the latency years in a state of effectiveness. Troubling events can be excluded from consciousness through the use of the structure of latency (see p. 107). This is an ego structure that induces repression of events and their fragmentation into parts, followed by a displacement that results in their return to consciousness through symbols organized into fantasies that hide the original events. A product of this ego structure for the child is a state of calm, quiet, and educability. This permits quiet in the classroom under the stress of humiliation. It also makes possible brutality on the part of parents that is tolerated to the point that the child's love for the parent can persist and preserve the child from confrontations that would disrupt the family.

Therapy sessions removed in time from such traumatic events are apt to reflect those repressions of experience that are so typical of early latency. Events have to be very recent to be recalled in therapy. Dreams are rarely told because they too fade in the path of the extensive use of repression. The ludic symbols of children who are capable of fantasy play absorb the energies that otherwise would have been invested in dreams and transference. For this reason it is a good idea to have parents report all dreams that have been told to them. As dreams go, so goes the fate of transference proper. Energies that might have gone into transference are absorbed into the symbols of play. Fantasy play becomes the source of information on the unconscious fantasy life of the child (see Chapter 6).

During the latency years, primal transference is developmentally a thing of the past. Primary transference can be seen when the child is in need, but it does not contribute a forceful impetus to the creation of the therapist as a valued source of needed help. Parents are better able and more appropriately suited to respond to such needs in the child.

The most important transference during early latency is that which can be studied as an epiphenomenon in the fantasy play in which the therapist is given a role to play. The nature of the role assigned can give a clue to the child's attitude toward the therapist as well as the way in which the child sees himself and his role in his fantasy of what the world is. For instance, a child who always assigned me the role of a subordinate in all his play fantasies, informed me, in reflecting on his life, that his mother was a general in their house and that he was one of her privates, since to be a general one must have privates to control. This opened the door to interpretations related to his feelings of low self-worth.

Because of the role of the structure of latency in dealing with recent events, the primary characters in children's fantasies tend to refer to parents, peers, and teachers rather than the therapist. Therapists come to the fore usually in situations in which the therapy session is scheduled at a time that interferes with some activity, a party, television show, or play date. Look for the therapist as symbol when the therapy intrudes on the reality of the child. A child who was angry at me for "making him come to therapy" could easily be directed to his mother's overprotectiveness, which interfered with all activities after school, as a factor in his life that heightened his sensitivity to the intruding role of the therapy in his daily round.

The therapist's passivity makes him a target for massive transference shifts. In response to humiliation, a child may in turn attempt to humiliate the therapist. A child given the silent treatment by a sibling may shift the hostility to the therapist and accord him the same silent treatment that he has received.

Some children keep their play to themselves, excluding the therapist in every way. One child shielded his play with his body. Another gave me a group of toys to play with and sent me to another part of the room. In each case the action was an expression of the evocative nature of the symbols in use, and evidence of poor object relations reflecting a psychotic process. This differential diagnosis should be kept in mind in therapeutic situations presenting such behavior.

LATTER LATENCY, FROM LUDIC DEMISE TO PUBERTY

From the standpoint of transference, the transition to the latter part of latency is marked by the occurrence of ludic demise and the shift from the primarily evocative to the primary communicative mode in the use of psychoanalytic symbols. Ludic demise refers to the gradual waning of the power of toys to serve as psychoanalytic symbols, which occurs around the 11th year of life. As this developmental situation unfolds, fantasy play becomes less and less effective as a pathway for drive discharge. Real objects are sought for the discharge of drives and recruited to play out roles in unconscious fantasies. Siblings and parents are excluded by incest barriers from manifest participation in these activities. Dreams take on the activity of fantasy discharge that had been the province of ludic play.

The stage seems set, as 11 years of age approaches, for transferences to the therapist to be generated. They are there. One must look hard for them, though, for with ludic demise the energies do not go toward the analyst but preferentially to peers, a phase-specific thrust of libido direction that serves species survival, supports removal (see below), and diminishes the amount of transference in adolescence. It also explains the acting-out tendency seen in adolescence as well as the phenomenon of reduced neurosis. This process diminishes with the increase in transference neuroses in the late teens and early twenties, and the reassertion of parental imagos at about 26 years of age.

For children who are driven to assert their individuality early on, the therapy situation can be interpreted by the child to be a manifestation of a relationship whose content and protagonists are separate from, and a secret to, the parents. This represents an early stage in the process of individuation that causes many youngsters to search for new identities and directions separate from those of their parents in the years of adolescence. One child who loved the dollhouse in my office asked her father to build one for her. The father agreed, and without contact with me, created a dollhouse with the same dimensions as mine. The child took this as a sign of contact between me and her parents that had been denied. Seeing us as fused, the child went into a furor, directing toward me the anger that she felt toward her somewhat uninterested parents but which she could not express to them because of a socially appropriate upbringing and the fear of loss of privileges should she become enraged at her father.

The nature of the interpretation of transference changes in late latency. The child's cognition in early latency requires that abstract interpretations be oft repeated and always be referred to a concrete example. As adolescence approaches, the operation of a memory organization that encodes abstract concepts becomes more and more effective. Eventually so many abstractions are encoded in memory that they can be evoked by the introduction of a related abstraction. In this way concepts can be introduced through interpretation that point out similarities and roots for transference not only in concrete experiences in the therapy situation, but also in memories and abstract reductions of repetitive life situations to recognizable patterns.

By the age of 8, there is a softening of the superego in the child. This is accompanied by the reappearance of frank sexual fantasies. The superego has less effect, making it possible for the growing child to explore the potentials of the body and world of the child. For instance masturbation becomes more direct and in evidence. Old superego restrictions are often projected onto the therapist. Guilt feelings in the sessions and robbery fantasies with capture and punishment are play activities that reflect this state of affairs.

The changes seen in late latency intensify in early adolescence.

TRANSFERENCE IN EARLY ADOLESCENT PSYCHOTHERAPY

Each of the types of transference I have described has a special vicissitude in early adolescence. Intensified drives and ludic demise give rise to an intensification of object-directed drive manifestations. The stage seems set for an intensification of all forms of transference. However, in reality, this does not take place in sustained form. Though the therapist has the opportunity to be a shaping first object who helps the fantasy take form by contributing examples, and contexts in loco parentis, the true arena for experiencing drive manifestations rests with interactions with peers. Drive is too strong and the call of peers too powerful. Drives do not become stuck in the transference. The therapist as transference object often is bypassed and limited to giving form and inspiration to the real-life adventures of the teenager. There is little to be gained from experiencing behavioral transference in fantasy in psychotherapy; there is hardly any transference proper to be encouraged in the hope that interpretation will bring insight to reinforce a conscious resolve to change.

Primal transference in principle can be observed when as a result of the burgeoning sexual drive pressures of the pubertal psyche, the patient may develop sexual fantasies which, though old in form, are new in strength. Rarely are these experienced by the early teenager consciously. Nonetheless the fantasies can be detected in their derivatives. The fantasies are primarily sexual. The aggressive drive does not intensify as strongly as the sexual drive. Depending on the respective sexes of the patient and the therapist, these latent fantasies, if not interpreted, can give rise to sexual acting out, unwanted pregnancies, or homosexual panic. It is therefore important to be on the lookout for signs of such transference, however fleeting, and to interpret them in the presence of hints that would not be considered justification for such comments in working with adults.

Primary transference takes the form of the therapist functioning as a lighthouse in a storm. The youngsters are apt to see a use for treatment when there is trouble in their lives, and to wonder why they are in treatment in periods of calm.

Characterological behavior increases. However, access to this activity as a source of insight is limited in many adolescents. There is a difficulty in engaging those whose immaturity is reflected in a failure to develop anxiety about their actions because they lack the perspective that comes with the ability to project the effects of one's actions into the future. This is more in evidence when an adolescent patient comes to psychotherapy only because he was sent by parents or by an institution. These patients would never seek treatment on their own. Therapeutic endeavors have to be aimed at the creation of a self-observing ego, which looks on from a watching post whose perspective is derived from the patient's expectations of adult life and its rewards.

Within this group of patients under duress, there is to be found a variant of transference rarely seen outside of child and adolescent psychotherapy. These patients are usually youngsters with severely antisocial behavior disorders. They suffer from variations and abnormalities in object constancy. They are unable to maintain a constant image of a libidinal object in their mind's eye. Clinically this results in a failure in superego development, since they do not develop a sustained image of a potentially punitive parental imago. Established superego demands are also difficult to maintain. Usually there is a history of an inconstant parental object (i.e., affect-starved children). Sometimes there appears to be a constitutional component contributing to this deficiency. Transference-oriented psychotherapies are of little value in the treatment of these children. They require corrective emotional experiences or structured environments to gain or survive. Transferences are not sufficiently sustained to make interpretations meaningful. Often in these therapies, the therapist is manipulated and used for something other than insight. Also there is failure to establish a transference object tie.

The form, shape, and usefulness of transference phenomena during late latency–early adolescence differ according to the nature of the past experience relived, and the level of maturation of the cognitive structures that both shape the manifestations of transference and provide the capacity to achieve insight and understanding. All transference manifestations have in common the psychotherapeutically useful characteristic that the patient's transference experience can be observed by both the therapist and the patient to be an incontrovertible example of a character trait of the patient, or an expression of a repressed drive derivative. In the presence of cognitive maturity (i.e., self-reflective awareness) that will make insight possible, examples can be used to link mutually observed transference experiences of the patient with related and similar experiences in the early life of the patient. In addition, the drives inherent in a fantasy (i.e., sexual urges) can be identified in the unconscious. One expects the patient to respond to the interpretation of such links with recollection of additional information that can be used in the therapy to understand many aspects of the patient's current behavior. It is possible that while a patient reviews and reports pertinent events in his life, he may gain intellectual insight into his idiosyncratic patterns of behavior. This provides only moderate therapeutically induced leverage in the direction of mastery of these patterns. Fantasy play contributes mastery through discharge and also to a small degree through such increased awareness of such patterns. Insight involving drives and the resolution of neurotic conflict is enhanced by the appearance of confirmatory data during the free association that follows a transference interpretation. Once this activity affords the patient experience of the origins of today's behavior patterns in drive-impelled memory traces from the formative years of life, it becomes possible to turn the exploration of current psychopathogenetic patterns of behavior into therapeutically effective working through of problem areas. Note that the same verbalizations on the part of the patient can be either conversation or psychotherapeutic working through. That which makes for psychotherapeutic working through is the creation of an awareness that transference behavior is a repetition on the time plane of the present of patterns from the past. One shows the patient in working through that a single episode of a given behavior does not serve the modern rationalization to which it has been assigned. The rationalization is an afterthought. It hides the fact demonstrated by its appearance in transference, that such behavior serves an internal and secret world of fantasy, which in turn mediates patterns of drives or of drive discharge established in early childhood. Certain fantasy components dominate the transference of adolescence. They are brought out under the pressure of the context of current adolescent object demands from a wider set of predisposing circumstances inspired by the events of early childhood.

TYPES OF TRANSFERENCES MET WITH IN ADOLESCENCE

Positive Transference Derived from Early Maternal Care

A child patient is primed to relate to the kindly ministrations of the therapist by a past experience of being able to turn to mother and have injuries soothed. The prior experience could be called the Band-Aid stage, and contributes to positive transference. This produces a state of expectant cooperation. Its existence should not be pointed out to the early adolescent unless it interferes with the treatment.

A 16-year-old girl with an acute phobic reaction found that she could travel anywhere as long as she had with her a pill which her therapist had given her. "It's like you are there with me," she would say.

Identification Transferences Based on Traumatic Experiences

Sometimes a look, a mannerism, or another type of casual characteristic can remind a patient of a past experience that was uncomfortable. The therapist can in this circumstance be identified with a hostile relative, for instance. The therapist is then reacted to as though he were the relative.

Repression Proper

Unfullfilled early infantile wishes that have been repressed grow in importance as sources of transference during adolescence. As an example, a small child's wishes for tender caresses, which have been thwarted by either a cruel or an emotionally distant parent, leave infantile needs unrequited. The establishment of internal prohibitions against the expression of such wishes results in inhibiting of their drive expression in the child. They are said to be in a state of repression. When manifestations of early experience of frustration of these wishes occur during psychotherapy sessions with adolescents, the phenomenon has a quality of transcience. It can be categorized as a form of transference proper. However, because its fleeting nature gives it distinct characteristics, it should be set apart and given the name *removal transference*.

In early adolescence, drive derivatives break free of the fantasy defenses of latency. They follow the shift of symbols away from fantastic referents and from the primary love objects (the parents) and settle for a moment on the therapist while on their way to peer objects and lasting relationships. This phenomenon is primarily a characteristic of the psychotherapy of early adolescence. It can be viewed as a phase in the process of removal (Katan 1937). Removal transference touches the therapist as it brushes by on the way from the parents to a peer. There is a remarkable similarity here to the "transitional object in statu nascendi" that was described by Winnicott (1953). A growing need comes from the increasing pressure of the drives as the result of weakening of symbol-based defenses and stronger hormonal influences. The therapist's role as the armature around which transferences are formed makes him the perfect foil for removal transferences. These transferences are particularly perilous events in early adolescent psychotherapy. The peril arises from the fact that the transferences serve as formative testing grounds for ensuing real-life experiences. Erotically tinged removal transferences can usher in sexual acting out with peers.

In addition, libidinal energies needed for the therapy can be withdrawn from the therapist when an erotically cathected peer appears. This can result in the decathexis of the therapist and a premature termination of the patient–therapist relationship.

Early Adolescent Pseudotransference

Because of structural immaturities there are psychotherapy situations involving the therapist that appear to be transference. The patient appears to be making fun of the therapist in what seems to be a transference. In actuality such situations are not the recreation of prior experience. Instead they are the products of the misunderstanding of the use of verbal communication. This can happen when the child feels that he can claim something to be a likeness of something, when it is not in any way a likeness of that which it is claimed to be. A prime example of this is the use of words as though they were capable of producing realities at the moment they are spoken.

Jim was 11 years of age. Strong of face and lean of limb, he actively voiced his preference for the playroom because "I feel more comfortable here." Yet he did not play out tales with the toys. Rather, he threw a ball or kicked a sack. In his mind he played out competitive ball games with peers or showed off to me his peerless skills. He was willing to talk freely about his problems with aggression control, which made life difficult for parents, neighbors, and schoolmates. His concomitant fear of thieves who might come at night (projection of aggression) was amply documented by his parents. When these were brought up, he discussed them freely. This resulted in a resolution of his fears, in that he was able to confront his anger as his own and thus master the need to project anger. There was marked improvement in his persecutory fantasies. They dwindled to a minor element in his symptom configuration. Soon he ceased to speak of his aggressive behavior. Therapy sessions threatened to become part of a fitness program for him. Then his mother called to tell that he had broken a window. When his mother's report was mentioned to him, he flushed and said, "She told you that. Damn, she told you that. Why did she have to tell you that. What a fool. If she tells you that, how can you believe me? Now you know that, I have to stay here longer. How long do I have to stay here now?"

Even though his mother wished the aggression to be brought into treatment, the child felt that if I were to say he was better, he would be "better" and could stop treatment without the bother of working through his aggressive behavior. "My mother says that when you say I'm done, I'll be all better." He interpreted this in the light of his own attitudes toward words. He felt that my word would be accepted as truth just as he expected his words to be accepted as truth. He had no conspiracy with his mother. Yet he depended on her for silence in support of his manipulative use of words to render his cause plausible.

It was explained to the boy that words cannot create reality, they can only reflect it. "When you say something, I don't listen for your words. I listen to what you are trying to tell me. It has to fit in your whole world, or I know it isn't true. Your world has your mother in it. What she says helps me to see the whole picture. You wouldn't be here if she wanted to help you fool me. If you could make up real things just by saying them, you would be very powerful. People who think they can do that get into trouble because they make up their own rules. Lots of times there is no room for such people. Then they get picked on and disliked."

While the therapist was alternately neighing and weighing the introduction of the proverb "If wishes were horses, beggars would ride" to a child whose thinking had not reached the level of abstract operations, the boy blurted out, "I used to think I came from another planet. I was so sure that I must have asked my mother a hundred times if I was adopted. That's why I always wanted to play 'Star Wars', when all the other kids wanted to play cops and robbers. I was waiting for my family to come and get me."

In the session, the therapeutic activity had been twofold. First, it served to modify the omnipotent use of words as magic instruments with an existence independent of the reality that all people test and share. Second, the therapist confronted and undermined the hypercathexis of fantasy, which is a manifestation of early adolescent reactive narcissism.

It is important to differentiate between manipulations that are expressions of transference proper and those manipulations that are attempts to trick the therapist through the use of words as magic instruments with an existence independent of reality. The latter reflects a stage in the emergence of mature cognition. The child was not acting out a wish to involve the therapist in a conspiracy; rather, he was exercising the use of the magic power of words. This reflected his interpretation of word use by adults. This interpretation is informed by early childhood experience with the magic power of words. Out of this he created a manipulation in the service of his narcissism, with the goal of achieving more free time and avoiding confrontation with unconscious material.

This manipulation could be conceived of as a form of primal transference. The child could be using the therapist as a foil for the exploration of the emergent cognitive dissonance that occurs between immature cognition and the developmental advance in abstract thinking that characterizes late latency–early adolescence. In adolescence, the child works on enhancing these skills and trying to comprehend their application. (Sarnoff 1987b). Mature cognition is characterized by the communicative use of consensually validated abstractions.

The child was not trying to involve the therapist or his mother in a conspiracy; rather, he did not understand the nature of truth. The therapist was aware that what his patient had told him was an anemnesis rather than history or a memory. If we define history as the story of what has happened as reported by many observers and as combed for contradictions and inconsistencies by many investigators, we can recognize the possibility of achieving an approximation of truth in the reporting of past events. If we define memory as all that a patient is capable of retaining of an experience, we recognize that even under the best of circumstances the whole truth is not available to the patient. And if we define anemnesis as a recollection which is an "excogitation of true things, or things similar to truth to render one's cause plausible" (Cicero, as quoted by Yates 1966, p. 8) we shall recognize that anemnesis can be a conflation of memory elements with the primitive thought processes that create truth out of words. This produces the primitive thought process of the preadolescent that makes overt discharge through fantasy possible and turns the therapeutic situation into a testing ground for exploring admixtures of the realm of reality and the realm of words. Such experiences within the "in vitro" tainted boundaries of the therapeutic situation challenge the assumption that any patient activities that engage the therapist are transference proper.

RECRUITMENT AND METAMORPHOSIS THROUGH TRANSFERENCE

Removal transference (defined above) is a stage in the establishment of object relations during early adolescence. The therapist often makes inroads into the patient's personality through his or her own behavior and thought style in addition to the use of interpretation in the service of insight.

J. T. was tall, willowy, winsome, and wise beyond her 16 years in the ways that women sway men. Her father, who was fascinated with her, could easily be made to "see the light" when she became flirtatious. She had been sent to therapy because of an unexplained drop in her grades that was directly relatable to clouding of thinking following marijuana use. A pout had crossed her face when she was told that the therapist would not call her parents to tell them that it was all right for her to sleep at a girlfriend's house the following weekend. As she got up at the end of the session, the pout turned into a sweet smile. She advanced toward the therapist. He moved back slightly and offered a handshake. "I only wanted to give you a hug and a kiss good-bye," she said.

"Kisses and hugs are parts of a different situation. Therapy has to do with thinking," said the therapist.

She had tried to recruit her therapist into an interpersonal interaction from a fantasy world informed by her relationship with her father. Through this act of transference she reached into the object world. The object world in the form of the therapist responded with an unexpected pattern of behavior, which offered a basis for a character metamorphosis.

S. P. was 10. It had already become apparent that the gracile young lad who spent hours in the playroom playing out brutal combats with toy soldiers felt no need to work diligently in school. His low marks had placed him in a remedial classroom where he was separated from his friends, whose level of intelligence and perspicacity he shared. He met with them after school. He felt left out of their school talk and was beginning to suspect that they were talking about these matters as a mean way of leaving him out of things. He had been sent to therapy because of disruption of the household produced by his constant provocations and fights with his mother. His mother contributed to the problem. She had difficulty in containing herself when he refused to clean up after his dog, left clothing on the bathroom floor, or left his socks and toe pickings on the living room cocktail table on the evening of a party she was giving for socially prominent people she had hoped to impress. He reported that he was often unable to do his homework because the fights with his mother upset him so that he could not settle down to study. He spent the time in his sessions playing out robberies and war games using toy soldiers. Though he spoke often with the therapist, psychotherapeutically effective communication was deflected by his immersion in evocative play. The therapist equated the distraction of the play with S.P.'s use of fights with his mother as a reason to avoid homework. The child made no verbal response. He just played on. There were no evidences of the gain of insight. The therapist began to think he was a very nice boy with a nagging mother and without an internalized tendency to become a partner in sadomasochistic wrangling. There was marked improvement in his behavior at home. This was at first attributed to discharge of drive tensions through the clash of toy armies in the playroom.

Concurrently, something strange was happening in the therapist's office. Not always, but often, the toilet paper in the bathroom became tied up in a knot. Sand deformed the soap. Emergency lighting fixtures became disconnected. Other children, taking heed of these events, began to engage in similar pursuits, so that identifying the culprit was difficult.

One day, when no other possible suspect had had a session, a telephone was found to be disconnected and a wad of paper placed so as to disrupt contact in an electric light socket. In the following session, the therapist described these events to the child, who responded with, "That's mean."

The therapist remained calm through the session. He checked the office before and after each of the patient's subsequent visits. It became clear that he was one of the sources of the problem, but not the only culprit. The therapist mentioned each damage to equipment and explained how he knew the child was at fault. "Gee!" said the child, "You don't get angry like my m— —[his words dwindled to a hum]."

"It's not something to be argued about. It's something to be settled."

After that the patient's contribution to the disorganization of the office disappeared. Concurrently he began to work on his lessons in the professed hope that he could regain his academic position and rejoin his friends.

One could construct a theory that he was in the process of moving his patterns of drive discharging from his family to the world. As part of this process he involved the therapist. Through provocations that disrupted the therapist's reality and set examples for other young patients to follow, he pushed the therapist toward a relationship that represented removal transference. Instead of finding a willing partner for sadomasochistic play as otherwise expressed in the battles of the toys, he found a therapist who diverted his energies toward useful interactions and provided him with a model for the handling of provocations that might come his way.

His foray into sadism was an attempt to recruit the therapist into a mutual interaction in the transference. The therapist's nonsadomasochistic response provided a model for a metamorphosis of behavior that enabled the exploration and establishment of new ways of relating to reality in place of old patterns of drive discharge.

THE APPEARANCE OF HOSTILE AFFECTS AND SEXUAL FEELINGS UNENCUMBERED BY THE STRUCTURE OF LATENCY IN EARLY ADOLESCENT PSYCHOTHERAPY

A unique characteristic of psychotherapy during late latency and early adolescence is the chance it offers to the therapist to confront therapeutic targets early in the life of the patient. Often the patient is seen just as new styles of thought are maturing or are just beginning to dominate. During early adolescence, libidinal and aggressive drives are briefly transferred onto the therapist. The passing touch of libido on the way to reality transfigures the transference in ways that can be enlisted for therapeutic insight. Because these transference-derived insights surface during a formative period, character patterns derived from roots shared with transference can be influenced. Aberrant behavior has the potential for transience, since secondary gain has not yet had a chance to lock a pathological pattern into place. As a result, therapy during this period of change should have great potential for shaping the personality at the start. During adolescence the child's personality is first emerging from the shell that had been provided by the inward turning generated by the narcissistic cathexes of latency. Reality looms larger. The therapist can observe the first experiences of confrontations between self and world in the absence of the protection of parents and the structure of latency. One is in a position to guide, interpret, and set examples while the structure of the personality is still flexible and more open to influence than when locked into place by an interdependence of defenses and secondary gains.

During the period of transition between latency and adolescence, the organization of defenses that supported states of latency falls away. The mechanisms that supported it are organized into new systems that carry the focus away from the egotism of latency toward the altruisms of adult life. The intermediate phase of transition between these two poles is adolescence. Anger, which had been siphoned off into displaced fantasy elements through the mediation of the structure of latency, is more immediately accessible.

The buffer of symbols is weak during the transition. The adult ego with its displacements, sublimations, fantasy, and symptoms must wait many years before it will be available to be interposed between the self that was the child and the people of the adult's world. During early adolescence, raw anger begins to stir, and for the first time for many of those who have been called by their parents "the best-behaved child I have ever known," rage appears to disturb their adjustment. Depression, projected anger, anxiety, unrest, and irritability when faced with passivity mark the period. They are the products of an attempt to forge a piece of the personality that can be used to modulate the impact of the drives. Affects that had been associated with drives during a healthy latency period are derived from the physiological manifestations of drives such as autonomic discharges, and from shame, guilt, fear of loss of love, longing, tumescence, and fear of ego dissolution or external forces of retribution. In early adolescence, the ego is not ready. Drive affects burst forth in a form and strength that cries for emergency relief and the development of a strong, long-term personality structure.

When children in this state (the struggle can contribute to discomfort and psychopathology from 11 years of age to the early twenties) come to psychotherapy, the problem is not how to get them "in touch with their feelings." Rather, it is to help them to deal with their very apparent feelings and to develop defenses to deal with levels of sexual drive and affect anger that they have never experienced before. The therapist is not protected by the presence in the patient of years of experience in dealing with such feelings in financially successful and independent adults. The children who are introduced to such unguarded anger for the first times cannot be depended upon after they have left the session to activate defenses that will result in "resetting" of the personality and a placing of anger on hold until the next session. The inadequately defended-against anger persists. It can mount in fury and give rise to fulminating rage and obsessing about remembered hurts and slights of childhood at the hands of parents and siblings. It draws vitally needed attention and energies from studies and work. Often the anger spills over into raging fights with parents, withdrawal from parents, and even suicide attempts.

In girls, removal transference carries libidinal feelings from the parent to the therapist on the way to the peer love partner. The lack of the incest barrier with the therapist results in an unnatural intensification of the sexual feelings, which can hurry interest and precipitate premature ventures into sexuality and pregnancy. Deferred angry feelings are similarly enhanced, when they are first intensely experienced in adolescent psychotherapy. Removal transference can open the floodgates to years of held-in rage directed at parents who by dint of their very presences and probity have controlled their child's affective life. The presence of a therapist as a transference object can serve as a catalyst that intensifies and focuses feelings of anger at parents. This can result in scenes, fights, and estrangements that disorganize the family and derail the life courses of the patient at a time when emotional pressures are high and the goal of the therapy is insight and the defusing of the negative aspects of drive pressures. Encouragement of transference and interpretation of its origin in interactions with the parents should be linked to an explanation that the goal of the therapy is understanding of the origins and resolution of the problem rather than an encouragement of a reign of terror aimed at revenge, rebellion, and too-early decisions about total independence from the parents. Failure to set this form of transference into the therapeutic context just described can result in deepening depression in reaction to rage, to which intransigent or distracted parents fail to respond. In the face of the adolescent sense that today is eternity, this depression, whose "poison roots" arise within the transference, can precipitate drug use, school dropouts, runaways, and suicidal threats, attempts, and finalities.

For example:

G. G., age 17, once said in a session, "I feel a dread within me. It comes over me from time to time. I feel depressed and frightened. I love my parents so that I can't stop coming here. Why are you emphasizing my mother so much? Why are you making me hate her?"

She had developed a fear of leaving her house without her mother or in the company of her friends. This fear had started when her friends had begun to speak about going away to college. She had asked her parents about possible colleges, and her parents told her that she would not have no choice but to go to the college they had chosen for her. Her father, an attorney, had sufficient funds to send her to any college, and the choice of a college of their religious denomination seemed arbitrary in the light of their lack of involvement in religious affairs. "They want me to marry a boy of the same religion, I think," she said wistfully in early sessions. As she said this, it seemed to be more an observation than a pivotal source of anger at passivity in the hands of overcontrolling parents.

In early sessions, she had reported fears of leaving her home because of a fear that she would become upset and not able to handle lonely feelings if her mother were not with her to comfort her. This gave the therapist a clue. Such a longing for a comforting companion is often evidence of conflict. It serves as a symbol of a repressed concern.

"What are the feelings you have that you fear?" asked the therapist.

"I get sad. I feel alone. I'm afraid I'm going to die. It's awful. Sometimes I feel I want to kill myself—I mean, go to sleep for a long time so I don't have to have these feelings for a while," she replied.

"The feelings are present always?" asked the therapist.

"No, only now and then. Most of the time I'm afraid they will come on, and that's bad too," she said. "I can hardly study. I spend so much time listening to records about lonely people. Gee, I wish I had a boyfriend." This is another clue to the therapist. Removal was not sufficiently far advanced for the patient to disengage her conflictual energies from her parents. The therapist knew that he should look for the source of the conflict in the relationships at home. He noted that questions that led away from family concerns led to answers that dwindled quickly.

In one session she came in reporting that she was depressed. "Depressed is anger turned on the self," stated the therapist. "When did the depression start?"

"On Saturday afternoon."

"What happened on Saturday?" the therapist asked.

"I had a fight with my mother," answered the girl. "I wanted to go out and I couldn't get my makeup. She spends 3 hours in the bathroom when she has to go, and nobody is allowed in there. Why did she have to use the one with my makeup? She sometimes isn't thoughtful. When I told her I wanted to go out, you'd think she would be happy. I wanted to go out and I wasn't scared. She wouldn't let me go cause she was going out to the library and she wanted me to stay home to make dinner for my father."

She began to feel angry at her mother and spoke of angry feelings, which were new to her. In the therapy, emphasis was placed by the therapist on ways of dealing with angry feelings rather than on encouraging the development of greater anger. The role of passivity in life was explored as a source of anger to be understood rather than to be reacted to.

PASSIVITY IN EARLY ADOLESCENCE

One of the primary sources of angry defiance in early adolescence is the experience of impotence in response to passivity at the hands of others who either by attitude or position in life take charge of one's life or give orders.

For example, a girl of 13, who walked on crutches because of an incapacitating bone pain for which no physical cause could be identified, reported a"hysterically funny" time at a big family party the Saturday night before her early Monday morning therapy session. The most fun came when the children began to "cheer wildly at the grandparents. They get so uncomfortable and embarrassed when we do that."

The therapist sensed that here was a role reversal, frequently seen at this age and of importance psychotherapeutically. He said, "You turned the tables."

"Most of the time you can't kid them," she answered.

"You are taught democracy, but when it comes down to it in your home, you get upset when you see how small your vote is," said the therapist.

She became heated in her discussion as she added, "My mother says, 'Clean up your room.'" I say, 'Why?' She says, 'Because I'm the adult.' Then I say, 'But Mom, it's not fair.' Before you know it we are having a small fight and I'm calling my friend to tell her what my mother is doing."

This interchange is perhaps the key to the conflict of generations that occurs in Western culture with its democratic traditions. In societies in which more authoritarian theories govern the relationship between children and family, conflicted early adolescence, with its defiance and rebellion, is not so much in evidence. Children are taught to revere the principle of equality amongst men. When they are old enough to think that they can function independently, they demand a vote in their daily destinies. Unfortunately for them, they find themselves confronted by "the tyranny of a gerontocracy, of old men who initiate the young men and forcibly impose the tradition of the tribe" (Harrison 1921, p. xxxvii). Children raised in the verbal traditions of democracy must learn that in the practical relationships of the home, "Parents lead. Children follow." The therapist would do well to be ever alert for signs of conflict reflecting this strain in the family interactions.

TRANSFERENCE AND THE MECHANISM OF CURE

Transference participates in the psychotherapeutic cure in two ways. One way is through insight. A second way derives gain from the mental process of transference itself. In the former, the transference experience adds a sense of reality to insight. In the latter, the process involved in the generation of transference contributes to progress.

Insight and Progress

The technique of psychotherapy requires that transference experiences be understood consciously for what they are. Freud (1909) described transference experiences as "feeling [in the therapy] which can only be traced back to old wishful phantasies of the patient's (sic) which have become unconscious" (p. 51). He later specified that feelings, to be transference, require that the ideas contained in the fantasy be characterized by a "special interest in the doctor" (1916–1917, p. 439). This special interest contains feelings and contents that "the patient has transfered without cause." He recommends that "we overcome the transference by pointing out to the patient [that the current experience does] not arise from the present situation and does not arise from the doctor but that they repeat something that happened to him earlier" (p. 444). We are advised to "interpret, discover, communicate" (p. 438) and "oblige [the patient] to transform his repetition into a memory" (p. 444). When the process and its contents become conscious, a sense of reality that confirms insight is added to awareness. As Freud (1909) saw it, transference brings conviction to insight. "It is only this reexperiencing in the 'transference' that convinces him of the existence and of the power of these unconscious sexual impulses" (p. 51). Freud (1916–1917) comments that "translation of what is unconscious into what is conscious" removes "the preconditions for the formation of symptoms" (p. 435). This can have far-reaching effects in the broader arena of the patient's life, wherever repetition of trauma or fantasy shapes the patient's choice of reactions and behavior. Freud (1914) reminds us that "the transference itself is itself only a piece of repetition, and that the repetition is a transference of the forgotten past not only onto the doctor, but also on to all the other aspects of the current situation," and "every other activity and relationship which may occupy his life at the time" (p. 151). In theory these other behaviors, symptoms, and reactions that are influenced by the repressed content may be affected positively by lifting the repression and gaining insight. Insight can be enhanced and can produce conscious distancing of oneself from drive-informed behavior. An interpretation of transference that is followed by recalls, play fantasies, memories, or dreams expands insight and makes conscious the mechanics of repression and the influence of drives on behavior.

Insight achieved through transference enhances knowledge of the unconscious early roots of behavior and gives access to a lattice into which to build conscious change.

Process and Progress

The very process of the development and encouragement of transference can give rise to progress without the interposition of conscious will. Abreaction reduces tension. There are unconscious metaphenomena produced during the evolving of a transference within therapy. Unconscious misperceptions when confronted with secondary-process cognition can be resolved through spontaneous reinterpretation and correction of ideas, and impressions on the part of the patient. Seeing earlier trauma or deprivation in the light of adult experience has the power to dissolve the influential memories and their behavioral products.

Abreaction refers to reexperiencing (reliving) past traumatic experiences and frustrations with full affect. Transference reactions have the quality of feeling real. The "special interest in the person of the doctor" (Freud 1916-1917, p. 439) which the patient has generated "without cause" (p. 444) feels real and is experienced as such. When tension is discharged in this way with diminution of immediate discomforts but no long-term effect, the process is called repetition compulsion. When the symbols of transference abreaction are part of a communicative process (communicative symbolization), repeated fantasy-based reexperiencing can result in working through and replacing fantasy with reality. This process is called reparative mastery. This is often seen as a result of the play of latency-age children both at home and in the office of a therapist. There are times when play therapy results in therapeutic gains with manifest changes in the fantasies that underlie play without the interposition of an interpretation.

In early adolescence, increased contact with new people in reality, plus recruitment and metamorphosis of elements of character from those people, results in improved ability to relate to others. This is achieved through the development of personalities that are reality related rather than influenced by drive-informed fantasy patterns. When play, fantasy, and reality objects involve reference to the analyst, the behavior is categorized as transference. As such, transference takes part in this automatic process of personality growth.

Insight produces emotional distance from behavior. This makes it possible to slow down automatic responses and to correct self-destructive activities. Under pressure of anxiety, remembered, present, and expected with apprehension, the application of more mature cognition to memories of motivating childhood experiences can change the content and result in modification of the fantasy structures.

During psychotherapy, other phenomena related to transference participate in cure through process and insight. These phenomena are fantasy play, dreams, fantasy, tales written or told, and actualization. They share with transference the ability to manifest, often in symbolic form, latent fantasy structures derived from drives and wish fantasies, which express unfulfilled childhood longings or serve to master the affects associated with early trauma. They differ from transference in that the manifest symbol is not the therapist. Instead the manifest symbols are the object of displacements from primary objects to forms within, upon, and beyond the boundary of the self, such as dreams, toys, and peers. In terms of therapeutic technique, one deals with these phenomena differently than one would deal with transference. Such phenomena and their handling will be dealt with in the next chapter.

REFERENCES

Abraham, K. (1924). A short study of the development of the libido. In *Selected Papers on Psychoanalysis*, pp. 418–501. New York: Basic Books, 1954.

Freud, S. (1909). Five lectures on psychoanalysis. (Lectures 5.) *Standard Edition* 2:49–55.

———— (1912a). The dynamics of transference. In *The Collected Papers of Sigmund Freud* 2:312–322. New York: Basic Books.

———— (1912b). The dynamics of transference. *Standard Edition* 12:97–108. London: Hogarth Press.

———— (1914). Remembering, repeating and working through. *Standard Edition* 12:145–156.

———— (1916–1917). Introductory lectures on psychoanalysis. (Lecture 27.) *Standard Edition* 16:431–447.

Harrison, J. E. (1921). *Epilogemina to the Study of Greek Religion*. New Hyde Park, NY: University Books, 1962.

Jones, E. (1916). The theory of symbolism. In *Papers on Psychoanalysis*, pp. 87–144. Baltimore, MD: Williams & Wilkins, 1948.

Katan, A. (1937). The role of "displacement" in agoraphobia. *International Journal of Psycho-Analysis* 32:41–50, 1951.

Laughlin, H. P. (1967). *The Neuroses*. Washington, DC: Butterworths.

Luria, A. (1968). *The Mind of a Mnemonist*. New York: Basic Books.

McCrone, J. (1991). *The Ape That Spoke*. New York: Morrow.

Neubauer, P. (1962). Personal communication.

Piaget, J. (1945). *Play Dreams and Imitation in Childhood*. New York: Dutton.

Sacks, O. (1989). *Hearing Voices*. Berkeley, CA: University of California Press.

Sarnoff, C. A. (1970). Symbols and symptoms. Phytophobia in a two-and-a-half-year-old girl. *Psychoanalytic Quarterly* 39:550–562.

———— (1976). *Latency*. Northvale, NJ: Jason Aronson.

———— (1987a). *Psychotherapeutic Strategies: The Latency Years*. Northvale, NJ: Jason Aronson.

_____ (1987b). *Psychotherapeutic Strategies: Late Latency Through Early Adolescence.* Northvale, NJ: Jason Aronson.

_____ (1989). Early psychic stress and psychosomatic disease: symbolic processes in psychosomatic disease. In *Psychosomatic Symptoms,* ed. C. P. Wilson and I. L. Mintz, pp. 83–104. Northvale, NJ: Jason Aronson.

Schachtel, E. (1949). On memory and childhood amnesia. In *A Study of Interpersonal Relations,* ed. P. Mullahy, pp. 7–50. New York: Heritage.

Winnicott, D. W. (1953). Transitional objects and transitional phenomena. *International Journal of Psycho- Analysis* 34:89–93.

_____ (1958). Transitional objects and transitional phenomena. (A paper based on Winnicott [1953]). In *Collected Papers: Through Paediatrics to Psycho-Analysis,* p. 239. New York: Basic Books.

Woodward, M. (1985). *Piaget's Theory, Modern Perspectives in Child Psychiatry.* Ed. J. G. Howell. Springfield, IL: Charles C Thomas.

Yates, P. A. (1988). *The Art of Memory.* Chicago IL: University of Chicago Press.

6

The Use of Fantasy, Dreams, and Play

Charles A. Sarnoff, M.D.

Latency is not a silent time for awaiting adolescence. It is not merely an adventitious element cast into the great sea of development. Latency is more than just a moment that leaves a little mark in passing. All of development must flow through the structures of latency. Adolescence evolves out of the cognitive transitions of latency. Psychotherapy for adolescents must be informed by knowledge of what can go wrong during these transitions. Psychotherapy during the latency years therefore affects not only immediate emotional problems, but also the long-range effects of distortions that occur during latency-age development. From the standpoint of pathological development the aspects of latency and adolescence that are most sensitive and most often in need of help are those functions that take part in the maturation of object relations, support the finding of comfort in fantasy, and grow as the result of the transformations in cognition that enhance reality testing.

The neuroses of the young come into being as a compromise between unconscious longings and the unbending demands of reality. Longings rise toward consciousness from zones where energies are free to seek discharge without restraint of object, place, time, or accidents of fate, only to be confronted with those stringent demands of reality that bind energies to obligations. The older the child, the stronger the influence of reality. Free energies run the errands of desire in pleasure palaces filled with fantasy. Bound energies bow to the harsh realities of adult size and knowledge acquisition that impinge on the small world of the humble child. Between the two extremes lie zones of fantasy-tinted compromise from which the neuroses of the young arise.

The neuroses of prelatency, latency, and early adolescence differ from adult neuroses in the degree to which they are influenced by maturation. With the exception of the intensification of obsessional defenses in the late twenties, the matrix of cognition of the adult is relatively fixed. By comparison, the underpinnings of neurosis in the young are in constant flux. One of the clinical products of this is the transient nature of neurotic symptoms in the young neurotic. There is an ebb and flow of drive energies and external pressures. Latent fantasy contents change in response to new siblings, humiliations, school challenges, and vicissitudes of parental adjustment beyond the control of the child. Rarely is the childhood neurosis an organizer of an ego splinter that by its very existence holds its finger in a dike, as it were, to counter inner pressures and permit the remaining ego some degree of autonomy, thus creating neutral ego functioning in the service of adaptation as adult neuroses and perversions sometimes do.

The childhood neurosis is evidence of a weak spot. Its presence is pervasively disorganizing. The therapist must be tuned in to many more factors than the adult therapist. He or she must be ever on the alert for alteration in the potential for neurotic symptom formation that is introduced by normal cognitive maturation, and persistent immaturities that spring into being when maturation fails to keep pace with the passing years. Childhood neurosis is like a volcanic island that grows by rising from the sea under pressure from afar, all the while adding to its bulk by eruptions. It has many sources for its features. The child therapist must be familiar with the sources of childhood neurosis, both the ebb and flow of life's tides and the somewhat eldritch isostacy engendered by cognitive transformations.

The neutral world of the child, supported by bound energies, can be approached through verbal exchanges in therapy sessions. This touches only the civilized crust of a child's existence. There are more personal zones of life. Drive derivatives do not gain easy entrance to reality interactions. Discharge of the drives is buffered by a recreation of the world through displacement of its elements into symbolic forms. Adjustment in large part revolves about the maintainance of a world of fantasy.

Though an adult who centers his life on fantastic evocations of his inner needs has lost his way, a child who treads the fantasy path is involved in acceptable behavior. Fantasy serves the satisfaction of needs in the world of childhood where there are no handholds in reality for inner wishes. A unique therapeutic approach must be developed to tap the world of unbound energies and unbound wishes locked up in the dreams, play, and latent fantasies of the latency child. Latent fantasies are the roots, manifest fantasies are the stalks and leaves, and dreams and play are fruits and flowers in the wishing bowers from which the symptoms of neurosis also grow. Neurotic symptoms are formed when the manifest symbols that represent these unconscious wishes are reshaped by cognitive structures of the ego that serve the moral and ethical demands of the outside world.

BEHAVIORAL NEOTENY

The maturation and development of children are influenced by a multitude of factors, each of which must be considered in understanding emotional growth errors that produce behavioral variants and pathologies in childhood and adolescence. Poor example setting can alter behavior. Strong affects can distract a child from the exercise of skills afforded by advancing cognition. Persistence in memory of early trauma and regression in the face of frustration can result in sustained immature behavior patterns. Innate potentials inherent in maturation are shaped by genetic forces. Juvenile cognition persisting through the achievement of adult form will produce an immature adult who cannot gain from social phase-specific educational opportunities. Darwin (1872) described the "loss of the adult stage of development" in species that reach reproductive potential "before they acquire their perfect characters" (p. 113). This process is known to biologists as neoteny. Budiansky (1991) has extended the concept to include behavioral characteristics and object relations. He points out that "variation within a species is normally limited . . . by basic rules of genetics and development. But there is one source of enormous variation within a species. . . . The range of variation in any adult population is minuscule compared with the differences that separate the average adult from the average juvenile. . . . If the genes that govern this development process change in such a way that adulthood is reached before the normal process of development is complete, youthful characteristics will be locked in. This process is called neoteny. . . ." (p. 20). Neoteny may be manifested by the presence of behavior that is derived from genetically controlled persistence of immature cognitive structure and function into adulthood, such as concrete thinking, magical thinking, narcissistic object relations, primary-process dominance, and dominance of the evocative pole in symbol formation. Budiansky (1991) illustrates this by referring to the persistence of dependency and ability for cross-species object ties as it exists in the object relationships of infantile forms of animals who become capable of domestication as adults.

The transient neurotic symptoms of childhood are products of ever-changing cognition. Such transformations of cognition characterize growing personalities. One manifestation of neoteny would be the potential to lock in immature forms of cognition and relatedness. When this is encouraged, either by genetic limitations on progress or by receptive parental or social attitudes, chronic persistence into adulthood occurs. On a species level this can produce large populations with maladaptive personality features, to which a tolerant and humane society may choose to adjust. In individual personalities this contributes to the formation of fixed immature cognitive structures. The fixed nature of these structures contributes to the chronic nature of neurotic symptoms in the adult. For this reason it is beneficial in child therapies to illustrate and encourage patterns of cognition (i.e., memory systems, symbolic forms, reality testing) that have enhanced adaptive potential in adulthood, in addition to interpretation and working through of fantasy.

FANTASY

There are thus two directions that therapy of children can take. One entails encouraging the maturation of cognition, especially in the areas of reality testing and the types of objects from which the symbolic forms of manifest fantasy are derived. The second entails resolution of latent fantasy and discharge of drives and tension through the encouragement and interpretation of fantasy.

It is natural and an occupier of much time for the child to engage in fantasy and fantasy play during waking life, as natural as it is for all ages to dream at night. In the child therapy session, it is possible to tap this process and adapt it to therapeutic growth, resulting in discharge of drives, resolution of fantasy structures, and encouragement of cognitive growth, freeing the child to enter adulthood unencumbered.

Biographies of writers describe the role of waking fantasy in the day-to-day adjustment of children outside the clinical setting. Kinkaid (1991), in reviewing a biography of the novelist Trollope by Hall (1991), describes Trollope as having a childhood where "humiliation loaded on the child through all his school years; the beatings and desolation; the turn of the heartsick and friendless little boy to an inward life of tale-spinning, where he could do clever things and win approval—where 'beautiful young women used to be fond of me' " (Kinkaid, p. 16, Hall, p. 30). As an adult, Trollope wrote forty-seven novels, which contain reflections of his childhood's pain.

Hoffman (1991), in reviewing a biography of Poe by Silverman (1991), tells us that "Poe's mother died when he was three years old. He never resolved his bereavement" (p. 17). Silverman describes the role of childhood trauma in determining adult psychopathology in what follows: "Much of Edgar's career, too, might be understood as a sort of prolonged mourning, an artistic brooding—on an assemblage of fantasies activated by an ever-living past. As no product of his imagination would put to right what had gone wrong or restore what he had once possessed, he would begin over and over, repeating in new forms, different imagery, and fresh characters and scenes of dilemma which he presented as the peculiar condition of his existence" (p. 78).

Fantasy in Latency

Latency is a magic road that wends its way through a landscape of fantasies. Of these fantasies, derivatives of the Oedipus complex loom like a mountain range running ever beside it. Tracing the same course, but as foothills, are anal-sadistic preoccupations. Scattered along the way, as the latency years unfold, is a march of fantasy responses to the challenges that accompany cognitive, physical, and social maturation. The challenges include humiliation, sibling rivalry, budding sexuality, and passivity.

The Age Frames of Fantasy

The Stage of Early Latency: Oedipality and Guilt

At the beginning of the latency period, before attendance at grade school begins (5 to 6 years of age), pleasing fantasy content is informed by the Oedipus complex. As the child reaches 6, the capacity to experience guilt develops. Then oedipal fantasies (taking the roles of either of the parents) cease to be the source of pleasant musings. Associated with guilt, their potential entry into consciousness generates fear. Guilt and expected retribution are transmuted into manifest fantasies of theft and imprisonment. Such fantasies discharge tension. In a part of the psyche sequestered from reality, they provide a sense of expiation or mastery for the feelings and situations involved. Such fantasies dominate the latency-age period.

Should these fantasies fail to resolve oedipal pressures, the ego responds with a regression that directs attention to anal-sadistic preoccupations, replacing the newer and more perilous Oedipus complex with an area that has already been dealt with in prior years—now to be confronted with a far more sophisticated and mature set of defenses. In the healthiest possible response, the anal-sadistic impulses are defended against by the mobilization of the mechanisms of restraint (reaction formation, symbolization, isolation, doing and undoing, and obsessive-compulsive defenses), which defuse the strength of the drives that impel the child to fantasy. The mechanisms of restraint produce a state of latency in the child. To the casual observer the child appears to have socially appropriate periods of calm, pliability, reasonableness, and educability during these states. These attributes underlie readiness for the activities of the elementary and junior high school years. Should drives be stirred by maturation or accidents of fate (physical and sexual growth, seduction, humiliation, losses), there is a danger that the potential for calm will be beyond the control of the mechanisms of restraint. This alternative is averted by the assertion of an organization of the ego with an unique association to latency. This is the *structure* of latency (Sarnoff 1976), which serves as a safety valve to preserve the state of latency. Through the action of the structure of latency, the offending reality stress is excluded from consciousness. Its content is fragmented, then displaced, and then represented by symbols that are organized into manifest fantasies that become the dream, play, and daydream fantasies of childhood. Often, the child, unequipped to deal with the dragons of reality, turns to victories in these fantasies as recompense and resolution for the problems of the day. This ego configuration provides alternative outlets for excess drive energies. By deflecting drive energies to oedipal level fantasy it diminishes the pressure of anal-sadistic energies on the static and brittle mechanisms of restraint. Lessening of their strength supports a successful defensive regression to anal-sadistic preoccupations. This regression obviates any need for conscious attention to oedipal concerns. Anal-sadistic preoccupations are squelched, defeated and diminished by the structure of latency. However, they are never vanquished and never fully disappear. Within cohorts of peers cloistered in the permissive zone found in the backseats of car pool vehicles, anal-sadistic ideation surface as children sing of doody and of a man with diarrhea.

With the passing of years, additional fantasy contents appear, resulting in a de-emphasis of oedipal fantasy in the middle and late latency years. These contents are responses to the problems presented to the child during the stage of latency-age development at which they occur.

The Stage of Middle Latency: Loneliness and Separation

A sense of independence from parents at about 7 or 8 years of age projects a child into a psychic reality in which he is all alone in the big world. Fear fantasies of being small and vulnerable follow. The impotence they feel may be symbolized by a dread of monsters, which not only represent what they fear but also serve as masking vehicles for projections of the child's own defensively mobilized aggression.

The Stage of Late Middle Latency: Passivity

Beyond the age of 9 or 10, the problem of passivity becomes a major issue. A sense of independence develops at this age and reaches a point at which children strongly wish to break free of parental control. They object to the passive role that they have to take in relation to the decision-making parent. This is in many ways a recapitulation of the 2-year-old's demand to know "who's the boss of me." These children would like to run their own lives. They object to parental control and interference on an ever-widening horizon of activities. Eventually this trend becomes so intense that they have little else on their minds. The child continually confronts the parent with "Don't treat me like a baby!" This is evidence of a child readying himself to turn his adaptive energies from inward-turning fantasies that solve problems through the manipulation of symbols, to demands and actions that will intrude on the world. The children become especially sensitive to situations in which their decisions are challenged or their immaturity emphasized.

The Stage of Late Latency: Ethical Individuation

Sensitivity to challenge to the child's social decisions leads to feelings of humiliation and inferiority, when ethical conflicts estrange them from their parents. This can include simple choices such as crossing the street alone or major decisions in response to peer pressure involving stealing, drugs, and sex. In defense the children generate fantasies about being movie stars, championship athletes, owning motorbikes, and so on. Some children who are conflicted about such confrontations deflect the challenge into fantasies of defiance. These can take the form of fantasies of theft and crime, which are at times acted out.

The Stage of Late Latency: Sexual Identity Crises

Awakening concern about sexual identity intensifies with the first growth spurt. This occurs at about 9 years of age. Body changes, though too slight to be detected by a casual observer, alert the child to pubertal changes. Children revive old concerns about sexual identity. They worry about what they'll look like as adults. It is not uncommon for boys to mistake breast buds as evidence of a sex change. This stirs up other fantasies and castration fears.

Conflicts of the prelatency and the latency years can be resolved through discharge and mastery using latency-age fantasy, or through reality interactions with parents that introduce clarity to thinking. Stresses that distorting and sensitizing fantasies bring to adolescent and adult life can be defused during these latency years. This is a natural process. Should this process fail, fantasy serves to deflect a child's attention from conflict-resolving realities. As a result there occurs a persistence of neurosogenic factors. Latency is a time when a reshaping of the self becomes possible. If, proverbially, "As the twig is bent, so grows the tree," then latency can be seen as a time for unbending.

THE MECHANISMS OF FANTASY

The fantasies produced by the structure of latency are highly symbolized, defensively constructed manifest fantasies. They are played out in symbolic latency fantasy play, and they mask latent fantasies. These are not just passive, unconscious symbol patterns, awaiting a cue to come forth and give some shape to the manifest fantasies of play. Their presence is part of a system of psychic forces that are ever ready to bring prior experiences, expectations, unresolved experiences, and traumas from the child's past into action in the child's interpretation and reaction to new experiences. An example of a preinformed expectation is illustrated by the experience of a prelatency youngster who was visiting his aunt. He asked for a cookie. There was no cookie in sight.

The aunt improvised with the offer of a cracker.

The child took it, bit into it, and finding that it did not give way to his teeth as a proper cookie should, announced, as he handed it back, "Aunt Carole, it doesn't work."

A child whose latent fantasies are influenced by sexual feelings for his parents will be apt to be stirred by seductive behavior to the point that the structure of latency will produce an oedipal fantasy-derivative in play. Failing this, there may be a shift in a regressive direction requiring the further mobilization of the mechanisms of restraint. The mechanisms of restraint deal primarily with regressions from oedipal fantasies. The latency defense of the structure of latency is less specific, since it is often called upon to deal with a multitude of possible complexes, sensitivities, instigators of anger, overwhelming excitements, humiliations, and the many put-downs to which the psyches of our patients as children are prone and heir.

The role of fantasy in the psychological life of the child extends much beyond serving as a place to hide from reality and feelings. Fantasy also helps to preserve family intactness. Fantasies can be used to discharge affects and tension. Manifest fantasy can be used to discharge, master, and resolve latent fantasies that serve as memory moieties, which carry into latency traumas and conflicts of infancy and the prelatency period that, if unresolved, threaten later life adjustments.

Fantasy and the Illusion of Knowledge

Anger at parents can be blunted by changing the topic in the mind's eye of the child. This is an example of self-distraction through fantasy. By substituting a symbol for a momentarily hated object, the child can produce a shift of cathexis (attention energy) from an emotionally uncomfortable area of contemplation to a more neutral one. The ego mechanism involved is called displacement. As a result of this phenomenon, the child produces for himself a life image that is shorn of painful reflections on the truth of the matter. A countercathectic "illusion of knowledge" (Boorstein 1983, p. 86) pervades memory supporting the myth of an idealized family relationship. One is reminded of the biblical proverb that tells of the stratagem of focusing on a fantasy of a dangerous beast in order to avoid admitting to a disinclination to work or progress: "The slothful man saith, There is a lion in the way; a lion is in the streets" (Proverbs 26:13).

Future Planning

When those whose fantasies are the product of an intact structure of latency reach adolescence, their capacity for future planning is strong. Early and middle latency fantasies are plans that bypass problems through distraction, drive discharge, and diminution of affect and mood. This is done through displacement from affect-charged latent symbols to manifest symbols that carry or attract less affect. The manifest symbols of early latency are selected from nonhuman unrealistic elements, which exist in a context of timelessness. As cognition matures, bringing latency to its end, there is a shift in the symbolic forms from which manifest forms are selected. Late latency manifest symbols include real people in real situations in a linear time frame. With this change in symbols, the structure of latency has the potential to convert from an ego structure to a personality skill. The latter solves reality problems through the creation of fantasies that plan for the future through the manipulation of the realities of the world. Thus does problem resolution evolve from alloplastic fantasy formation to auto-plastic future planning. Enhanced reality testing runs parallel to this process. The more reality influenced are the symbols used in fantasy, and the more that ludic symbols give way to real creatures in the daydreams of the young, the greater is the chance that the daydreams and play fantasies of childhood will be gratified through their new role as patterns and as guides to fulfillment in shaping adult life. This insight was acutely perceived by Rabindranath Tagore (1936) in his poem "The Beginning":

"Where have I come from, where did you pick me up?" the baby asked its
   mother.
She answered half crying, half laughing, and clasping the baby to her
   breast, —
"You were hidden in my heart as its desire, my darling. You were in the
   dolls of my childhood's games; . . ." [p. 14]

Fantasy as Reparative Mastery

Ordinary daily events, when interpreted in the light of the charged memories that they call forth, can generate distortions of reality and misunderstandings. Such sources of tension can be reduced in a child by the defusing of these memories through discharge of linked affects in fantasy-dominated play. Rage released in a fantasy locale reduces tension at home, in school, and in other forms of play. Affects can be neutralized by displacement of activities to zones of calm where mastery can be assured.

Not only do events evoke conflicts. Conflicts can seek out events. The forces of mastery and repetition seek successful new experiences in reality to serve the same purpose as the generation of manifest fantasies that heal through discharge, reassurance, and the resolution of past traumas. As a result, latent fantasies, which carry old imbalances in drive pressures into contemporary situations, are reduced. Cognitive transformations, which are slowed by distractions and anxiety, can then progress.

Fantasy as a Manifestation of Compulsion to Repeat

Not all fantasy activity achieves resolution through discharge in manifest latency fantasy. Typical of this is the persecutory fantasy, which in latency depicts a cruel monster attacking the child, and which in later life, when real people are recruited to populate fantasies, takes the form of recurrent experiences of being treated cruelly by peers and lovers. Manifest fantasy content is synthesized from age-appropriate symbolic forms associated with levels of development reached as the result of the cognitive transformations of latency. Repetition in fantasy and reality that fails to resolve the conflicts associated with latent fantasy are manifestations of the repetition compulsion. The distinct nature of child and early adolescent psychotherapy is mandated by three pathological elements that produce these observations. These are (1) failure of fantasy or behavior to relieve instinctual pressures (repetition compulsion), (2) failure to progress to age-appropriate symbolic forms, and (3) interference with object relations on a reality level by instinctual pressures that seek expression of fantasy through the manipulative use of real objects. Psychotherapeutic strategies in the treatment of neurosis in the young require techniques that remediate these problem areas. To be able to do this, the therapist must have an understanding of the disorders of age-appropriate cognitive transformation that produce such pathologies.

THE ROLE OF FANTASY IN THERAPY AND ADJUSTMENT

The encouragement of fantasy during psychotherapy enhances the effectiveness of an important developmental task of latency, namely, the resolution and defusing of the impact of persistent memory of fantasy and trauma that occurred as prelatency experience. Fantasy play makes a contribution to this process by enabling the child to discharge tension and master trauma through catharsis and reliving. Fantasy in the growing child is normally manifested in thought and in words, in dreams and in play. In large measure, psychotherapy of the young adapts such normal fantasy to the goals of therapy. For the fantasy-rich child, this is done through encouraging fantasy play. For the child poor in capacity for the formation of fantasy and symbol, one attempts to enhance skill in the use of words and symbols (see Chapter 5, the case of Roy). Once fantasy can be introduced into therapy, it becomes possible to encourage its use as a medium for the discharge of tension. Tension discharge can be achieved without interventions or interpretations by the therapist. In a similar way, fantasy play can be used for mastery of current trauma.

Dynamic interpretation can harness fantasy play to therapeutic goals on a more complex level. Interpretation of experiences, unconscious fantasy, and symbol content can bring latent conflicts into awareness. This enhances the effectiveness of psychotherapy by making unconscious content available for discussion. In this way, impact of past and current traumas can be defused through confrontation with reality.

Fantasy during latency contributes to adjustment in later years. It serves as a proving ground for the role of trial action (thought) in solving problems. As the symbolizing function matures, reality objects serve as sources of the symbol content of fantasies. This enhances the application of reality testing in judging the appropriateness of efforts at problem solving. In this way, the trial action that is implied in thought and fantasy grows to be future planning. Failure of this natural developmental step during latency produces an individual who thinks in an egocentric, nonlinear manner, as seen in amotivational syndromes and adolescent drug users (Pittell 1973).

Two kinds of experience can encourage this developmental shortfall. The first is severe trauma that shatters the effectiveness of the structure of latency. The second is the presence in reality of events that may be interpreted as fantasy come true. The latter leads to an obliteration of the fantasy–reality boundary. This becomes especially a problem in regard to the sensitizing fantasies that create distortions through expectation in adult life. Fantasy-come-true experiences result in a stripping away of the influence of reality and a regression to primary process in fantasy-oriented thinking. The child is left with the impression that if fantasies can come true, there is no telling what can happen. "If wishes were horses, beggars would ride" ceases to be an admonition in favor of restraint. Instead, wishes and fantasies make things to be feared and programs for progress that summon vast energies to the pursuit of hollow crowns and nonexistent castles set in clouds that ignore the wind.

The mastery of fantasy through play permits discharge and mastery of stress. Stress can be the product of immediate pressures, or the result of unresolved conflicts. The more a child can use communicative symbols in the development of fantasy, play, or dream, the more effective is the mastery of stress. Therefore, the encouragement of communicative symbols is therapeutic. They help to achieve resolution of sensitizing fantasies through communicative mastery. Communicative symbols bring problems into an arena of consciousness shared by therapist and child. Where there is a misunderstanding or a fantasy distortion or a sense of deprivation or a misinterpretation because of drive-dominated wishes, communication with the analyst can establish a zone of interaction in which to introduce realistic understanding and resolution of the situation to which the child is sensitive. In the case of Roy (see Chapter 5), discharge in play was effective in lessening his aberrant behavior. Only when he was able to communicate through the symbol "king" could his motivations be placed in consciousness and challenged and diminished. Only insight could diminish the slant of his beliefs to bring them into line with reality. Freud (1909) noted the "psychological differences between the conscious and the unconscious" (p. 176). He noted that "everything conscious was subject to a process of wearing-away, while what was unconscious was relatively unchangeable" (p. 176). As will be noted more fully below in the section on Primary and Secondary Process, in order for what is unconscious to become conscious, rules must be followed that insist that contexts of reality be admixed.

Fantasy formation during latency derives its contents from many sources. Recent events, comic book characters, culture heroes, and the villains of history all take their places—in the helter-skelter palimpsest that is human memory—upon, above, around, and below the emotional complexes of early childhood. Subliminal impressions beguile the ears and eyes of the therapist, distorting the message. Similarities between memory elements cause fusions in recall that establish symbollike forms that lead the therapist astray. They are subject to all the failings that befall the communication of things past and remembered. Such complexities add difficulty to child therapy. The cognitive organization of memory in the child is so different from that of the literate adult that special listening skills must be developed. The child in fantasy play is harder to understand than the adult who remembers. Fantasy play and dreaming are memory modalities that share qualities with free association. However, because of the primitive nature of thought process in the child, the associations are looser. There is more primary process involved (see below). The wandering mind of the child may easily set the therapist to wandering as well. This is especially disconcerting when one's free-floating attention, an informative study of one's own reactions to the associations of the patient, drifts unguided in presence of the excessively disconnected symbolic elements in the fantasies of the child. Free-floating attention becomes less of a source of information. Instead it becomes a target for attention that takes the therapist's attention on an inner-directed track away from the child. In the meantime the child too drifts. His mind follows source elements other than the progenitors of his problems. The therapist is suffering from "lulling" (Sarnoff 1976, pp. 243–246). When the child finally comes to a word or situation that could be interpreted, the therapist, his mind elsewhere, is not ready to make the intervention. The therapist must train himself to attend to the child's mental content in the same way that a baseball outfielder must not let up for a moment, though a ball may come his way only once an hour. A poor defense taken against lulling is active participation by the therapist in the child's play on the level of the child. This contaminates content. An useful approach to lulling is the continuous diagnosis of fantasy content, psychosexual regressions, and cognitive changes during the child's play. A search for the stimuli that give rise to such changes initiates forays into free-floating attention, ever refreshed by the input of the child's productions.

Fantasy formation is the core of the process that produces manifest fantasy, play, and dreams. As such, fantasy was presented here first. The structures of all three products undergo developmental changes. The predominant theme in this process is the movement of sources of manifest symbolic forms from the fantastic to the real. This is a part of the late latency–early adolescent maturational process that draws the attention of consciousness away from the fantasy of the subject and toward the reality of the object. The child rises to adulthood on such wings of reality. There are both normal and pathological aspects to the cognitive growth process. The degree to which reality testing replaces the sense of reality defines the success of the maturation and development of reality testing. The therapeutic approach to abnormal behavior must take into account both the content of fantasy and cognitive aberrations of symbolic form that force a breach in reality judgments. For instance, a child who acts out his fantasies because of poor symbol formation, and who cannot use fantasy to achieve comfort or delay, becomes a behavior problem. On the other hand, a child gifted in fantasy play, and with a similar latent fantasy, is seen as creative.

We turn now to a study of this cognitive growth process. There will be two emphases: first will be an emphasis on the development of reality testing as a means of adaptation. Second will be an emphasis on cognitive transformations that expand the roles of fantasy, play, and dream from sources of comfort to effective tools in the mastery of such functions as developing future planning and exploring abstract truths. Immaturities, aberrations, and failures to grow contribute to knowledge of the origins of pathogenetic form and content in both reality-testing fantasy formation and behavior. This, in turn, makes possible an understanding of the foundations of effective psychotherapeutic strategies. Once we have completed this task, we will proceed to the study of use of the dream in therapy of the young and the use of play in latency-age children.

THE COGNITIVE GROWTH PROCESS

Cognitive Transformations

The cognitive transformations of the latency years produce a capacity to deal with reality commensurate with changes in size and strength in the growing child. They also accomplish a shift in object relatedness necessary for finding mates.

Immaturities in latency-age cognitive transformations produce cognitive defects. Drives that underlie fantasy find their way to expression through twisted channels. This contributes to psychopathology.

Failure of the symbolizing function to mature interferes with the search for an object in reality with whom to share the expression of drives (see below). This gives rise to a persistence of the evocative pole in symbol formation. Symbols fail to go from amorphous to human manifest forms. The outcome is animals, plants, things, and situations instead of people in the manifest symbols that take part in neurotic symptoms.

Primary- and secondary-process thinking develop in parallel. During development, secondary process may fail to outstrip primary-process thinking as they vie for the attention of consciousness. This can be the result of a defect in the development of repression, with a concomitant failure of symbols to fullfill their role. That role includes the socialization of the manifestations of the drives. Impaired reality testing results. This is manifested in the ascendance of a personalized sense of reality in place of mature socially shared reality testing (i.e., in these people the reality one feels outweighs the reality that all can touch).

Disordered memory systems leave false traces of experience. This alters later interpretations of perceptions. The results are perceptual and interpretive distortions (see below).

Failure to move from preoperational to operational thinking in achieving the interpretation of concrete perceptions results in action orientation and narcissistic (symbolic and intuitive) thinking. This undermines reality testing. An example of disregard for reality in a 7-year-old can be seen in the straight-faced pronouncement that is quoted here: "Dr. Sarnoff, a strange thing happened as I came into your office. I got all better—so I don't have to come back here anymore."

COGNITIVE DEVELOPMENT

The development of the way that reality is perceived, remembered, and understood is incomplete when a child reaches the age of 6. Piaget has described the development of the capacity to interpret observed phenomena during the latency-age period, and Freud has described the cognitive structures necessary for the acquisition of socially acceptable behavior during latency. Their contributions fit into a context of widely extensive cognitive changes that can be organized into three periods.

The Cognitive Organizing Periods

Each cognitive organizing period (Sarnoff 1976) represents years during which specific cognitive skills mature and develop. When immature skills reach a high level of effectiveness, they coordinate to produce a demonstrable alteration in general behavior, which initiates a new phase of development.

In relation to latency, the first such period occurs between 2 and 6 years of age. The effectiveness of latency-age fantasy, in producing a state of calm, pliability, and educability during the latency years, depends on the adequacy of development of the symbolizing function, repression, verbal-conceptual memory organization, and behavioral constancy (the ability to recognize clues to appropriate behavior) in the prelatency period.

The second cognitive organizing period occurs between 7½ and 8½ years of age. The cognitive abilities maturing during this period include concrete operational thinking, abstract conceptual memory organization, the shift in fantasy content from thoughts about fantasy objects to thoughts about reality objects, and reorganization of superego contents in the direction of ethical individuation (in which the child's own motivations begin to dominate and contents derived from parental demands have less impact). The maturation and coordination of these cognitive skills become manifest clinically at about 8½ years of age. This is the age that, for most clinicians, separates early from late latency.

The third cognitive organizing period occurs from ages 10 to 13 years. Cognitive growth during this period is involved in achieving a shift from a mental life that focuses on personalized fantasy to a mental life that places emphasis on reality knowledge of the world and the search for a love object in reality. The events in development relating to cognition that characterize this period are the preadolescent vicissitudes of projection, body image changes associated with pubertal body changes, object-oriented shifts in the direction of object relatedness, intensification of narcissistic investment of the libido in fantasy structures (the content of the fantasies changes to reality objects, but the fantasy remains an important factor), and a shift from the evocative to the communicative mode in the selection of symbolic forms (Sarnoff 1987b).

A fourth cognitive organizing period can be identified during the transition to adolescence. It is dominated by the theme of the completion of the transition to object relatedness. Impelled by the loss of the symbolizing function as a primary organ for sexual discharge and encouraged by the impact of menarche and the first ejaculation to seek libidinal objects in reality, the child builds a bridge to the object world. The bridge is built by a shift of secondary-process requirements (see below) from an emphasis on reality testing to an emphasis on the needs of the loved and sought partner. An observing object in the mind's eye begins to review fantasy and future planning with the needs of the object as the criteria for acceptability. The ability to fall into altruistic love is pendant to this development. This developmental step is built around the maturation of the use of communicative mode symbols. These are also at the core of aesthetics, creativity, and future planning. A shift to this more mature form of symbol is a sign of emotional health. Underlying the strengthening of the communicative symbol is the development of communicative speech (Kraus and Glucksberg 1977), which begins to gain priority at 12 years of age. This refers to the development of verbalization tuned to the needs of the listener for clarity, empathy, and completeness on the part of the speaker. A third element in the underpinnings of the capacity to fall in love is tertiary elaboration. This refers to the unconscious reorganization of verbalizations to align content with knowledge of the background, point of view, and philosophy of the listener (Hoffer 1978).

The most important of the cognitive transitions, from the standpoint of psychopathology and psychotherapy, involves memory organizations and symbolic forms, mental operations, and the primary-process/secondary-process synergism. The first two will be described in the following section. Mental operations and the primary-process/secondary-process synergism will be discussed in the subsequent two sections.

MEMORY ORGANIZATIONS

Vygotsky (Luria 1976) said in the early 1920s, "Although a young child thinks by remembering, an adolescent remembers by thinking" (p. 11).

The cognitive organizations involved in this change are named, in order of increasing maturation: affecto-motor memory organization, verbal conceptual memory organization, and abstract conceptual memory organization. These are the primary conduits through which the world of experience is apprehended and carried forward in time by memory. When one considers that the definition of consciousness that character-izes the theory of psychotherapy revolves about awareness of percep-tion in the context of prior experiences of the perception and future implications of the perception, one must reach the conclusion that pathological turnings in the ways of memory are central to the under-standing of pathological behavior and symptoms.

Affecto-Motor Memory Organization

The affecto-motor memory organization begins in life's first years. It consists of two components, motor and affective. The motor compo-nent, the first to be acquired, consists of purposefully modified patterns of motor activity. Essentially, the contents of memory of this component are syntaxes consisting of interrelating motor components.

The affect component of the affecto-motor memory organization is made up of the ability to evoke recall of learned patterns in the form of affects, perceptions, and bodily postures associated with an initial experience. It represents the ability to organize recall about sensory experiences. These are usually recalled in their entirety.

Conceptual Memory

Conceptual memory is defined as the ability to evoke recall of learned patterns in the form of verbal signifiers such as words and related symbols. Conceptual memory can be divided into the earlier-appearing verbal conceptual memory and the relatively late-appearing abstract conceptual memory.

Verbal Conceptual Memory Organization

Verbal conceptual memory organization is able to be operative by the third year of life at the latest. It is not the primary means of memory used until about 6 years of age. That is when latency begins. The extent to which it is activated is determined by environmental and social factors.

Abstract Conceptual Memory Organization

Abstract conceptual memory organization refers to a maturationally based modification of conceptual memory. It appears first between 7½ and 8½ years of age. It consists of the skill of interpreting events in terms of their intrinsic nature and retaining the substance of this in memory through abstractions with or without words (Sarnoff 1976, 1987). The usual area of childhood activity in which such interpretation takes place is in "getting the main idea" during reading. By the age of 12, accumulation of abstractions in memory should have reached the point at which abstractions can be applied to the interpretation of other abstractions. Children who fail to achieve this have trouble getting the main idea in reading, doing reports that require summaries of multiple sources, and three-part word problems in math.

SYMBOLIC FORMS

Symbols are created at the interface between cognitive functions and the world. Drive energies can be masked when they find acceptable form through symbolization. The strength of secondary-process thinking (see below) depends on the ability of symbols to limit displacements to representations with low valence for attracting affect. Psychoanalytic symbols (called "secondary symbols" by Piaget [1951]) are symbols whose abstract link to the concept or thing that they represent has succumbed to repression. This begins at about 26 months. There is a march of symbolic forms that can well be studied in the objects chosen to populate persecutory fantasies. At first, states of being such as loneliness and darkness are directly expressed. During the third year of life, hostile wishes directed at loved ones are denied and projected (displaced) onto plants and animals. With the onset of the latency years, amorphous forms such as goblins and ghosts predominate. At about 8 years of age, humanoid forms such as witches are called upon to represent persecutors. At 11, the small play figures (ludic symbols) used in fantasy play give way to full-sized objects (peers and adults) who by their power features or personality can be invested with protagonist membership in the child's world of inner fears. In late latency, peers begin to be recruited in reality to play out roles in scenarios derived from the latency fantasies of the child.

Running parallel to these events is a shift in emphasis in the selection of symbols from those that merely evoke inner affects (evocative pole symbols) to those symbols which play a dual role (communicative pole symbols). The latter serve both the evocation of memory and trauma, and mastery of trauma through the communication of information in a context of comprehension of the needs of others (Sarnoff 1987).

Intrinsic to the nature of evocative symbols is the selection of a symbolic signifier to represent unconscious content without regard for the communicative or aesthetic value that it has for an audience. Often when a trauma or affect-laden fantasy figure has been repressed, the affect remains free-floating in the memory systems. Freud (1909) noted that in that circumstance "we are not used to feeling strong affects without their having any ideational content, and therefore, if the content is missing, we seize as a substitute some other content which is in some way or other suitable" (p. 176). Highly personal and idiosyncratic symbolic forms selected in this way hide the identity of the latent content. These symbolic signifiers evoke—for the benefit of the egocentric aspects of the individual—inner feelings and experiences. In each case, already mastered fantasies and feelings are reexperienced at the expense of reality. Evocative symbols represent a victory for narcissism. The product of this repetition is momentary mastery through gratifying play based on prior successful experiences.

Intrinsic to the communicative symbol is selection of representation based on the needs of the listener. Communicative symbols represent a victory for reality testing, altruism, and nonegocentric influences. These symbolic signifiers work for the benefit of object relations. The transformation of fantasies by changing symbol content and symbolic forms to match the ways of the world enhances object relations. Through such fantasies, contact with the reality of the therapist can be achieved, interpretations made, and discussion initiated. Working through then becomes possible. Past traumas can be de-emphasized and reparatively mastered and processed. A psychotherapeutic strategy that encourages the development of mature symbols and symbolic fantasy play in therapy sessions results from these theoretical considerations. (By way of example, see the case of little Roy in Chapter 4.)

When the march of symbols has reached the point that real figures can be recruited to populate fantasies, the communicative pole dominates selection of symbols, and situations are constructed and interpreted on the basis of reality testing derived from operational thinking, the cognitive underpinnings of the ability to fall in love have been achieved and the task of latency has been completed. In working with early adolescents in therapy, the therapist must evaluate the child's level of attainment in these areas. Psychotherapeutic strategies should be developed that will enhance these cognitive skills (Sarnoff 1987b).

FROM PREOPERATIONAL THINKING TO ABSTRACT OPERATIONAL THINKING

A maturational shift underlies the enhancement of reality testing during latency and early adolescence. This shift entails the increased use of external cues in place of memory and intuition in the interpretation of new experiences and stimuli. It parallels the observations of Jean Piaget on the thought processes that are used in the interpretation of the perception of reality. The terms *preoperational thinking* and *operational thinking* are used in those writings of Piaget (1951) that describe these changes. Preoperational thinking (concrete interpretations of perceptions and experiences) uses sensorimotor intelligence. Operational thinking (abstract interpretations of perceptions and experiences) uses conceptual intelligence. The shift from primary emphasis in thinking from sensorimotor intelligence to conceptual intelligence takes place in early latency (from 6 to 7½ years of age).

Preoperational Thinking

Preoperational thinking has two stages (sensorimotor thinking and symbolic intuitive thinking). The first is an expression solely of a sensorimotor intelligence based on a memory system that encodes sensation and motor schemata. The second begins after 26 months. It adds unconscious idiosyncratic symbolic interpretation of occurrences to thinking.

Sensorimotor Thinking

At first, preoperational thinking consists of the establishment of isolated linkages between successive perceptions and movements. There is a failure to place the current experience in a total context, consisting of a predisposing past and a sense of implications for the future of the event at hand. As Piaget (1951) describes it, sensorimotor motor intelligence "functions like a slow-motion film, representing one static image after another without achieving a fusion of the images" (p. 238). This is an intelligence that is "lived and not thought" (p. 238). Only motor and perceptual events inform this intelligence. Potentially related signs, symbols, and other verbal concepts are excluded. Because such intelligence lacks verbal representations that would make possible the efficient storage of information, verbal communication of consensually validatable interpretations of perception and experience within a context of a time sense are not available. The sensorimotor intellectual experience is limited to the moment of experiencing and to the observer alone. It lacks potential for a social organization of shared knowledge.

Toward the end of the first year of life, a second stage comes into view. The mind is ready to understand words. This readiness is played upon by social interactions such as parental insistence on word use. Verbal concepts are introduced at this point. Then words can be used to represent schemata of experience and action. Classifications and relationships between experiences can now be frozen into consistent verbal form, stored in verbal memory systems established in the child's mind. Narcissism in the very young child is expressed in a tendency to assimilate all new experience to preestablished conceptions that have been codified in this way.

Intuitive Thinking and Symbolic Reasoning

Such personalized interpretations of events, unmoored to reality limitations, tend to acquire associations through displacements and condensations that link them to uncomfortable affects. Repression, which becomes available at 24 months, permits the production of substitute formations (symbols) with diminished affects. Symbols, in turn, introduce a memory function that permits the child to encounter perceptions and experiences that have the power to stir uncomfortable affects, with associations that diminish the chance for a realistic interpretation of the event at the same time that they make the confrontation tolerable. Comfort is achieved at the cost of diminished reality perception. At this point in development, repression and symbol formation become the basis for intuitive thinking and symbolic reasoning. This begins at about 26 months (Piaget 1951, Sarnoff 1970). Symbolic reasoning is dominated by personal influences, which limit pragmatic reality pressures that would limit latitude in the free creation of concepts. Personalized symbols become the basis for recall. Perceptions and combinations of images are organized into exotic entities that correspond more to the child's desires than they do to the realities of form (Piaget 1951). This state dominates during early childhood and the first years of latency.

Percepts remembered through words do not become fully integrated into a verbal memory system until 6 years of age (Sarnoff 1976). Constant reworking of concepts through verbal interaction in an interpersonal setting and through testing impressions against pragmatic imperatives spawned by reality diminishes the strength of symbols and intuition, and creates definitions, classifications, and relationships that are shared in society. Thus individual thought is accommodated to the influence of "a common, objective reality" (Piaget 1951, p. 239). In this way the verbal conceptual memory organization evolves. It can support conceptual intelligence. Conceptual intelligence, in turn, supports the development of concrete operational thinking, which ripens at about 7 years of age.

Concrete Operational Thinking

Concrete operational thinking is characterized by interpretation of perceived concrete events in light of preconceived socially or observationally validated concepts. Such "concepts are either systems of classes, sets of objects grouped according to relations between wholes and parts, or systems of particular relations grouped according to their symmetrical or asymmetrical nature" (Piaget 1951, p. 218). This intellectual process gives rise to growth. Implied in the establishment of these clusters of concept is a step in development in which assimilation to previously established conceptions gives way to accommodation to "the qualities of the objects composing the groups whether or not the child himself and his own activity are also involved" (p. 218). Concrete operations serve reality in areas where bound energies contribute to adaptation, such as academic work. Accommodation to qualities of objects rather than to intuitive interpretations becomes stronger and stronger as latency progresses.

Concrete operations help in the creation of a socially agreed-upon milieu in which definitions are established that create a boundary for the meanings conveyed by word use and signs. Thus, social conventions and agreed-upon realities are established. This is the cognition that accepts myths and social regulations, whose validity lies more in agreements and conventions of society than in the intrinsic nature of things. With the advance of primacy for concrete operations, intuitive word use and idiosyncratic symbols in waking life give way to the properly social signifier. The persistence of secondary (psychoanalytic) symbols subverts this process. In the form of dream (oneiric) symbols and play (ludic) symbols, secondary symbols support a process that undermines the move toward accommodation to reality in waking life. Ludic symbols (e.g., a toy used to play out an unconscious fantasy concept) have a mobility of potential meaning that provides for the persistence of intuitive and symbolic thinking. During the latency period, they provide a safety valve for the discharge of unbound energies and the mastery of emotional stresses, both real and the result of intrusions from the unconscious. The ludic symbol survives until it is extinguished (called ludic demise) at 10 to 12 years of age (Sarnoff 1987a).

A small but not inconsiderable percentage of children fail to develop full capacity to use words and symbols, including ludic symbols. Such youngsters have little in the way of imagination. For their outlets they prefer physical activity such as sports. Under stress, their decompensations take the form of somatic symptoms and action-oriented behavior (Kernberg 1991).

Between 7 and 8 years of age, the "assimilation" of perceptions to idiosyncratic preconceptions is balanced by the "accommodation" of a child's understanding to socially defined concepts of objects. At the point in development, established impressions or interpretations of observations by a child can be altered by reality. The process, the achievement of dominant influence by external influences, is called reversal. When reversal is operative, the child's capacity to be influenced by reality is enhanced. The assimilation of perceptions to idiosyncratic preconceptions can also be balanced by an accommodation of the child's understanding to a remembered, socially defined concept of an object. At this point a shift occurs in which the object itself comes to serve as an example of the concept rather than as the source of the definition (Piaget 1951). This is a developmental advance in abstract thinking. This process supports the development of concrete operations.

When internalized definitions that were learned from others come to dominate the interpretation of perceptions, a form of assimilation is produced that has the potential to counter the strengthening of reality testing provided by accommodation. This process perpetuates and supports the myths of culture, producing socially influenced and consensually validated concepts that can distort interpretations of new experiences and indications of intrinsic realities. Social identity is enhanced by fixation at this mythogenic cognitive level of organization. The responses are socially shared and reflect previously injected influences of society. As such, they may be considered to be a priori social accommodations to reality and an adaptive manifestation of reversal.

The ability to separate words from things and organize them into concepts makes it possible to establish categories that are independent of individual percepts. Once established (about age 8), such thought and memory groupings, often shared by society, offer a medium for memory that permits the storage of abstract concepts—the abstract conceptual memory organization (see Sarnoff 1976, p. 117). At first, only the interpretation of those events and things that can be seen concretely contribute to these abstract conceptualizations (concrete operations). By age 12, this memory skill can have grown sufficiently so that verbal abstractions and the intrinsic nature of events can be comprehended and the knowledge so gained applied to new situations (abstract operations).

Clincial Considerations

Failure of cognitive development to proceed beyond sensorimotor thinking can be seen as a symptom congruent with states of infantile autism. There is a natural unfolding of cognition up to the level of concrete operations in healthy children. Development beyond that is mediated by social custom. Concrete operation supports tribal living, whereas adaption to industrial society requires abstract operations (Nurcombe 1976). Although this circumstance is not included under the rubric of pathology, youngsters, who are limited to concrete operations, can easily be seen as potentially dysfunctional underachievers, prone to the influence of myth and unable to deal with failures of social function based on the intrinsic nature of industrial or social processes. The development of abstract operations is accompanied at the age of 11 by the ability to interpret proverbs. It is at that age that one uses concrete thinking on tests of proverb interpretation as evidence of persistence of the predominance of concrete operations.

A knowledge of Piaget's understanding of the interpretation of perceptions is important in the psychotherapy of latency-age and early adolescent children. For one thing, interpretations have to be geared to the child's ability to share ways of interpreting meaning and the stability of definition that the child brings to word use. The more involved is a child in concrete operations, the more necessary is it to repeat topics and interpretations. Concretely experienced events and perceptions can be understood abstractly by a child who has attained the level of concrete operations. There is no guarantee that these insights will be remembered if the abstract conceptual memory has not yet been reached. Repetition enhances the function of this memory system in youngsters early in the process of developing it. The misinterpretation of cues from the world, based on memory elements that are used to explain new phenomena, is an intrinsic element in the origins of pathological processes. So is the creation of new situations based on old personal myths and misconceptions. Reality testing develops as the result of a maturation of skills that give accommodation to new inputs, priority in greeting new experiences. The therapist must be on the alert to differentiate between the child whose prior experiences have taught fear in meeting new situations, and the child whose new experiences are interpreted in terms of the assimilation of new events to fantasies formed from their own hostile affects (a form of projection). Once this differentiation is made, the therapist can choose whether to help the child to improve his ability to test reality, in the case of the child with weak reversal; or to help the child to accept the reality of the past and be guided by the realities of the present and future, in the child with normal capacity to accommodate to the world.

PROCESS THINKING DURING LATENCY AND EARLY ADOLESCENCE

Piaget's studies deal with the development of the role of reality in the interpretation of perceptions and phenomena. His theory describes the process and the timing of the acquisition of knowledge of reality. The study of the development of memory systems (Sarnoff 1976, 1987a) describes the process by which this knowledge of reality becomes encoded in memory to serve for later interpretation of perceptions as well as a guide to compromise formations (i.e., symbols). In maturity the latter consist of reality-oriented manifestations of drives. The way in which remembered reality comes to influence compromise formations and ride herd on drives seeking discharge was outlined by Freud in his description of primary and secondary process. In Freud's theory the secondary process, which guides the drives to expressions in reality, does not finally become sharply differentiated until puberty. This differentiation—syncretic with the development of reality testing and the ascendance of the reality principle in late latency—can be viewed as a manifestation of a shift from primary-process thinking to secondary-process thinking. In the absence of this step in a child, psychotherapy must take on as a goal the development of mature secondary-process thinking.

These terms, primary process and secondary process, were first used in those contributions of Freud (1900, 1915) that describe cognitive changes that give credence to external realities at the expense of memories and reminiscences. The reality testing that is attained through the influence of secondary process is shaped by pragmatic imperatives placed in a child's path by objective reality. The devaluation of an immature sense of reality, informed by hopes and wishes, is achieved at the expense of the pleasure principle.

Primary Process and Secondary Process

Freud first introduced the terms "two systems," or primary and secondary process, in *The Interpretation of Dreams* (1900, p. 603). They formed an integral part of the topographic theory, an early Freudian theory in which the areas of mental functioning, namely, the system unconscious (Ucs), the system preconscious (Pcs), and the system consciousness (Cs), are organized according to their availability to self-reflexive awareness and illustrated in a topographic map. Two types of psychic energies, unbound and bound, were identified as fueling the topographic systems. Unbound energies characterized unconscious processes (system Ucs). Bound energies characterized conscious processes (system Cs).

The context of mechanisms that characterizes unconconscious mental life was called primary process by Freud (1900, p. 603). It is characterized by free energy expressing uninhibited motivations. The context of mechanisms that police the passage of unconscious contents into consciousness was called secondary process by Freud (1900). Secondary process is characterized by a search for internal consistency in conscious thought and the formation of acceptable substitutes for primitive wishes. Of the substitute formations, the foremost are communicative symbols. Communicative symbols consist of passions of the mind clothed in the uniforms of culture.

The inhibitory nature of the secondary process was clearly stated by Freud (1900) when he wrote, "I propose to describe the psychical process of which the first system alone admits as the 'primary process', and the process which results from the inhibition imposed by the second system as the 'secondary process' " (p. 601). The role of substitute formations (e.g., symbols) in executing the inhibiting requirements of reality and the system consciousness appears in the phrase, "loose connections are merely obligatory substitutes for others which are valid and significant" (p. 591).

Primary process refers to the characteristics of the area of the mind which Freud (1915) called "the unconscious." These characteristics are:

Cathexes (energized attentions) are mobile. This is achieved through displacement and condensation. (These mechanisms are sometimes considered to be all that there is to the primary process.) Energy cathexes can be shifted from one idea or object to another. Cathexes associated with many ideas can be funneled into one idea. Drive energies can be shifted in the direction of a new idea or object in a way that results in repression of the original ideas or objects to which attention cathexes had been directed.

The unconscious is under the sway of the pleasure principle.

There is little influence from objective reality.

There are wish impulses that "exist independently side by side, and are exempt from mutual contradiction" (p. 186). There is no negation, no varying degree of certainty.

There is timelessness (pp. 186–187).

Secondary process refers to the characteristics of the structure through which the preconscious guards the gates of consciousness. The activities of this structure are:

Inhibition of drive discharge.

Exclusion of displacement and condensation.

Enablement of communication between ideas to permit them to modify and influence one another.

Introduction of time constraints on the discharge of wish impulses.

Establishment of a censorship that will affect both social and personal inhibitions of direct expression of wish impulses.

Establishment of conscious memory.

Organization of a testing of reality that is based on the influence of objectivity and socially organized ideation (p. 188).

Substitute Formations—Symbols

Drives, wishes, and passions are not ignored as the result of the strengthening of secondary-process mechanisms that occurs during the latency years. Standing athwart the gulf between what primary process proposes and what secondary process can allow as final disposition are compromise formations. Free displacement and condensation in primary process permits the selection of substitute representations. Substitute formations serve as realistically acceptable objects for drive discharge when the desired object would be an unrealistic or even dangerous choice. The inhibition that guides secondary-process function limits the choice to safe compromises. Of all the substitute formations produced by this interaction, symbols serve best as vehicles to bring wish fantasies within grasp of a world of actuality from which wishing can dare to wrest gratification. Reality-oriented substitutes (symbols) represent drive derivatives at the same time that they protect the system consciousness from unmodified incursions of the same drives that, by their nature, would challenge reality and instigate peril.

Though the formation of symbols requires mechanisms with the characteristics of the primary process, especially displacement and condensation, the final form of the symbol is influenced by the adaptations to reality needs that are the hallmark of secondary process. Symbols are a safe-conduct pass through which unconscious content can travel freely and unencumbered within the precincts of consciousness.

A shift from primary to secondary process is only apparent. Both processes persist into adult life. There is really no shift between the two processes. Rather, enhanced reality testing and a shift to the use of communicative symbols and the selection of symbol representation from elements of external reality strengthens secondary process and makes it easier to differentiate from primary process. This differentiation between the two processes evolves during latency.

As an expression of the differentiation, primary process persists in dreams, fantasies, and neurotic symptom formation, whereas secondary process persists in functions that free the ego to take part in the adaptive commerce of daily interactions. The apparent shift between processes represents a change in the level of maturity of the symbolic forms used. The more realistic are the sources used as symbol, the more realistic do the fantasies appear, and the more is the impression given that a shift has taken place.

Symbols themselves undergo a maturation and development that color the communication between unconscious wishes and the world. An example of primary process expressed through dominance of immature symbolic forms, enhancing intuitive interpretation of phenomena, follows.

The 6-year-old boy feared a new unknown, subway travel. In the face of the roar of the train and the rush of people leaving the station, he asked, "Daddy, if this isn't a cave and that [sound] isn't a dragon, why are all those people running?"

Regression to primary process–driven fantasy can occur in adults exposed to unexplained dangers. This has been described insightfully by Tasso (1581) in a stanza from "Jerusalem Delivered" (13:18) in which men confronted by an enchanted wood find that they have not courage.

As an innocent child has not the courage to look where he has a foreboding of strange spirits, or as in shadowy night he is afraid,

imagining monsters and prodigies still, so did they fear without knowing
what it can be for which they feel such terror—except that their fear creates
for their senses prodigies greater than chimaera or sphinx. [p. 284]

Two developmental tracks traced by the maturation of symbols serve
to strengthen secondary process and reality testing. The first is the
march of symbolic forms from distorted images to real people, which is
most sharply detectable in persecutory fantasies. The second is a shift
from the evocative pole to the communicative pole in the selection of
symbols by the symbolizing function (Sarnoff 1987b). As symbolic
representation comes more and more to be shaped by communicative
needs and justice for partners in drive discharge, the more does it
appear that a shift to secondary process (greater influence of reality on
the form taken by drive discharge) has occurred.

Failure to achieve maturation of symbolic forms in secondary-process
functioning permits a hegemony of the system unconscious, which is a
state congruent with psychosis. This maturation is expected to take
place in late latency–early adolescence. Therefore during the latency
years and in states of latency, manifest fantasies that contain primary-
process thinking and symbols that are idiosyncratic to the subject are not
considered to be pathological. Such conscious thinking is considered to
be pathological, however, in the waking fantasies and fears of early and
late adolescence. Primary-process thinking is acceptable in dreams of all
ages. Clinical concomitants of these observations are the rarity of
adultiform content in psychoses before the age of 12 and the loss of play
in adolescence; the emergent importance of dreams in therapy with
adolescents; ludic demise and the loss of fantasy play with ludic
symbols in adolescent therapy; and difficulty and shame in reporting
daydreams beyond the latency years. The blurred boundaries between
primary- and secondary-process thinking during waking fantasy in
latency-age children was implied by Freud's (1915) comment that "a
sharp and final division of the contents of the two systems does not . . .
take place until puberty" (p. 195).

FANTASY AND COGNITION, PLAY AND DREAM

The characteristics of psychopathology change for each stage of life.
Persistent fantasy informs content consistently; changing cognition
determines metamorphoses of form. Latency and early adolescence
contribute to this process, with cognitions that are transient. New forms

of cognition modify their psychopathologies as emergence toward adulthood unfolds. Both fantasy and cognition can be influenced during the latency years by therapy as well as by certain reality influences on the child.

In the latency-age child, the ability to tell fantasy from reality is influenced by overstimulation, such as seduction, family tragedy, and the occurrence of events that are so close to the fantasy that they blur the boundaries between fantasy and reality for the child. These reality events, in addition to producing a failure in the cognitive maturation of symbolic forms, and failure in the development of reality testing, lead to the persistence of fantasy as a mechanism of adjustment in adolescence and adulthood. Psychopathogenetic fantasy content is resolved through abreaction in play and dream; by communication as in therapeutic interaction; and through passive participation in shared fantasy, as in reading, hearing bedtime tales, and attending plays and films. A decay of fantasy occurs with the enhancement of reality testing that occurs when increased size provides reality gratifications to replace fantasy goals. Fantasy that is unresolved in these ways persists into adolescence. Cognitive changes shape new forms of psychopathology to represent these fantasies during adolescence.

Cognitive growth in the latency years is influenced by environmental and genetic factors. Overstimulation and excess affect, such as fear and anxiety that occur in interpersonal interactions, can leave little time for the development of natural potentials to develop mature symbolic forms and reality testing. Psychotherapy directed at fantasy and cognition results in resolution of symptoms in the young in a manner that clears the way for healthy functioning in the adolescent and adult. Time in its passing resolves these symptoms as well. This results only in an apparent gain, for fantasy persists. New pathologies evolve, forged in the fires of adolescent drive. They take their shape from new cognitions informed by persistent fantasies.

Prelatency fantasies flow through latency into adolescence. Old wine finds its way to new bottles. Should cognition fail to mature, poor reality testing and immature symbolic forms are produced in the adolescent and the adult. This projects into life situations both neurotic symptoms and a psychotic sense of reality that values memory and idiosyncratic thought content above all other inputs. When drive-propelled wish fantasies fail to be resolved in latency, they persist to color the content of fate neuroses, neurotic symptoms, and psychoses. Child therapy is capable of correcting immediate symptoms and affecting adult psychopathology as well by resolving fantasy and guiding cognitive growth.

Failure to negotiate the cognitive transitions of latency is a prelude to the establishment of a pathogenetic competition between early childhood memories and reality for control over individual human existences.

Maturation itself can be influenced by predestined genetic limitations, such as genetic variation in the potential strength of a given level of immaturity to persist into adulthood. This process may be described as a neoteny (defined as a genetically determined persistence of childhood cognition into physical maturity, creating biologically mature individuals with maladaptive cognitive styles).

The natural resolution of immaturities in fantasy, symbolizing function, and reality testing falls into the temporal province of the latency years. Many can be approached psychotherapeutically during latency and early adolescence. At these ages, because of immature cognition, psychotherapeutic process differs from that seen in working with adults. The manifestations of fantasy and free association are different, especially as expressed in fantasy play and dreams. This requires modification of psychotherapeutic techniques, as discussed in subsequent sections of this chapter.

DREAMS AND PLAY IN THE TREATMENT OF NEUROSIS IN THE YOUNG

Symbols, fantasy, and cognition are the building blocks through which the elements of unconscious mental life such as latent fantasy can be shaped into conscious representations. Latent fantasy can be held in memory for extended periods of time, making it possible to transport early life experience to the present, whence it can influence normal and pathological manifest forms of behavior in childhood. Normal behavior includes dreams, play, and transference (see Chapter 5). Aberrant behavior includes symptoms and characterological behavior. The fantasy antecedents of aberrant behavior and of play, dreams, and transference are shared. A key to understanding characterological pathology and symptoms should be discoverable in the latent fantasies which are shared by both healthy and pathological derivatives. Latent fantasy can be discerned in the stories and symbols of play and dreams. The nature of latent fantasy has already been described in early sections of this chapter.

Both cognition and fantasy combine to produce pathology. Aberrations in cognitive function create aberrant behavioral forms. Latent fantasy contributes content. Cognitive function influences the choice of current manifestation of fantasy from among such possibilities as symptoms, play, dreams, or behavior. Therapy of children should be geared to the treatment of pathological content as well as pathological form in the psychopathology of childhood. The goal of therapy in dealing with the neuroses of the young is to relieve psychopathogenetic current distress while enhancing the natural growth of the personality. The therapist attempts to move the child towards an ability to test reality so well that his adult life will not be lived far removed from fact; and he will be able to deal with reality directly rather than through misinterpreting it.

To understand the manifestations of the unconscious as they impact on the psychotherapeutic situation in the young, the development of that aspect of cognition (symbol formation, fantasizing function, and cognition function) that reworks content into cryptic forms must be at the therapist's fingertips. There is no time to "look it up" while conducting psychotherapy sessions. This knowledge offers a basis for identifying change in behavior, symbol, fantasy, or symptom that has been produced by interpretation, as differentiated from changes that are the result of maturation of cognitive function. This differentiation provides guidelines for increasing therapeutic emphasis on altering cognition and enhancing reality testing. These are important additions to interpretation of the content of latent fantasy in the psychotherapy of the latency and late latency–early adolescent child.

A study of the development of symbol function, fantasy formation, cognition, and reality testing has already been presented earlier in this chapter. We now turn to the therapeutic use of this information in understanding dreams and play in the young.

DREAMS IN PSYCHOTHERAPY DURING THE LATENCY YEARS

Limitations on Dream Reporting During the Early Latency Years

The early latency child can express his conflicts and drives through fantasy play. Although fantasy play symbols are secondary-process phenomena, which in adult form will be involved with reality events and neutralized energies (use of the couch in adult free associations permits a related regression of symbolic forms to these early latency levels), the immaturity of these symbolic forms available in early latency creates fantasies that are sufficiently like primary-process products for them to be used like dreams. They can be interpreted as dreams are. In like manner, they can serve as a tool for trauma mastery through vicarious living-through, either by catharsis or through the mental experience of a corrective object relationship. Therefore, in child therapy, fantasy play functions as a dream equivalent. Its use obviates the need for expression of drive derivatives through the direct reporting of dreams to the therapist. Hence, spontaneous dream reporting in children in psychotherapy during the early and midlatency years is rare. Dream interpretation at this age has been discussed by Anna Freud (1926), Lippman (1956), Sterba (1955), Sarnoff (1976), and Voth (1978).

Sterba (1955), in a study of spontaneous dream reporting, found that in 1,000 treatment hours with five phobic children, only three spontaneously reported dreams appeared. She concluded that dreams "are found to play a surprisingly insignificant role in the treatment of children" (p. 130). Drawing on her experience, she noted one exception to this. "One may see repetitive dreams around one subject, such as, for example, dreams of water or fire in (bed) wetters . . ." (p. 131). Dream reporting is uncommon in child therapy sessions, though they occur frequently in certain groups such as bed wetters.

What is the clinical usefulness of the dreams that are reported? Voth (1978) implied an unequivocally positive impression about the usefulness of dreams. He described a patient who was able to free-associate to dreams verbally and to search out unconscious meanings. I (1976) have noted that there are some children who can cooperate in this way, but that such talent is not universal. Voth has suggested that the primary factor to be considered in explaining this difference is age. He states that "it may well be that younger patients do not associate as well as did this very bright eleven year old boy" (Voth 1978, p. 255). Age and levels of cognitive skill are important in determining how well a child can free-associate on a cognitive level of codification for recall that matches that of an adult in therapy.

Anna Freud's (1926) contribution is extracted here.

[We] have in dream interpretation a field in which we can apply unchanged to children the methods of analysis of adults. During analysis the child dreams neither less nor more than the grownup, the transparency or obscurity of the dream content conforms as in the case of adults to the strength of the resistance. Children's dreams are certainly easier to interpret. We find in them every such distortion of wish fulfillment as corresponds to the complicated neurotic organization of the childish patient. But there is nothing easier to make the child grasp than dream interpretation. At the first account of a dream I say "No dream can make itself out of nothing; it must be fetched every bit from somewhere"—and I then set off with the child in search of its origins. The child . . . follows up the separate images or words into real life with great satisfaction. I have conducted . . . analyses [of unintelligent children] almost exclusively using dreams. [p. 18]

However, Miss Freud (1926) soon thereafter described clinical incidents in which latency-age children in therapy reported dreams following which "associations to the dreams fail to appear" (p. 18).

The ability of the child to express his conflicts through fantasy play using dreamlike symbolism produces a dream equivalent. Both play and dreams in the child utilize symbols of such primitiveness and immaturity that they may be used both for discharge and for mastery clothed in a cryptic guise. In this way ancient hurts come to rest in the psychological equivalent of an unmarked grave. Preservation of the hiding place encourages suppression of dream reporting. In addition, there is a tendency to tell the dreams to parents, resulting in an attenuation of the energies needed to keep the dream in consciousness. As a result the pressure to express drive derivatives through spontaneous dream reporting during therapy sessions is lessened.

Dream equivalent play is based on fantasy activity available from 3 years of age until ludic demise at the end of latency. During this period, drive energies seeking outlets through symbols derived from the idiosyncracies and intuitions of the child (symbol-producing subject) can find an effective outlet through the use of the evocative psychoanalyic symbols that dot the fabric of the early latency child's play. A marker for onset of psychoanalytic symbol use is the appearance during ontogenetic development of distortion dreams. As noted in Sarnoff (1976),

Dreams which contain psychoanalytic symbols have not been reported prior to the first half of the third year of life. Until then, there is no distortion in dreams. Before twenty-six months, dreams are primarily wish-fulfilling dreams. Anxiety dreams occurring before this time contain direct reproductions of anxiety-causing situations met in recent daytime experience. The appearance of these events in dreams is an attempt at a mastery through repetition identical to that which is seen during traumatic neuroses in adulthood and latency. [p. 278]

Wish-fulfilling dreams appear throughout life. As children grow and symbolic forms mature, the characteristics of dreams and play diverge. The symbols of play fantasies take on more and more communicative characteristics. Manifest symbolic forms find expression in elements of shared reality. The more that fantasy content is colored by reality, the closer it comes to becoming future planning and the closer does its role shift from solving problems in timeless magic realms to addressing problems within the linear time frame of reality.

Distortion and symbol formation contribute to dreams and fantasy beginning with the third year. Maturation of the cognitive skills that support adjustment through fantasy and the development of the state of latency provide a drive outlet through the use of primary-process–like symbols in fantasy play. This persists and may divert energies from dream reporting until further maturation strips fantasy of much of its discharge potential during late latency. This later step in maturation moves dreaming for the first time into a position of primacy as the vehicle through which the evocative symbol is borne to the therapist. It explains the relative paucity of dream reporting in the psychotherapy of early latency-age children. It leaves unanswered the question, Why do many children who have spontaneously reported dreams fail to associate to the dreams verbally? The answer lies in the nature of the symbols used. When one asks a patient to free-associate to a dream element, one is asking that dream content be passed through the seine of secondary-process thinking. In children, tertiary elaboration is limited. Secondary process, called upon to associate to dreams, utilizes symbols that are tinged by assimilation. The personalized quality (intuitive and relatively free use of condensation and displacement) found in these symbols interferes with their communicative value. In essence, the secondary process of the child appears as a pseudoprimary process. As such it is a step on the way to reality testing. From the standpoint of placing dream contents in a context of a self-awareness consciousness consisting of an appreciation of a symbolic content in terms of its origin in the past and its implications for future adjustment, dream recall fails. Dream symbols of the latency-age child preserve an emphasis on their purpose as cryptic encoders that defer energies from insight and problem solving, even when recalled.

Before the capacity to use verbalized abstraction appears in late latency, children tell the therapist latent memory contents, through dream equivalent symbols produced during play. In creating dreams and play in early latency, the fantasizing function can use primary process in creating children's dreams because there is no reality limitation on dream content. Fantasy play symbols, however, are limited to available toys and games. This forced accommodation superimposes a reality element on the sources of symbols. For this reason, games with rules and playing pieces stifle the appearance of fantasy, whereas unworked clay, wood, or paper encourage creative play less encumbered by extraneous influences of place, time, or circumstances. Primary process in dreaming and pseudoprimary process in fantasy play are equally effective mechanisms for cryptic drive discharge. (It should be noted that, to a limited extent, light dreaming sleep can become subject to accommodation [see "The Effect of Myths about Dreams on Dream Content" in Sarnoff in press].)

Fantasy symbols in play form predominate in the associations of the early latency-age child while awake. The younger the child, the more is he apt to be sucessful in presenting his associations to dreams in direct fantasy symbols and activities requiring play objects rather than words, in creating contexts for the expression of his latent concepts. Older children who are in states of anxiety can regress to the use of earlier modes of cognition such as fantasy play. This produces patterns of behavior in psychotherapy sessions that appear to be failures of free association. In actuality, what occurs is a failure to produce adult-style verbal free associations. The unwary therapist of adults can miss such content if he fails to realize that even in adults an occasional gesture, organ response, or mention of an object can be an association on a regressed cognitive level; witness Ferenczi's (1913) description of a 5-year-old boy who crowed like a cock. This is one of the earliest references in the literature to the poor skills of verbal free association to be found in early latency-age youngsters.

Ferenczi reported that

immediately on entering my room his attention was attracted by a small bronze mountain cock among the numerous other objects lying about; he brought it to me and asked, "Will you give it to me?" I gave him some paper and a pencil and he immediately drew a cock. . . . But he was already bored and wanted to go back to his toys. Direct psychoanalytic investigation was therefore impossible. [p. 244]

Unfortunately, Ferenczi did not follow up the other conclusion to be drawn from his description. Children have other ways of remembering and therefore associating to concepts and memories. Among these are the capacity to play out or draw pictures of the concepts and memories.

Play and fantasy symbols produced during these processes are rich in reflections of latent content associated to a problem of the day or a dream that has been reported. Knowledge of the nature of these symbolic forms can help in understanding the flow of a child's thoughts and in the analysis of his dreams.

Through insight on the part of a therapist into the intricacies of symbol production, a child can be helped to expand the expression of his associations.

Since spontaneous dream reporting is rare, it is wise for the therapist to ask parents to report dreams told to them by the child. Also, with insight into the nature of the child's cognition, any dream fragment can be expanded upon by having the child draw a picture of that which was seen in dreams. In drawing the dream and talking about the picture drawn, it is often possible to obtain additional details and associations to the dream. In working with latency-age children, dream interpretation yields little if one waits for the child to associate to individual symbols. If a symbol can be made into a cardboard figure and introduced as a toy, the fantasies built about the cardboard figure can be seen as dream associations. For instance, a child who had dreamed of a snakelike monster was encouraged to extend her associations to the dream by making a hardened clay representation of the monster. This play symbol was then used in session after session to produce a multitude of fantasies and contexts, which expanded insight both for her and for the therapist (Sarnoff 1976). A 9-year-old boy reported a dream of "only snow." He was known to talk little. It had been inferred that he had relatedness problems. When he was asked to draw the dream, a dark shadow to the side turned out to be a house filled with neighbors. Another technique of encouraging the translation of the verbalized dream into ludic concrete symbols is to encourage the child to draw the dream, preferably in the form of a storyboard that permits the depiction of the passage of time. Then cut out the figures from the drawings and glue them to a piece of cardboard. Make a stand and encourage the child to use the figures produced as playthings or puppets to play out and expand on the dream. The early latency child's ability at abstract interpretations of concrete representations (concrete operational thinking) responds to such a toy. A dream told through a toy meets the child's mind where it dwells. Abstract interpretations about concretely represented dreams can be understood at this age, adding a resource to the abreaction that is experienced during play by the prelatency child. Because of the relative weakness of verbal concept memory and abstract concept memory at this time, retention of insights transmitted in this way requires that the interpretations be repeated in future sessions.

DREAMS IN PSYCHOTHERAPY DURING ADOLESCENCE

The adolescent psychotherapy patient differs from the latency-age patient. Ludic demise has come and gone. Ludic symbols play no important part in his or her associations. This is a rather obvious difference, which dictates that play therapy is inappropriate for the adolescent age group.

The transition from play to talk as the primary mode of communication is not a sharp one. Over a period of months, the child shifts between talks in the consultation room and toys or constructions in the playroom. Late in the process, choice of the playroom comes to represent a reaction to stress. The therapist should see this reaction as a regression and should search for the stressing problem in the same way that one would look for a day residue in working with adult dreams. Silence or slowness in working in either mode of expression (play or talk) should be responded to with the suggestion that the other mode be used. In the early adolescent, spontaneous dream reporting of rather extended dreams comes to the fore in parallel with the loss of play as a conduit to carry psychoanalytic symbols in their role as memory moieties for the recall of fantasy and trauma.

The difference between the early adolescent and the older adolescent, when considered as participant in psychotherapy, is more subtle. The cognitively mature adolescent who willingly seeks therapy, who is verbal, and who is psychologically minded is likely to benefit from the free-association-based interpretive process that works well in the form of psychoanalytically oriented psychotherapy for adults. Dreams reported are shorter and the interpretation of dream symbols is often seen as an interesting exercise in the exploration of adult experience. Unfortunately, few early adolescents fit into this category.

Transitional characteristics typical of the late latency–early adolescent phase contribute to dream content. These characteristics include removal of fantasy expression from parents to peer objects, conflict about sexual identity, castration anxieties, omnipotence, resentment of passivity in relation to parents, oedipal involvements and pressures, and persistence of evocative polarities in symbolic usages. The last is of special concern in therapy, since it limits the direct communicative value of free association in determining the latent meaning of a dream symbol. For the most part, work with the dreams of early adolescents requires psychotherapeutic strategies that take into account immature thought processes. Thought disorders, such as impaired object–ground differentiation in social situations, leading to poor personal priorities and difficulty with giving up present pleasures for future gains, can often be detected in difficulty in differentiation between "split life" dreams (see below) and future planning. Reactions to emerging physiology and new and enhanced object relations influence adolescent dreams, giving their content phase-specific characteristics. Manifestations of and reactions to the internal physiological, instinctual, and cognitive changes of youth often enter therapy packaged in a dream.

The starting point for many of the characteristic experiences of adult dreaming occurs in early adolescence. Erotic dreams become far more frequent, their content more frank. In erotic dreaming, an exception occurs in the characteristic blocking of pathways to motor expression of dream content, in which dreamers walk in dreams while lying still. Sexual excitement finds glandular expression with a flow of fluids, especially the nocturnal emissions (ejaculations) of boys. Exploration of associated erotic dream content can bring into therapy prelatency fantasies. Such fantasies have evaded attrition associated with the constant working through and discharge that is the effect of latency-age play. Such erotic dreams are manifestations of puberty along with menarche and the first ejaculation (Sarnoff 1976). These phenomena are markers for a maturational enhancement of object relations. They indicate changes in the direction of maturity for the organs that discharge drives. The development of the capacity for orgasm propels the child toward the search for love objects. The search de-emphasizes discharge under the condition that personal fantasy be satisfied, while enhancing the power of discharge patterns that derive form from the needs of the partner in courtship.

The content of erotic dreams can reveal evidences of unresolved unconscious infantile fantasy wishes that could undermine reality-based object seeking, or reveal ambivalences toward such wishes. For instance, a girl who dreamed of being raped revealed through her dream her rejection of self-initiated sexuality. Yet the choice of activity in a dream is the choice of the dreamer alone. The dream of a young man, in which the barrel of his rifle melted before the entrance to a cave that harbored a big cat, suggests sexual ambivalence.

Unresolved early fantasy, detectable in erotic dreams, is ascribable more strongly to a child's drives than to reality experience at this young age. Evidence of such fantasies in dreams should alert the therapist to detect similar content in a child's description of films, stories, and people. What appears to be only the reporting of daily events in adolescence is likely to be fantasy associations. The adult talks of neurotic situations he has brought upon himself. The adolescent has hardly had time—and certainly has hardly the power—to impair his erotic relationships, though he can create chaos with parents, school, and sibs. Fantasy that will soon influence life at first influences dream content in early adolescence.

In addition, such fantasy influences the selection for inclusion in therapeutic associations of interactions amongst the many couplings encountered in school those stories which can be seen to represent mythic traditions. Their stories vibrate in harmony with their personal patterns of unconscious fantasy. Here are life plots that catch the mind's attention because they offer a way to liberate memories that have been held captive by repression. Through them can be expressed universal unconscious content. Of all the interactions between the heroes and leaders of ancient times, why are there so few remembered, and those few shaped into a few plots that are burned into the consciousness of a culture? The content of these traditions is infused with the makings of the family romance, the oedipal phase, masturbatory and core fantasies. They resonate with repressed memories of the child. They echo the content of an unrest that cries for resolution. Repressed memories and the personal fantasy life of the child guide in the selection of topics in free association, recall of school social life and dreams. They indicate where psychotherapeutic work need be done.

"Split life dreams" refers to a phenomenon in dreaming in which relationships are preserved through the restriction of the expression in dreams of drive energies (hostilities) which would break up a primary waking relationship. For instance, a late adolescent had a much older boyfriend who had taken up her time and talked of a lifetime relationship. However, he showed no inclination to seek, or ability to hold, a job. She clung to him and their shared hopes while in her dream life she dissipated her anger through dreams of meetings and marriage ceremonies from which all overt traces of the boyfriend were banished. Such integrations of dreaming and adjustment can be seen at any age. They tend to be frequent in adolescence because of the lack of life skills for dealing with incompetent peers.

In the latency-age child, such a use of fantasy is certainly present in dreaming. Fantasy play offers an arena for substitute fulfillments and tension discharges that are unattainable. For the child, it is a familiar part of the daily round. Ludic demise (Sarnoff 1987a), which deprives the child of such waking outlets, shifts the burden of carrying this task to dream symbols, resulting in an intensification of this activity in adolescence. The possibility that this outlet will become the cornerstone of a character trait of manifest paralysis in dealing with real problems requires that the process be explained to the child in any therapy in which it is found.

The Interpretation of Dreams in Early Adolescence

The use and effectiveness of dreams as discharge or communicative psychological instruments undergoes a transition as the result of the cognitive changes of late latency–early adolescence. As in work with adults, dynamic psychotherapy with adolescents uses specific interventions in the interpretation of dreams. There is the technique of asking the patient to look for elements (the day residue) in recent days' events of which the dream reminds one. This establishes a link between the dream content and unprocessed daytime stresses, the mastery of which requires more work. There is the technique of asking the patient to respond to each dream symbol by instructing him to say whatever comes into his mind while associating to the symbol. There is the technique whereby the therapist avoids focusing on the dream. In this approach, the therapist seeks enlightenment by considering the session's entire contents to be dream associations.

In work with early adolescents, one may ask about day residues and pursue the use of the session as an association to the dream, as is done with adults. Limitation on ability with abstractions during early adolescence makes free association to dream symbols a relatively unproductive activity. The pursuit of themes that tie together content (secondary elaboration) can be useful in giving clues to problem areas that define goals for therapy.

At times little is produced by these approaches to dreams in the adolescent. Often the adolescent has little curiosity about his dreams and seems to associate with few apparent symbols. The patient appears to be bringing in no depth material. Yet the latent fantasies are there. They must be looked for with insight into the way the adolescent manifests latent content. The plots of movies and the lives of peers that the patient describes are chosen because they resonate with latent fantasy. Clues to the nature of these fantasies can be found in the patient's dreams—more specifically, in the context that organizes the dream symbols into a meaningful tale for the dreamer. For this the therapist turns to the organizing story that ties together the dream elements into what appears to be a coherent story for the dreamer (secondary elaboration) and tries to see if there is a typical core fantasy, which in adolescents often needs resolution. Such content alerts the therapist to the dreamer's problem fantasies.

For instance, an immature 19-year-old man had never lived away from his mother's home. His parents were estranged and had lived apart for years. He was very attached to his mother and tried his best to substitute for his father. He tried to be the man of the house. During a period prior to his parents' reconciliation he had the following dream:

He was in Russia—with his mother—and two brothers—they ran as they were being pursued—his mother fell a couple of times—each time, he picked her up.

Ignoring the idea that an organized story had been told, the therapist inquired about each individual unit of the dream. There were no associations. The patient expressed wonderment at the flimsy connection between each unit of the dream and that which he knew about himself. The family came originally from France. The dream consisted of symbols selected from realistic representations. It was fantastic in quality of content when considered in the context of the patient's waking life. No day residue could be uncovered. If the dream content were to be viewed as a symbolic representation of the life of an oedipally involved young man, one could see parallels in his current life situation and problems. The boys are in a strange land with the mother. Someone pursues (guilt—the father?). The mother's falls could be interpreted as ambivalence about returning to the father. The boy reinforces her flight by helping her up. The individual elements of the dream are not interrelated. Each can exist on its own. Put together as they are by the dreamer, they seem to conform to a familiar theme, the Oedipus complex.

What can be done by the dream interpreter faced with a dream having so few associations? One could make an educated guess at the nature of the core fantasy that predicts and shapes the boy's fate. An oedipal fantasy is one of the usual fantasies active at this age in young men who have failed to achieve removal. There is no certainty that this is the operative fantasy. However, in the absence of associations to the dream, the oedipal fantasy can be used for the formulation of theories, not as a lead to interpretations but as a source of a call to alertness on the part of the therapist for similar themes that would offer confirmatory associations derived from stories or tales about the adventures of peers.

THE USE OF PLAY IN THE PSYCHOTHERAPY OF THE NEUROSES IN THE YOUNG

For the developmental reason that play symbols lose strength with the advent of adolescence, ludic play as a therapeutic modality is restricted to early childhood and the latency years. In fact, psychotherapy during the period from the first appearance of psychoanalytic symbols until late latency (from 2 through 11 years of age) is distinguishable by emphasis on play in therapy sessions. In psychotherapy at all ages, fantasy can be expressed through dreams, daydreams, and verbalized reworkings of reality. During prelatency and latency, the expression of fantasy is augmented, and in many youngsters overshadowed, by play. Special techniques are needed to deal with play as an expression of the unconscious fantasy life of the child.

Though the therapist may cooperate in play, he should not truly be a play partner for a child patient in therapy. The therapist must be careful not to intrude his own ideas into the initiation and content of the play interaction. Rather, the therapist should participate as a willing accessory in the expression through play of the child's fantasy and will. Providing equipment, toys, and raw material serves this role. Carving, pasting, and building play characters and making devices such as cars and houses enhance this role. Excluding structured games encourages fantasy with roots in the child's memory. The introduction of reality limits is served by the nature and quantity of toys available. In large part one augments the ego of the child by contributing an adult bridge of mature powers and skills over which an expression of the child's fantasy life can connect with the real world.

Mature skills serve expression of fantasy wishes in a real-world context, while introducing the modulating influences of realities and possibilities. The adult reality testing of the therapist limits possible contexts of expression where safety is a question, and enforces recognition of reality limitations. This encourages two concurrent processes. The first is expression of fantasy in a way that makes interpretation possible. The second is a limiting experiencing of reality that hurries accommodation. Concurrently there is a shift to the use of reality-based symbols in secondary-process thinking. This step in the development of reality testing underlies the development of future planning and love object finding.

Play is more than a fantasy derivative that provides for discharge of tension and the practice of socialization skills. It also serves as a conduit for the expression of infantile drives and the recall and mastery of infantile stresses and traumas. In order for the therapist to use this process therapeutically, play must be recognized to be a moiety that codifies memories for conscious expression, albeit masked, that bypasses confrontation with reality. Play is a secret form of drive derivative. Decoding of play is a psychotherapeutic technique, which opens the door to indentifying latent fantasy. In the case of little Roy (see Chapter 5), the patient's play and attitudes, revealed in aside comments, opened the way to his latent fantasy of being a person of power who had the right to defecate at will at any time or place.

During late latency, when the symbols used to express waking fantasy become more socially communicative and selected from full-sized elements in reality (ludic demise), play ceases its role as the primary carrier of fantasy. Dreams are not so time-limited. Dreams enhance their role as a primary conduit for fantasy, a role that continues throughout life. Toys (play symbols) are three-dimensional, consciously controlled, and small. As such they fail to serve when reality testing at the service of intensified instinctual needs rejects play symbols that realistically cannot satisfy.

The effectiveness of the use of play in child therapy depends on the memory organization in use by the patient, coupled with the therapist's awareness of its associated limitations. This is especially so when the operative level of memory function of the child is on an affecto-motor level. At this level symbols can represent events and trauma without the interposition of verbal memory elements. In the case of little Roy, this permitted him to act without the limiting inhibition that verbal self-reflective awareness would have provided. Codification in words brings to bear social challenges and validation of behavior through linkage to intensified memory storage of inhibitions. When this happens on a level that is sufficiently verbal, it can be challenged logically. Failure to be able to encode abstract interpretations in memory interferes with the ability of the child to carry insight from one session to the next. In the early latency-age child, abstract interpretations have to be repeated during many sessions.

Free association in children does not occur in the manifest form that one finds in adults. In adults, conscious effort can be enlisted to encourage verbalization of insights into self, memories, latent contents, the past, and verbalized abstractions. Free association in words reflects unconscious motivation and is determined by psychic factors. The stream of consciousness thus produced bears the imprint of the inner workings of the personality. In children, in the presence of a weak ability to use words in this way, play becomes a preferred means for the expression of fantasy. In the transition to adolescence, play (ludic) symbols mature with age, becoming less evocative and more communicative, and eventually give way to peers as symbols. As a result, in adolescence free association shifts its zone of action from play to verbalization.

PLAY

Fantasy Play

The latent content of fantasy is manifested in toys as symbols during fantasy play, where toys and full body action take the role in fantasy play that visual imagery takes in dreams. The contextual flow of fantasy play consists of expressions of latent fantasy content influenced by current stresses and modulated by reactive regressions. For the most part the manifest symbolic forms of childhood play hide their latent meanings from the child who plays.

Knowledge of the development and nature of the symbolic forms produced by the immature symbolizing function of the latency ego can help the therapist to introduce fantasy play in therapy. Drawings, toys, and dolls can serve as ludic symbols to elborate insight, create extended contexts, recreate affects, and reactivate the quickly repressed fantasies that appear and then seem to disappear at the time of major stresses. For instance:

A midlatency child found herself at a loss for words in describing threatening experiences while in school. She was able to reveal a fantasy of an armed murderous revolt against the teacher when encouraged to draw pictures of the participants. The pictures were cut out, glued on boards, and turned into puppets. These could be used session after session to reflect her unfolding day-by-day experiences.

Conversion of a dream element into a toy can be used to extend the associations to a dream. For instance:

A child of 7 who dreamed of a snakelike monster but could give few verbal associations was encouraged to extend her associations to the dream by being asked to make a clay monster. The dream symbol, now a toy, was then used in subsequent sessions to produce fantasies and contexts that enhanced the understanding of the dream and the child (Sarnoff 1976).

At times children in therapy pursue such a conversion from dream symbol to play symbol without the intervention of the therapist. For instance:

A 7½-year-old boy had precipitated a physical attack from his father because of parental refusal to purchase an expensive electronic toy. Eventually the parents responded to the depression and despair of the child and acquiesced to the purchase. For weeks after, the child was beset by a mixture of preoccupation with his new toy and resolution of the humiliation felt in response to his impotence before the might and power of adults. In two consecutive sessions during this period, he presented first a dream and then a fantasy. On Tuesday, he spontaneously reported that "I had a dream that my friend was driving a car. I told my mother that I wanted to drive a car too. She said no. I kicked her hard in the behind. She let me drive."

On Thursday, he began the session by picking up a piece of balsa wood and asking me to carve a switchblade knife for him. I asked him to draw the knife he wanted. His drawing was vague; however, the type of knife that he wished soon assumed sufficient shape for me to begin to carve under his guidance. A knife was produced, which he began to brandish and throw about the playroom. "Whom would you want to use the knife on?" I asked. He answered, illustrating his fantasy with full body movements and gestures, "I'd stick my dad, if he didn't give me what I want. I'd stick him in the behind." By way of illustration, he turned the knife on himself and directed its penetration toward his own anus.

Note the use by the child of anal-sadistic fantasy content in response to feelings of humiliation. An oedipal content of the fantasy is clear. The typical latency-age anal regression in response to overwhelming oedipal tingeing of facts and perceptions is illustrated. The latent content of both dream and fantasy bear the impress of the same psychodynamic context. There was more here than a request for a toy. Children naturally employ toys and dream symbols interchangeably as manifest symbolic forms to be used to express latent content. The therapist's encouragement of play with toys or dream symbols takes advantage of the existence of common roots below the arborization of symbolic forms. The therapist does not play with the child but rather places at the child's disposal adult cognition and manual skills to be used in the creation of symbolic forms that can serve as conduits for the communication of a child's inner life.

This approach becomes less appropriate in the late latency child who is beginning to seek objects for the discharge of his drives in real action with real objects in his peer group. The more verbal older child in therapy tends to stop and think about what has happened and then to bring verbal memories of it to therapy. Should this not suffice, the therapist can encourage fantasy play as an extension of free association.

Memory Function in Play Therapy

The link between past experience and current recall is memory. The moieties that codify memory for current recall in child therapy differ from those of later years. The difference is the presence of psychoanalytic symbols in the play of child therapy.

Memory function influences psychotherapy twice over. Recall of past events, either in reporting or in free association, depends on memory. Without memory there would be no insight therapy. The recall of insight and interpretations encountered during therapy is also a function of memory. A child who has not yet attained a level of memory organization that will permit the retention of abstract concepts may nod his head in agreement to an interpretation framed with such thought, but will be unable to understand and to retain the concepts for use in comprehending future behavior or holding insight.

Spontaneous Recall

Free association depends on spontaneous recall. Spontaneous recall is best illustrated by "fill-in-the-blanks" questions on tests. This should be differentiated from multiple choice recall through recognition. Spontaneous recall can occur without external prompting, as happens when a tune is suddenly recalled, an unaccomplished responsibility pops into mind, or during free association in the course of one of the psychotherapies. Spontaneous recall can also occur in response to a suggestion or request that something be recalled. Such is the case in the fill-in-the-blanks questions mentioned above and in the response to a question or interpretation by a therapist. There are other forms of recall, such as recognition recall, in which a representation of the experience or the thing to be recalled is shown to the subject and is recognized as part of a prior experience. Recognition recall may be used to activate spontaneous recall. Spontaneous recall is the activity involved when the nonintrusive therapist permits the patient to free-associate. Free associations are spontaneously recalled thought elements.

The nature of spontaneous recall is shaped by the media for representing past experiences, appropriate to the situation, age, and culture of the subject. These may be actions (as in fate neuroses), words (as in adult analyses), affects (as in mourning), and symbols (as in dreams and fantasy play). There appears to be compulsion to repeat prior experiences (Freud, 1926). This is especially so in response to experiences that have been uncomfortable, traumatic, humiliating, or incomplete (Zygarnik effect). The repetition attempts to serve a mastery function. For instance:

A 10-year-old boy came for his appointment within an hour after two older boys had demanded that he buy marijuana from them. They threatened to kill him if he told anyone. He told his parents, after hiding for half an hour. Pressure to master the experience caused him to present himself as a hero. He left out the part of the story in which he hid in fear.

Movement, Affect, and Play Symbols as Free Association

The following clinical vignettes illustrate the therapeutic approach to the child who is capable of verbal recall but who has made a defensive shift to free association mediated through a system of recall that is immersed in movement, affect, and ludic (play) symbols. Note that the main thrust of the technique is to get the child to use a more mature verbal form of communication and memory organization in generating associations.

Converting Action Into Fantasy

A youngster, age 9, stopped talking to the therapist and began to bounce a ball against the playroom wall. The therapist watched for evidences of fantasy. He searched for evidences reflecting any associated thought content. He noticed that the child was saying numbers as he played. "What are you playing?" the therapist asked. "Are you keeping score in a game with you or with someone else?"

"With my father," the child said. "Quiet, I'm winning."

Unlocking the Fantasy to Reveal the Problem Within

A 10-year-old boy in the third year of treatment began a session by picking up sticks and guns from all over the playroom. He locked some play money in a box and hid it. He announced that it was a box of doubloons. He gave the therapist a gun and told him that they were going to rob the bank where the doubloons are kept. Stories of robberies and being captured were standard fare for this child. They usually occurred when he felt guilty about something. The therapist asked about this. The boy explained, "I really like stories about robberies and being captured. Nothing special happened (to stimulate the fantasy)." He then proceeded with the story, in which he played the chief and I a henchman. In the course of preparations for the robbery, he walked from the playroom into my office, where he planned the crime while sitting at my desk and swiveling in my chair. This was a change from the routine story. I pointed it out.

"I'm the Godfather," said he. "I need a big desk."

I pointed out that I've noticed that people his age often go to my chair when they come into the room. What did he think the reason was?

He explained, "When I was little I could use the table in there as a desk." He then described in detail his need for objects in reality to fulfill his fantasies. "Now when I want to feel like a big shot, I have to have a real desk."

I asked, "What else do you do when you need to feel like a big shot?"

"Have some gum," he said.

"You chew gum?" I asked.

"Sure, said he, "did you ever smoke?"

"No," was my reply.

"I'm going to smoke," he said, "'cause then I'll feel sharp like a grownup and when I'm twenty I'm going to buy a stick of marijuana and try it. Do you know what marijuana looks like? Today someone said, 'A penny apiece or 100 for a dollar.' I bought one." He went to his coat pocket and took out a "punk" and asked if it were marijuana. He seemed relieved when I told him it was not. We spoke about drugs till the end of the session.

Though the boy began the session by playing out a fantasy, the therapist was able to bring the child to a discussion of developmental changes in his defenses as well as bringing into focus the question of fear of drug use, which was the problem behind the evoked fantasy. He had mobilized fantasy as a defense (one of the functions of the structure of latency). The original conflict of the day was reconstituted by calling attention to a change in the content of an oft-repeated fantasy. The stress of the conflict had resulted, in this lad, with an obviously well-organized abstract conceptual memory organization, in a regression to affecto-motor expression as a defense against feelings of guilt and smallness. He chose action involving the desk, chair, and role of the Godfather. This was associated with chewing gum, which symbolized adult-type relief from tension in the form of smoking. The therapist's verbalization encouraged the child to shift to verbalization. His concern that his search to feel like an adult would lead him to drug use could then be pursued on the level of verbal abstraction.

Converting Verbal Conceptual Memory Elements into Meaningful Communication

Now let us turn to the impact on the activity of the therapist of the comprehension of a child's level of cognitive function during an initial interview in a 7-year-old whose mental life has achieved only the level of verbal conceptual memory. This illustrates the modification of approach required to put the therapist in touch with the cognitive level of a patient who has learned to remember by rote the essential nature of the experience remembered, but without necessarily comprehending its intrinsic nature on an abstract level.

A 7-year-old boy was brought for evaluation because of anxiety, hyperactivity, and excessive anger. At the beginning of the session I asked why he had come. He explained that he had "behavior problems."

"What are they?" I asked. He had difficulty with this, finally explaining that he knows what to do, but it just comes out bad. He answered questions freely, and in a short time I had determined that he heard his own voice telling him to misbehave. It seems that words like "behavior problem," "excitement," and "I want to do better" were rote repetitions of things he had heard his parents say. Not knowing of the voice, they had theorized an explanation, which they called "behavior problem." The child knew that he would be rewarded if he used the words of the explanation. However, he could not explain the abstract meaning of the phrases as they had been used. When asked, "What will you do when you are doing better?" he answered, "I forget what I do wrong. I never done it twice. I try not to do it."

"What?" I asked

"I want to behave better," said he. He could not tell what that meant or when he had misbehaved or what he had done. He could use words for effect, but not for meaning. He said his mother said he misbehaves when he is "excited." I then asked him, "Do you know what it means to be excited?" He tried to find words. He had a concept but no words. He began to jump up and down. He stepped aside and, pointing at the place in which he had been jumping, said, "Like that." Thenceforth he said, "you jump up and down," whenever he wanted to say excitement. By using the same phrase, I was able to question him about situations that excite him and the things he does when he "jumps up and down."

He could not recall his "make-believes," but he did remember that he had dreams of monsters. He said, "I pretend monsters come in dreams and kill me." I asked what a monster looked like. He said that he didn't know. He could feel the monster but not see it. I asked him to draw it. He said, "I can dream a monster, but I can't draw it."

I asked, "Can you make one out of clay?"

"Sure," he responded.

I gave him Play-Doh. He made two pylons, then another two. These, he explained, were legs. He made two more legs and began to make a body to put on them. As the clay monster took form, he became scared of it. He could not continue his work on it. I found that although he feared the three-dimensional figure, he could continue to work with a less threatening two-dimensional picture. I had drawn a picture of the legs of the clay figure. He looked at it and, peering at the clay figure, drew into my sketch a body and head.

These vignettes from an initial interview illustrate

1. The affecto-motor recollection of a concept (jumping for excitement) followed by the establishment of a verbal description as a signifier of the concrete act. The verbal conceptual mode of expression was then used to explore the experience of excitement. Surely this is a child who thinks by remembering.

2. The observation I have noted repeatedly: that an early latency-age child can draw what he has difficulty describing and can mold what he has difficulty drawing, and that a child who cannot draw may be able to fill in another's drawing. This may be used by a therapist in encouraging an otherwise noncommunicative child to associate further when blocked. This is done by using phase-compatible materials to encourage associative expression.

Treatment of the Child with Delayed Abstract Conceptual Memory

We now turn to the problem of the late latency-age child who has not achieved full usage of abstract concepts as the medium for retention in memory. The goal of the therapist is twofold. In addition to seeking phrasings for interpretations that are compatible with the patient's style of thought and memory function, the therapist should also seek to help the child achieve an abstract-conceptual memory organization, so as to enhance retention of interpretations. By helping the child to develop the capacity to store abstractions in memory, the therapist helps the child to gather a context of abstractions through which to interpret his own behavior. Strengthening of these functions furthers the results of child therapy.

To some extent this problem may be found in each child who has recently entered the late latency phase. Insofar as this is so, the brief recommendations presented below are applicable in many cases. One should be especially on the alert for this condition in youngsters who present with symptoms based on the use of motor function and body organs or orifices. Such conditions as enuresis, stuttering, encopresis, and thumb-sucking have in my experience often been accompanied by difficulty in schoolwork and limitation in the abstract conceptual memory organization. A cardinal sign indicating the presence of this condition is a combination of extended fantasy play with answers to questions that consist of the word "fine" or a distracted grunt. Other clues are extended and detailed reports of dreams or television shows. The latter reflects the presence of an extraordinary verbal memory, which, when coupled with difficulty in abstraction, resembles Luria's (1968) mnemonist.

One such youngster, 10 years old, asked me if I had seen the film, *The Wizard of Oz*. I asked him to tell me about it. To my amazement, he presented the script, or so it seemed, almost verbatim. He took two sessions to do it. When I asked him afterwards what the story was about, he could not tell me.

In dealing with youngsters with this problem, one should constantly refer back to earlier fantasies or events that can be described using abbreviated phrases. In essence, one lends ego by introducing an "abstract" or symbol that the child will be able to recognize as a part of the whole. Sometimes the child is so delayed in the development of abstraction that word exercises are not sufficient. In that case it is best to use a medium for recall that the child is literally capable of handling physically, such as clay figures, dolls, or drawings. Such concrete objects must be presented in a context from which abstractions can be developed. Here one creates a relationship between concrete objects and an abstraction. This mimics, as paradigm, Piaget's concrete operational thinking (see above)—that is, the ability to make an abstract interpretation of something concretely experienced.

Clay figures can be made that represent an element in a fantasy. The tendency to forget abstract concepts can be overcome by preserving the objects for future sessions. They become touchstones through which recognition recall can make memory for abstractions therapeutically viable. Such objects should be kept in a safe place. They can be brought out in session after session repeatedly, and can be used as reminders of earlier and similar fantasies when a derivative fantasy based on the same latent fantasy as the earlier one is presented. Pictures can be used in the same way with children who are at the level at which two-dimensional items can be used for activating spontaneous recall. Often, a bulletin board to which drawings can be stuck can be used as a substitute memory. The figures can be used to remind the child of an interpretation. When they are accompanied by words, the use of words for transmitting abstractions in memory is reinforced and furthered. For instance:

A 10-year-old boy had a fantasy about an army tank. He was not capable of elaborating on it. I suggested that he make one for us to use so that he could tell me about the fantasy by acting it out. The next session, he brought in two enormous shipping crates from which he built the tank. He was so concrete in the memory organization used in his fantasies and free associations that he could not play out his fantasies with the slight degree of abstraction needed to reduce the tank in size. When he found his "tank" unwieldly, he welcomed my drawing of a tank and went on from there.

In youngsters such as this, who have difficulty in creating word representations and drawings, it can be useful to draw a background of houses or the out-of-doors and to place figures in the picture, inviting the child to add his own answering figures. The fantasies involved here are not necessarily the child's alone. They are influenced by the therapist (forced fantasies). As such, interpretations derived from them are not strongly valid. The process by which the therapist forces fantasy is not aimed at uncovering material. Instead it aims at developing new skills in the retrieval and presentation of memories. Thus, one encourages free association through offering communicative tools. An example of this therapeutic technique of enhancing ego skills follows in the case of Paul.

Paul, age 10, who had diurnal enuresis, was subject to episodes of breaking things. He drew some pictures of "the breaker" when asked why he wet. He could tell no more than this. He had a year of therapy in which techniques were used that enhanced the formulation and verbalization of memory recalls which dealt with abstract relationships. Emphasis was placed on verbalization of abstractions about figure drawings based on dream elements or presented in episodes of play. He was encouraged to relate puppets based on his drawing to each other through storytelling through puppet plays. There were exercises in drawing figures based on the integration into the whole of parts of animals, which were lined up but not in appropriate spatial relation to one another. After a year, the child was able to apply his expanded ability to create contexts to creating a connection between his wetting and the breaker. When I pointed to a picture of the breaker (I had cut it out and, with a firm backing, pinned it to the wall), he could explain that he that he heard the voice of the breaker telling him to "break" whenever he wet and broke things.

There could be no resolution of the symptom until it could be described in its entirety. Only when "it" (voice and action) could be identified, could we expand insight into the life context in which wetting occurred. The child was able to identify what he was doing. He was able to relate his behavior to parental punishment. Then it could be explained to him that the voice was a projection of his wish to revenge himself on his father whenever the father scolded him, and that the wetting and breaking were actions that started within him.

In the case of Roy (see Chapter 5), the concept of king could be kept in play in the therapy as the result of keeping the golden crown in the playroom for weeks after. With the same goal of enhancing the operational use of ideas as though we were working with a mature memory, I tend to keep broken items around to illustrate aggression, teasing, or destructive tendencies. In one case, I left a tear in the bathroom wallpaper for 2 years.

A state of doubt in the face of aggressive parental figures who interfere with the child's comfortable expression of phallic competitive strivings is a prime psychological factor in the retardation of maturation of the abstract conceptual memory organization. It should be looked for in such cases. Interpretation at the child's level of memory organization will enhance abstract memory as well as correct pathology.

Treatment When the Child Has a Competent Abstract Conceptual Memory Organization

In treating the child with abstract conceptual memory skills, the approach is similar to that of the treatment of adults. Both groups "remember by thinking." Until about 12 years of age, abstract concepts normally can be applied to concrete events. At 12, there is the development, as observed by Piaget, of abstract operational thinking. Application of remembered abstract insights to abstract situations can then be expected and utilized.

THE CONFLICTING ROLES OF PSYCHOANALYTIC SYMBOLS IN CHILD THERAPY

The Therapist and the Symbol

The relationship of the therapist to the symbol during child therapy has conflicting aspects. On the one hand, the therapist weakens the effectiveness of symbols in his role of helping to make the unconscious conscious. The child therapist interprets the underlying meaning of the symbol of the moment. In this way symbols are undone, and trauma and fantasies are brought to the surface for insight that can lead to conscious working through. With this activity the therapist helps the child undermine symptoms, as well as master the occult roots of intrusions from his or her past. In addition, the therapist aids in the ontogenesis of adolescence by changing the nature of latency-age symbolic forms. To do this, he undermines the work of symbols by encouraging the late latency-age child to use reality elements to replace the chain of imaginary symbolic forms from which latency-age fantasy is wrought (see above sections on Symbols and Secondary Process).

On the other hand, the therapist works to strengthen and preserve ludic symbols through therapeutic techniques that parallel a natural process, which is the resolution of trauma and latent fantasy through manifest symbolic play. Symbols need to be preserved to encourage such discharge through the cathartic role of symbolic play.

Strengthening the Use of Symbols

During the onset of latency and throughout its course there is an ongoing process of resolution of prelatency and infantile internalized conflicts by "working through" using the medium of symbolic play. The psychotherapy of prelatency children requires that ego functions supportive of the conflict-resolution function of fantasy during latency be developed. These include verbal-concept memory and the capacity to develop and use psychoanalytic symbols. What is achieved is resolution and mastery of trauma and latent fantasy, without insight, through play.

Latent fantasies manifested in psychoanalytic symbols can self-dissolve through catharsis and living through. This capacity gives rise to a therapeutic technique that achieves resolution of false realities and limits the ability of infantile wishes to distort "fact" and distract the child from more mature pursuits.

Verbalization in children enhances the working through of, and disenabling of, fantasy contents that are destined to underlie transference wishes in adults. Communicative discharge and confrontation become possible with the development of speech and the evolving of decipherable cryptic symbols. This permits the interpretation of infantile sexual wish-informed fantasy in child therapy. The appearance of, encouragement of, and interpretation of symbols in child therapy results in controlled reparative mastery, working through, and a confrontation of the "sense of reality" with reality testing.

Psychoanalytic symbolic language systems express concepts that would otherwise be lost in the presence of the lacuna-riddled memory created by the many forms of repression and exclusions from consciousness that accompany the development of verbal conceptual memory. Conceptualization and the systematizing power of language give the therapist tools for strengthening reality testing, sublimation, further working through using fantasy, and reparative mastery.

Psychoanalytic symbols arise as a mechanism for resolving or processing, and thus reducing, affects associated with the drear recalls of yesteryear and the guessing and fear that the thought of tomorrow may bring. This is achieved by substituting items taken from a network of related words and ideas, the outer reaches of which have less valence for attracting affect. The further removed are these semiotic items, the less recognizable they are and the less affect is felt. These substitute items become the manifest psychoanalytic symbols.

Psychoanalytic symbols alter conscious naming and awareness of realities, perceived or remembered, producing elements that, collectively, we call the system unconscious. Psychoanalytic symbol–dominated experience undermines the potential for lucid living. Play fantasies are created out of psychoanalytic symbols. Through them, drives that impel unconscious affect-laden concepts can be discharged.

Weakening the Use of Symbols Enhances Reality Testing and Secondary-Process Thinking

Psychoanalytic symbols work to counter lucidity and to blur the understanding of meaning in play and dreams. They blur the meaning of ludic play and work toward counteracting lucidity in dream meaning. What is more, psychoanalytic symbols impair self-reflective awareness. A subcategory of this impairment is an absent capacity for the perception of a relationship between that which represents and that which is represented.

Blurring of meaning produced by the cryptic nature of psychoanalytic symbols interferes with the development in late latency of a network of abstract concepts of self. If the use of waking symbols remains strong, there is impairment of the production of an extended and coherent awareness of self in the context of time, place, and the social order. This awareness is necessary for adolescent and adult adjustment. The obscuring capacity of waking symbols must be obtunded if reality testing is to be enhanced. It is part of the psychotherapy of the young to encourage the replacement of fantastic elements with realistic elements in the sources from which symbolic forms are selected.

Interpretation reverses the symbolizing process, introducing awareness of deeper meaning into the mélange of confusing cues produced by ludic symbols. Therapy gains through reflection on the connection of ludic symbols to waking experience. Roy, whose case was discussed in the preceding chapter, came into therapy with insufficient verbal self-awareness of his grandiose latent fantasy life to be able to correct his impressions by a confrontation with reality. His symbolizing function was weak, and so he discharged his rage through organ language (encopresis) and characterological behavior (rage episodes, demandingness). Psychoanalytic symbols were actively developed or enhanced by the therapy. This made him more comfortable by giving him symbols through which to represent his latent fantasy in play. At the same time, the displaced nature of his play distracted his attention from his mother's demeaning attitude towards him. Discharge of drive tensions was made possible by his newly organized powerful -person fantasy. The possibility of discharge did not aid insight, however. When he involved the therapist in the role of a person demeaned, and was able to produce the word "king" to describe his power, a communicative verbal link was added to the conjoint memory of Roy and the therapist. The golden crown added a visual dimension. Once insight into the meaning of the symbol was possible, the symbols were devalued in favor of a search for meaning that would bring Roy into contact with the devastation that his latent fantasy of power was bringing to his daily life. Symbols provided a key to the cryptic door to insight. Interpretation and discussion turned the key.

GOALS AND MECHANISMS OF CHILD THERAPY

Making the Unconscious Conscious; Freeing the Child to Confront Reality

Making the unconscious conscious entails more than the disclosure of hidden meanings by putting them into words. Consciousness implies understanding perceptions (recalled or newly experienced) in terms of how the past influences a current interpretation of a fact and the meaning of a current perception for future life.

Unconscious tensions and drive derivatives that have been displaced to symbols, and fantasies and problems that have found expression in cryptic manifestations, can be addressed directly through the interpretation of symbols. Once revealed to awareness, the problem of intrusions from the past becomes opened to inspection and resolution. This frees the personality to recognize reality stresses and to deal with the future. When one realizes that unconscious elements intrude on the interpretation of perception to alter one's reality, it is possible to appreciate reality better and to deal with it more effectively. Maturation and therapy replace the symbolic elements in fantasy with reality elements. This converts fantasy resolutions for problems into future planning, and it widens the child's perspective on reality to include facts and realities that can be responded to and worked on in therapy.

Unconscious content falls into two categories. There are elements for which no words have been assigned during the shift from affecto-motor to verbal-concept memory; and there are elements so strongly linked to uncomfortable affects that verbal elements to represent them must be avoided. Psychoanalytic symbols provide an intermediate pathway for the entrance of the latter into consciousness. These are verbal or visual representations sufficiently removed from the original concept that is represented, to assure that the affect associated with the original is diminished. In the case of Roy (see Chapter 5), it was necessary to help him to create such symbols in order to give the interpreter something to interpret. Interpretation of the symbol then opened the door to the mental content that had influenced behavior, but whose context was not available to consciousness, reflection, and discussion. Once the concept could be represented through a symbol and then, through interpretation, could be opened to a lucid and more complete view of his behavior, a self-observing object could be established in his mind's eye that could go wherever he went, as it were, and help his inner speech (Vygotsky 1934) to correct self-discomforting behavior.

In achieving self-awareness, Roy followed a course of development that retraces a stage in the evolution of consciousness. He moved from an existence as a primitive slave to instinct, a life of the moment, to that of a person who understood his behavior within a linear context of past, future, moral values, and facts. He gained enough knowledge of what was going on in his life to be able to control what went on in it. Another trace of that stage in modern man is the lucid dream, in which, by definition, the dreamer is aware that he is dreaming and can control what happens in the dream. The lucid dream is a rare type of dream in our culture (Sarnoff in press). Lucid dreaming (LaBarge 1990) is an example of self-reflective awareness refined to the point that words can be utilized to crystallize dream experiences into a matrix of sustained simultaneous understandings of sensations, associations, prior experiences, and future implications during dreaming (REM) sleep. During lucid dreaming there is no sensory contact with the waking world, but there is awareness that one is dreaming, and within the dream one is capable of making changes in dream content and events. One can initiate movement within such a dream and alter the course of the dream to avoid unwanted outcomes. Such an awareness while awake—which can grant access to and control of reality by putting aside the strength of symbols for a patient—is a goal of psychotherapy. The closer a representation comes to reality, the more does secondary-process thinking move toward its mature form.

A major transition in a child's orientation to his life occurs when, as a result of maturation, words representing abstractions can be associated with percepts and affects and other experiences that previously only called for reflex responses and symbols. Abstraction expands awareness to encompass past and future, giving meaning involving a sustained longitudinal history to new experience. Such awareness brings insight into consciousness. Psychotherapeutic interpretation expands the arena for this memory resonance. Potential for such self-directed awareness in an abstract context involving past, present, and future converts the child's awareness from a point existence in time to a linear phenomenon. A linear concept of life is necessary for survival in modern society. Tolerance for the uncertainties of the present and the future, and for the pain of the past, is part of adult adjustment to reality. One of the roles of therapy is to prepare the child to tolerate this by helping the child replace manifest symbols with the facts they coyly hide and represent, so that problems and latent fantasies may then be addressed directly. The role of memory-resonant consciousness in creating the discomforting affects of men and women was succinctly and well put by Robert Burns (1786) in "To a Wee Mousie." On disturbing the house of a wee small mouse, the poet begged the frightened tiny creature's pardon with these words:

Still thou art blessed compared with me!
The present only toucheth thee:
But, Oh! I backward cast my eye on prospects drear!
And forward, though I cannot see, I guess and fear.

SUMMARY

Fantasies, dreams, and play are organizations of symbols that offer useful sources of information during the psychotherapy of neuroses in the young. They carry content about latent fantasy, drives, and affects. Fantasy, dream, and play offer excellent vehicles for transference and hidden meanings. There are developmental cognitive aspects to latency and adolescent psychopathology, which sets it apart from psychopathology in the adult. For this reason the therapist should be tuned to aberrations of form as well as content, and should be aware that what appears to be therapeutic gain can actually be developmental in origin. At any age, symbols can be used to encourage fantasy discharge and expression, and then interpreted in the search for insight. During early latency, with its scant outlets, it is advantageous to the child for the therapist to encourage symbol formation to strengthen discharge pathways. In late latency–early adolescence, with the increase of reality potentials, reality testing and mature secondary-process thinking are enhanced by the weakening of symbols through interpretation and through encouraging reality elements in place of fantastic elements for use as symbols.

REFERENCES

Boorstein, D. J. (1983). *The Discoverers*. New York: Random House.

Budiansky, S. (1991). In from the cold. *The New York Times Magazine*, Section 6, December 22, p. 20.

Burns, R. (1786). To A wee mousie. In *My Heart's in the Highlands*. . . . Norwich, CT: Jarrold, 1980.

Darwin, C. (1872). *Origin of Species*. New York: Hill and Wang, 1979.

Ferenczi, S. (1913). A little Chanticleer. In *The Selected Papers of Sandor Ferenczi*, vol. 1, pp. 240–252. New York: Basic Books, 1950.

Freud, A. (1926). *The Psychoanalytic Treatment of Children*. New York: International Universities Press, 1946.

Freud, S. (1900). The interpretation of dreams. *Standard Edition* 5.

——— (1909). Notes upon a case of obsessional neurosis. *Standard Edition* 10:153–250.

——— (1915). The unconscious. *Standard Edition* 14:156–216.

——— (1926). Beyond the pleasure principle. *Standard Edition* 18:3–66.

Hall, N. J.(1991). *Trollope*. New York: Clarendon/Oxford University Press.

Hoffer, W. (1978). *Early Development and Education of the Child*. Northvale, NJ: Jason Aronson.

Hoffman, D. (1991). Review of Silverman, Kenneth. *New York Times Book Review*, December 22, p. 1.

Kernberg, P. (1991). *Children with Conduct Disorders*. New York: Basic Books.

Kincaid, J. R. (1991). Review of Hall, N. John. "Trollope." *New York Times Book Review*, December 22, p. 1.

Krauss, R. M., and Glucksberg, S. (1977). Social and non-social speech. *Scientific American* 236:100–106.

LaBerge, S. (1990). Lucid dreaming: psychophysiological studies of consciousness during REM sleep. In *Sleep and Cognition*, ed. R. Bootzin, J. Kihlstrom, and D. Schachter, pp. 109–126. Washington, DC: American Psychological Association Press.

Lippman, H. S. (1956). Panel: the dream in the practice of psychoanalysis. L. Rangell, reporter. *Journal of the American Psychoanalytic Association* 4: 132.

Luria, A. R. (1976). *Cognitive Development: Its Cultural and Social Foundations*. Boston: Harvard University Press.

_____ (1968). *The Mind of a Mnemonist*. New York: Basic Books.

Nurcombe, B. (1976). *Children of the Dispossessed*. Honolulu: University of Hawaii Press, 1976.

Piaget, J. (1951). *Play Dreams and Imitation in Childhood*. New York: W. W. Norton, 1962.

Pittell, S. (1973). The etiology of youthful drug involvement. In *Drug Use in America: Problems in Perspective: Technical Papers*. Vol. 1; *Patterns and Consequences of Drug Use*. Washington, DC: U.S. Government Printing Office.

Sarnoff, C. A. (1970). Symbols and symptoms, phytophobia in a two-year-old-girl. *Psychoanalytic Quarterly* 39:550–562.

_____ (1976). *Latency*. Northvale, NJ: Jason Aronson.

_____ (1987a). *Psychotherapeutic Strategies in the Latency Years*. Northvale, NJ: Jason Aronson.

_____ (1987b). Shifting symbolic forms during late latency-early adolescence. In *Psychotherapeutic Strategies in Late Latency through Early Adolescence*, pp. 47–67. Northvale, NJ: Jason Aronson.

_____ (in press). *Symbols—In Structure and Function*. Northvale, NJ: Jason Aronson.

Silverman, K. (1991). *Edgar A. Poe*. New York: Harper Collins.

Sterba, E. (1955). *Panel: The Dream in the Practice of Psychoanalysis*. L. Rangell, reporter. *Journal of the American Psychoanalytic Association* 4: 131.

Tasso, T. (1575/1581). *Jerusalem Delivered*. Detroit, MI: Wayne State University Press, 1987.

Tagore, R. (1936). The beginning. In *The Crescent Moon*, pp. 14–15. New York: Macmillan.

Voth, H. H. (1978). Dream analysis in the treatment of an eleven-year-old boy. *International Journal of Psychoanalytic Psychotherapy* 7:254–274.

Vygotsky, L. (1934). *Thought and Language*. Cambridge, MA: MIT Press.

7

Resistance

G. Pirooz Sholevar, M.D.

The resistance accompanies the treatment step by step. Every single association, every act of the person under treatment must reckon with the resistance and represents a compromise between the forces that are striving toward recovery and the opposing ones.

Freud 1912, p. 103

Psychoanalytic pioneers assumed that the analytic process could be established and the unconscious material accessed more easily with children than with adult patients because the child's unconscious and conscious mental activities were less strictly separated than those of adults. The analytic situation was hoped to activate the instinctual derivatives and enable them to emerge to the surface relatively easily because there would be fewer forces opposing the analytic process. In reality, the above expectations proved incorrect, and the forces opposing the analysis of children at times have proven stronger than with adult patients for a variety of reasons. Analysis of resistance with children remains the most exacting part of clinical analytic work, partly because resistance bars the way to the analysis of significant life-historical material and its own analysis through "resistance against analysis of resistance" (Sandler and A. Freud 1985, Schafer 1973).

Initially, the phenomenon of resistance was considered a barrier to the achievement of the analytic goal of gaining insight. More recently, the *positive* aspect of the resistance has been emphasized, which allows the patient to remain in analysis and become engaged in the psychoanalytic process (Schafer 1973). Therefore, resistance is currently viewed as *compromises* made by patients with free association in order to allay anxiety and maintain their tie to the analytic process by setting some comforting conditions under which they can proceed with the task of analysis (Morgenstern 1991).

DEFINITION

Resistance is a paradoxical phenomenon regularly encountered in the course of psychoanalytic psychotherapy, particularly psychoanalysis. The patient, who has willingly asked for treatment to resolve neurotic problems, opposes the process in a variety of ways that would serve to defeat the objective of change (Moore and Fine 1990). Resistance may take the form of attitudes, verbalizations, and actions that prevent awareness of a perception, feeling, idea, or memory that might serve to establish a connection with earlier experiences and bring about insight into the nature of unconscious conflicts. Though often evidenced by an avoidance of free association, resistance in a broader sense encompasses all of a patient's defensive efforts to avoid self-knowledge. Usually unconscious at first, it may persist long after it is consciously recognized (Stone 1973).

The analyst helps the analysand achieve increased comprehension of his or her life history, and especially of his or her psychological difficulties in this life—historical context as a basis for psychological change. By resisting, the patient exhibits that he or she is simultaneously engaged in two opposing or contradictory actions, although one action might be done more insistently. Therefore, we consider that the resistance is stronger in one case in contrast to the next case or next stage where the drive is stronger (Schafer 1973).

Resistance is pervasive in every analysis. It varies in form and intensity from patient to patient and in the same patient at different stages in the analysis. Analytic process threatens to bring into awareness through free association and other means repressed childhood wishes, fantasies, and impulses that would produce painful affect. Resistance represents the ego's defensive efforts against this possibility by opposing the analysis itself (Moore and Fine 1990).

Resisting is engaging in actions contrary to analysis while also engaging in analysis itself. It is the patient contradicting himself in action; it is analytic *counteraction*. Resisting or resistance is something one does, and one might do it more resolutely or effectively than one does the work of collaborating in any ordinary sense of that word (Schafer 1973). The statements such as "can't," "won't" and "don't" refer to *disclaimed action* and are manifestations of resistance or a force or entity that renders the person unable to proceed with the work of analysis. Disclaimed action is itself a form of resisting, and when it is the very action of resisting that has been disclaimed, we have an instance of the so-called resistance against analysis of resistance (Schafer 1973).

Resistance manifests itself against the progress of analytic process and the perceived pressure from the analyst. In reality, the object of the resistance is not the person's own rejected unconscious wishes or the perceived pressure from the analyst, but the patient himself is the object of the verb "to resist" (Schafer 1973).

Resistance is a defense against gaining insight (Rangell 1983). The forces of resistance prevent the patient from producing derivatives from the unconscious and protect the repression of intrapsychic conflict by barring it from consciousness. In addition to interference with free association, resistance cancels out the emotional impact and the consequences of most penetrating interpretations, including the interpretation of transference. Resistance stops the patient from putting into practice the understanding he has gained, thereby continuing his repetitive acting out (Schafer 1973). In the psychoanalysis of adults, resistance manifests itself as barriers to free association—the potential road to the recognition of unconscious mental activities. In child analysis, other modes of psychic expression and communication, such as playing, are blocked to prevent insight formation. The knowledge that is kept unconscious is maintained out of reach by virtue of its unacceptability to the ego (Rangell 1983).

Pearson (1968) has provided a broader definition of resistance in child analysis: Resistance in child analysis refers to "all forces which prevent the child from producing derivatives from the unconscious, *plus the conscious resisting of the child and/or parents* and [the] analyst's own unresolved conflicts concerning children" (p. 357). "Resisting treatment" and "resistive behavior" has been defined as behavior that is generally present prior to the patient entering psychoanalytic treatment.

Resistance is defined differently in behavioral and interpersonal psychotherapies, where it is primarily viewed as a reaction to the therapeutic situation and intervention.

HISTORY

Resistance has played a central role in the development of psychoanalytic technique and theory. Initially, Freud (1912) considered resistance simply an *obstacle*, such as in the case of the patient's defiance of the analyst's authority by violating the fundamental rule. He thought of it as an automatic defense against remembering the repressed memories of traumatic events that had led to the symptom formation. His concept of resistance shaded over into the concept of negative transference. Freud (1912) thought this internal opposition to permitting into consciousness dynamically unconscious material should be overcome by the authority and persuasion of the analyst. When he discovered that resistance operated unconsciously, he noted that its appearance, recognition, and interpretation were essential to the work of analysis. Analysis of the resistance and the transference then became the hallmark of psychoanalytic treatment. Freud (1923, 1926) later discovered that resistance stemmed primarily from the defensive efforts of the ego. However, he also believed that the id provided its own resistance by continuing the operation of the repetition compulsion beyond the achievement of insight. The superego contributes its share of resistance, which emanates from a sense of guilt or need for punishment. This element of punishment serves to prevent the patient from achieving the success of recovery through analysis; it thus is the basis for a potential negative therapeutic reaction (Moore and Fine 1990).

In the early days of psychoanalysis, psychoanalysts relied heavily on free association to discover the resistances. Free association was considered the patient's primary and essential task. It was not uncommon then for an analyst to give up a patient if he or she did not agree to free-associate. Today, most analysts consider asking the patient to readily undertake free association as undue interference with the orderly progress of the analytic process, and they leave it up to the patient to say what he or she wants to say and to retain what he or she does not want to say (Sandler and A. Freud 1985).

RESISTANCE IN PSYCHOANALYSIS OF ADULTS

In the psychoanalysis of adults, resistances are usually viewed according to the inner agencies that give rise to them. The ego resists the psychoanalytic process by siding with the defenses in order to ward off unpleasure, anxiety, and guilt feelings. The superego, threatened by the emergence of fantasies, thoughts, and feelings, opposes their admission into consciousness. Drive derivatives, which are released by the analytic process, act as resistances by pressing for fulfillment in reality and in action rather than being used to gain insight. The id resistances oppose the changes in behavior and thoughts and tend to endorse the principle of repetition (Pearson 1968).

In the psychoanalysis of adults, *five* sources of resistances are encountered: three from the ego, one from id, and one from superego.

Resistances arising from the ego are:
Repression resistance
Transference resistance
Secondary gain from the illness

Resistances arising from the id:
 Id resistances requiring "working through"
Resistances arising from the superego:
 Sense of guilt or need for punishment.

Defense and Resistance

There is a pervasive relationship between resistance and defense. Generally, resistance occurs in analysis; defense occurs in life. However, defenses can be strengthened or can arise during the course of analysis, and resistances can occur in life situations as well as in analysis (Rangell 1983).

In the classical view, one treats resistances as manifestations of defenses and interprets them. Conceptually, what is generally referred to as *defense analysis* may be somewhat misleading, because from a technical point of view the emphasis is more on the *analysis of resistances* than on particular defenses. The defenses are only interpreted in the context of whatever is being defended against (Sandler and A. Freud 1985). One arrives at the understanding of the defenses by watching for their appearance as resistance in analysis.

The term *defense analysis* was introduced and elaborated clearly in child analysis by Berta Bornstein (1949), who emphasized the necessity to analyze the defenses first. This guiding principle to analytic technique was, however, previously practiced by some psychoanalysts. In the analysis of the resistances or of specific defenses, the analyst is interpreting the patient's conflict or anxiety in order for the patient to feel freer to release the repressed material.

Conscious Withholding and Resistance

Conscious withholding of material should be differentiated from the phenomenon of resistance, which is withholding based on the patient's defenses. Conscious withholding or "willful withholding" refers to a disregard of free association or of the analytic contract. Here the patient opts out of the obligation to speak the truth and to say what is on his mind (Anna Freud in Sandler and A. Freud 1985). The patient may withhold thoughts about the analyst, information about his sexual life, or money because they may be considered rude or embarrassing. In complete conscious withholding the patient does not mention such phenomena to the analyst at all.

One can deal with the partial conscious withholding by saying, "Well, if you can't talk about this subject, there must be a good reason, and perhaps we should look at the reason." If the patient states that "I can't say what I thought about you, I am too embarrassed to say it," one could say, "Why should you be so embarrassed? Do you have any idea why you are so embarrassed?" In this way, one would try to stimulate associations to the resistance (Sandler, in Sandler and A. Freud 1985). One could also deal with partial conscious withholding by saying, "It is a very good sign that you told me so soon that you cannot talk about [a subject], because that means that you will mention it very soon" (Sandler, in Sandler and A. Freud 1985, p. 9).

Both conscious and unconscious withholding could be based on transference feelings. Hellman (1985) refers to a patient who would not discuss her sexual feelings based on the transference feeling that the analyst was a malevolent and destructive person and therefore that good things should be hidden from her (Hellman, in Sandler and Freud 1985).

Conscious withholding, just like silence in analysis, can have an anal and aggressive cause and may be related to preoedipal pathology. The patient's withholding or refusing to free-associate may be rooted in envy or in anal conflicts. While the ability to speak is certainly under ego control, what seems important is that such patients cannot let themselves speak.

There is always a level of resistance in the analytic work that fluctuates because of the need for the individual to maintain psychic equilibrium. If there is a complete absence of resistance in the patient or a sudden flow of the unconscious material, this may be an ominous sign and often means an unwelcome breakthrough. However, analytic students who are in analysis can use this form of resistance by showing no apparent resistance. At that point, one wonders what is being hidden (A. Freud, in Sandler and A. Freud 1985).

Working Through

Once the patient's unconscious conflicts have been uncovered and some insight obtained, resistance may lead to delay or even failure to progress, reflecting an unconsciously determined reluctance to give up inappropriate childhood wishes and their maladaptive, defensively distorted expressions in symptoms, character, or behavior. Moreover, the relief or mental equilibrium that the neurotic symptoms has achieved for the individual is hard to give up. The many factors contributing to resistance make the process of working through an essential part of analytic work.

Technical advances in psychoanalysis have demonstrated that the simple uncovering of unconscious material and thorough understanding of the defenses exhibited by the child in different situations such as home, school, play, or in transference does not automatically result in insight formation. The analytic process has made us fully aware of the presence of a counterforce, an anticathexis of the ego that we would term "resistance" or repression resistance, which can result in the emergence of a new defense following the delineation and interpretation of the old one. The new defense has the function of protecting the repression. For example, when a latency age child's need to blame everyone else except himself for his shortcomings was interpreted to him, he exhibited a prolonged period of boredom in treatment and complained to his parents about it. The interpretation of the boredom to him and to the parents (who also tended to side with him) resulted in the emergence of feelings of inadequacy centered around his concept of having a small penis inherited from his father. This was a source of great embarrassment to him (Pearson 1968).

Transference Resistance

Of particular importance are the resistances that emerge in the sphere of the transference, that is, transference resistance. Fundamentally, transference should be considered as a form of resistance by which the patient defends against remembering and discussing his infantile conflicts by insisting on reliving them through the analyst with more satisfaction than he had experienced in childhood. Transference resistance manifests itself through the emergence of powerful affects such as anxiety and joy, particularly directed toward the analyst. The patient may misconstrue the analytic situation and develop strong feelings for nonexistent reasons. The patient's affect may be in contradiction to what is happening in analysis, such as hating the analyst for helping him or loving him for imposing an unpleasant restriction (Fenichel 1945). The transference is considered a resistance, inasmuch as the patient endeavors thereby to gratify his or her narcissistic, erotic, or aggressive wishes in the present rather than remember their origins in past object relationships. Hence, acting out may function as a major and serious resistance. One form of early resistance against transference is by the patient forming a strong relationship outside of analysis with someone else as a "resistance against transference."

In a general sense, all transference is resistance, all resistance is transference, and both are a repetition. Transferred resistances may take the form of defenses against awareness of transference wishes, fantasies, and thoughts. Once in awareness, transference wishes and attitudes also may become so intense as to interfere with the progress of the analysis. One set of transference wishes and attitudes may operate as a profound resistance against awareness of some other, more threatening set (Moore and Fine 1990).

RESISTANCE IN CHILD ANALYSIS

In child analysis all types of resistances exhibited in the psychoanalysis of adults are present, but they assume intensified or varied forms. Additionally, children exhibit specific resistances characteristic of them. Anna Freud (1965), in *Normality and Pathology in Childhood*, has listed *eight* types of resistances in children. She has particularly emphasized the urge to outgrow and reject the past, which can function as a strong resistance to the progression of analysis. This resistance is particularly apparent in the transitional phases from oedipal to latency period and during the adolescence. The eight types of resistances in children described by Anna Freud (1965) and summarized by Pearson (1968) are:

1. The child does not enter analysis on his own motivation and does not feel bound by a contractual arrangement with the analyst to follow the analytic rules.
2. The child is more motivated to relieve the short-term discomfort and anxiety of the treatment situation and does not consider a long-term view of treatment.
3. Acting out is the more age-appropriate form of behavior for the children than talking and reflecting on one's verbal productions.
4. The insecure balance between the internal and external pressures in the child makes him adhere rigidly to his defenses. The defensiveness is further intensified with the emergence of adolescence, which increases drive activity.
5. During childhood, the more primitive defense mechanisms continue to operate alongside the more mature ones. The increased number of defenses tends to make the child more defensive and therefore resistant in the analytic situation.
6. The ego tends to habitually side with resistance at the time of heightened pressure from unconscious material and negative trans-

ference. Therefore, the active support of the parents is necessary to make the child stay in treatment.

7. The urge to outgrow and reject the past is strong during childhood and is particularly strong during the adolescent years. Therefore, children tend to reject the analytic process, which encourages an open communication with the past.

8. Children tend to externalize their conflicts in the form of finding environmental irritants and prefer to search for external solutions. The child's preference for looking for external rather than internal changes can be mistaken for "negative transference," which refers to a different phenomena.

The combination of the above factors can make the analytic situation a difficult encounter for the psychoanalyst and tax his or her skills. The "difficulty can reach the point that for long stretches of the analysis, [the analyst] has to manage without active assistance from his patient" (A. Freud 1965).

Pearson (1968) has expanded the concept of resistance in child psychoanalysis by stating that the definition of resistance in children should include not only the types of resistances in adult psychoanalysis but also:

the resistance of the *child before and during* treatment,
the resistance of the *parents before and during* treatment,
all *conscious* wishes of the child and parents to resist treatment, and
the resistance of the analyst.

The Child's Resistance Prior to Analysis

Pearson (1968) has described the child's resistance to entering treatment or "resisting treatment" according to the child's developmental stage. He describes the following stage-related phenomena:

During *prelatency*, the child may become very anxious if the mother is not present during the sessions. The child analyst may feel uncomfortable about the presence of the mother in the playroom and may discourage her presence. This may be based on the analyst's own unresolved conflicts. However, if the mother is included in the treatment, she may be able to learn about the nature of the child's play and continue to interpret to the child following the session. She may also express empathy for what has happened. With the mother present, the young child's resistances to play may vanish. Transference resistance hardly develops and acting out is virtually absent during this developmental phase.

During the *latency* phase, the conscious resistance is widened. The child generally reveals or exhibits no anxiety in treatment about his daytime or night fears, or compulsions. He acts as if the symptoms are the concerns of his parents and they hardly bother him. The child's resistances are further heightened by the feelings of embarrassment about coming for treatment. He may be afraid of the analyst reading his mind and consequently looks away from the doctor.

Transference reactions develop in the latency period, and the child may run away from strong erotic and aggressive feelings toward the analyst by becoming more resistant toward treatment.

During *prepuberty*, the child's masturbation becomes an important conscious resistance. He is afraid of the analyst (and his parents) discovering it and denies or minimizes his masturbation by saying that he has never, or seldom, engaged in this activity. Another source of resistant behavior in the prepubertal child is his/her constant tendency toward activity, which may be very extreme and interfere with the analyst's attention to the child's production.

Many of the above resistances may be consciously experienced by the child before he or she enters the analyst's office. They may also become manifest after entering treatment. The child's commitment at this stage to say what comes to mind is significantly below what is experienced in adult analysis.

In *puberty* or *adolescence*, a major source of resistance is the child's fear that the analyst is an ally of the parents, who would like to make him over into the kind of the child his parents desire. This attitude requires frequent clarifications from the analyst to distance himself from the parents and underline his job, which is to help the child understand himself and to arrive at better solutions for his life.

A major source of resistive behavior during puberty is the embarrassment to talk about sexual thoughts and feelings by attempting to keep them out of treatment for a long time. Transference resistances become stronger during this period of development. The adolescent frequently finds it impossible to directly discuss his or her feelings toward the analyst, and acting out in the transference is regularly observed.

Resistive behavior should be differentiated from the resistances in the treatment situation, which are generally based on the defense mechanisms. As a result of treatment, the child's defenses and attitudes change. However, the continuation of the symptoms in face of seemingly effective analytic work may indicate that more resistances are interfering with the resolution of intrapsychic conflicts.

The Child's Resistance in the Course of Treatment

The conscious resistances predating the initiation of treatment continue during the treatment phase, too (Pearson 1968). Such conscious resistances may include the child's reluctance to tell the analyst and other people about "bad" things he does, mixed loyalties about telling the analyst what he doesn't tell his parents, or reporting parental conflicts occurring at home. The analyst should reassure the child of the confidentiality of the material, but also should ask the parents to repeatedly state to the child that it is alright to report to the analyst everything that happens and to hold nothing back.

Another source of conscious resistance is the attempt to keep frightening thoughts and feelings out of consciousness. The child may frequently tell the analyst to "shut up" and threaten to walk out of the office or not to return for treatment if the analyst continues to talk about unpleasant feelings.

Secondary gains from the symptoms are also a source of resistance in treatment. For example, the interpretation of the school phobia and separation anxiety based on aggressive fantasies toward the mother may not stop the child from staying home, which can gratify his passive feelings. The analytic work requires consistent and persistent interpretations, and working through of the child's reaction formations and conflicts in a way similar to that in psychoanalysis of adults.

The Parents' Resistance During Treatment

The parents' resistance to bringing their child to treatment is also significant. They may feel embarrassed about having a child with emotional problems or feel guilty and responsible for their own part in the illness. They may be reluctant to spend a significant amount of money to undertake the treatment. They frequently resist treatment by asserting that the child will grow out of his difficulty by himself.

Parents' psychological reactions to their children's illness take many forms. Guilt feelings are paramount among the parental reactions to the child's symptomatology and illness. Parental guilt tends initially to facilitate the parents' seeking treatment, but it acts in the service of resistance after the treatment starts, and frequently continues long after the child has been in analysis. Parental guilt may assume many forms, including the complaint that the child is getting worse instead of better; and the persistence of an ambivalent attitude toward treatment, as seen in "forgetting" sessions and undermining the treatment in a variety of other ways. Unconscious resentment about the analyst succeeding where they have failed, and the unconscious need to have the child remain infantile for a variety of reasons, including parental masochism, are frequent findings. The financial difficulties about continuing the treatment is a frequent excuse for interrupting the treatment of the child (Pearson 1968).

The Analyst's Resistance During the Course of Analysis: Countertransference

Resistance in the analytic situation does not emanate exclusively from the patient; it may also reflect the state of the analytic dyad, which is profoundly affected by the analyst's style, personality, and countertransference problems. Technical misjudgments, such as inappropriate timing of transference interpretations, have been observed to contribute to resistance, particularly in the form of acting out (Pearson 1968).

The resistance of the analyst is understood as *countertransference*, based on the unresolved conflicts of the analyst concerning children. This definition has later been expanded to also include the analyst's attitudes and feelings toward the parents of the child, which may be displaced onto the patient in the analytic situation.

Child analysts generally have many characteristics that have allowed them to undertake the difficult profession of child analysis. They are generally able to endure bad behavior, physical contact, getting on the floor, and engaging in endless play that may be more enjoyable to the child. In order to function adequately, the analysts should have succeeded in analyzing their own passivity and defenses against masochism. They should be able to tolerate the parental ambivalence toward the child's treatment, particularly its cost. The analyst's resolution of his own conflict over passivity is necessary to help him or her refrain from giving advice to the parents that may aid or abet defenses that actually require changing the external situation at home. He must avoid getting involved in treating them. From the therapeutic point of view, it would be more helpful to refer the parents for their own treatment, which would help them with their difficulties and which may, in turn, influence the welfare of their child (Pearson 1968). An exploratory but neutral attitude toward parents would allow parental conflicts to come out into the open during the child's treatment and hence be explored and understood.

A REVISED CONCEPTUALIZATION OF
RESISTANCE: "ACTION LANGUAGE"

Roy Schafer (1973) has proposed that resistance can be best understood within the framework of "action language," a new proposed reconceptualization of psychoanalysis that consists of a set of concepts organized around the idea of action. Action is construed in a special sense and encompasses all human psychological activities in contrast to conventional use of the word *action*, which refers to motivated motoric behavior. Schafer's proposal is partly based on the observation that the analysts treat thought as action. Being conscious of something is also viewed as an action.

Schafer asserts that resistance should be described as "action language," in contrast to the mechanistic language of traditional metapsychology. Second, he considers the concept of *self-deception* as the key to understanding all defensive activities of which resistance is the major instance. The concept of self-deception refers to faulty observation where one erroneously observes one's own actual or conditional actions. Third, he proposes that the model for conceptualization of resistance should add the place of the mother systematically to the classical Freudian patriarchal view of resistance, which has been based on positive oedipal conflict between the fathers, sons, and daughters. Fourth, he suggests that affirmations (see Negative and Affirmative Language, below) must be understood as part of the theory of resistance rather than viewing resistance as a negative phenomenon.

Self-Deception

The concept of self-deception (Schafer 1973) refers to a type of reflective activity by which the patient somehow continues to keep the many truths from himself or herself. It consists of some account of the following:

1. One does not know about all of his or her actions,
2. One gives signs of not wanting to know about all of them, and
3. One is successful in actively preventing his or her knowing all that might be known in this regard.

Self-deception refers to an incorrect or faulty way of observing one's own actions or remembering, anticipating, and judging events, contexts, implications, or alternatives. In faulty self-observation, there is an ignorance or unreadiness to observe one's actions. The person is avoiding experiencing his or her actions anxiously due to anxiety, guilt, shame, or some other painful emotions. In self-deception, the person is both the subject or agent as well as the object of the specific actions done by that person.

Self-deception or faulty self-observation relates to one of two possibilities: either one is carrying out actions inattentively or one is remaining ignorant of actions one would do were one not engaged in effective counteractions of some sorts. The person can be selectively inattentive and ignorant. In psychoanalytic investigation, the analyst explores these actions and their modes in order to gain access to the dynamic unconscious. The actions refer to infantile psychosexual activities such as impulses, drives, and defensive counteractions.

The person may take actions against investigation of the reasons and the modes of his or her actions and therefore become engaged in "resistance against the analysis of resistance" (Freud 1923, 1937). The analyst counts on the surfacing of resisting, and he is never disappointed. The psychoanalytic investigation begins with the analysis of resistance where resistance is consciously affirmed, even if this effort at analysis may not advance very far (Schafer 1973).

Resisting Maternal and Paternal Authority

Freud viewed resistance in the analytic relationship in terms of relationship between the father, the son, and daughter—all involved in positive oedipal striving (Schafer 1973). The mother remained absent in Freud's formulation of resistance. Freud's view of the parent–child relationship in terms of the struggle with patriarchal authority excluded the role of the relationship with the mother in resistance, because the mother was considered as a loving parent, in contrast to the forbidding patriarch, within the context of positive oedipal relationship. Therefore, his principal explanatory tool remained the positive Oedipus complex of the boy (Schafer 1973).

Schafer (1973) proposes a developmental theory of resistance that is more complex and complete and closer to actual contemporary clinical work. According to this model, the patient can be seen as equally defiant of the archaic mother's authority and striving to differentiate himself from his mother. By his strivings, the child establishes and maintains differentiation and wards off the mutual attempts at merging initiated by the child and the mother. The blocking of the influence of the interpretation (not swallowing and digesting them) and maintaining a detached, aloof, bitter, mistrustful attitude toward the analyst may represent some aspect of preoedipal resisting. Here in a constipated, anal way, the patient disappoints the analyst-mother of the toilet training period (Schafer 1973).

Negative and Affirmative Language

The clinical analysis eventuates in investigation of affirmations such as wish fulfillment. This is the final goal of the analysis of resistance and defense. The patients gradually reveal that unconsciously, they take a steady and exclusive view of the analytic situation representing one dangerous instinctual situation (Schafer 1973). By the analysis of resistance, the phenomenal world of the patient is reconstructed and the patient discovers the reasons for his mounting opposition. This process results in the expansion of the patient's views, actions, fantasies, and their underlying wishes. Although the opposition and resistances have their negative aspects, they also have affirmative, even constructive sides, such as protecting relationships, being faithful to ideals, maintaining pride and autonomy, and achieving mastery. By analyzing all that the person does not wish to be or do, we analyze, too, everything that he or she wants (Schafer 1973).

CASE EXAMPLE: THE ANALYSIS OF A NEUROTIC BOY

The following is a summary of the analysis by Colarusso (1991) of Jim, a 10-year-old neurotic boy. The detailed report of Jim's analysis as summarized succinctly by Glenn (1991) and Sholevar (1991) has served as the basis of this summary. In this case report we see the balance shifting from the emergence and interpretation of resistance and defenses to the interpretation of drive derivatives as each facet becomes more prominent. Other aspects of the analytic process are clear as well. Often a particular unconscious conflict first manifests itself in reference to feelings toward the analyst and then appears to be derived from feelings toward Jim's actual parents. Eventually transference from the parents of yesteryear becomes clear.

Jim was a 10-year-old boy with symptoms of unhappiness, temper tantrums, and difficulty making friends. He was eager to be cured of his symptoms and quickly got the idea of how analysis could help him. Although Jim reported his fear of snakes and feelings about his parents in the early sessions, he quickly became silent. The analyst's response to the prolonged silences was a suggestion that he enter the playroom; that it might be helpful and fun as well if he spent some of his time playing. This was an effort to circumvent the resistance through action rather than interpretation. Jim's silence occurred after expressing anger and referring back to his earlier statement that "adults don't know how children think," which left the door open to discussing his guilt and anxiety about angry thoughts.

Jim started by talking and then retreated to coloring a book. As the analyst encouraged him to play, he engaged a full range of communication with his analyst, interrupted at times by anxiety.

Early in analysis, Jim expressed the fear of the analyst getting angry with him for dirtying his walls, which was interpreted. He then became aggressive toward the analyst but defended it by the feeling of boredom and attempted to join the analyst rather than compete with him. The fear of aggression was interpreted. Jim then resorted to compulsive drawing.

Having been instructed to play, Jim chose to dramatize his angry fantasies of destroying his home and family. In an early session, in response to the analyst asking whether Jim thought the analyst was angry, Jim responded by saying that he doesn't understand why the analyst lets him play like that when his parents don't. Jim's hesitation to mess in the playroom was seen as a displacement to the analyst of inhibition because his parents, especially father, objected to it. Later his fear of his father, and hence of the analyst, could be seen as a result of anger toward his father, an anger traced to sexual wishes toward mother. The boy said this even though the analyst had explained to Jim that his playing was a form of communication, which would help the analyst understand the reason for the boy's worries.

Following the analyst's interpretation of Jim's fear that the analyst would become angry if Jim dirtied his wall, Jim's play became more aggressive and he even attacked the analyst. Defenses against aggression manifested themselves as resistances in the sessions as the patient became bored and joined the analyst as an ally in play. Interpretation of these resistances and defenses led to a brief engagement in compulsive drawing and then a new means of communication: Jim brought playing cards into the sessions, a phenomenon the analyst did not interpret as a resistance but rather as a means by which Jim could express conflicts over competition and aggression.

Jim cheated in order to beat the analyst but became anxious and briefly employed regression to anality. Things became a bit complicated when the analyst, in response to Jim's questions, acknowledged that he knew the patient was cheating and added that Jim did this to feel big and strong. Jim became sad, and before long the analyst realized Jim felt tricked and defeated by the analyst. The analyst interjected this outcome, thereby releasing the patient from his distress. A minor complication occurred when the analyst went further than the patient could go. He showed the patient that Jim wanted to order his parents around and control them, not simply because he felt they did it to him and wanted to keep him weak, but because of his own aggression. Possibly this early drive interpretation was premature, but after the analyst repeated it a second time, Jim agreed.

Jim was now making his own observations, even when he cheated. He introduced a new game, which the analyst could interpret. He played king to the analyst's slave or general to the analyst's private soldier. The analyst felt that he, the analyst, represented the patient and made interpretations about the patient's bad feelings about feeling weak, bad feelings that included anger and led to fear. This allowed Jim to attack the analyst through bringing in anti-Italian jokes, but the attack led to fear of retaliation, which the analyst then interpreted. The analyst explicitly stated that Jim felt afraid when he attacked him, and this enabled Jim to go further and *kill* the analyst in a game and then cut off all appendages, except his penis. When the analyst observed that one part was not destroyed, Jim agreed that he had spared the penis. The displacement had defended against his expressing his aggression fully.

Now Jim could talk of penises with relative safety, but a degree of displacement was necessary. He talked of the movie, *The Towering Inferno*, and stole a lighter. Soon he came to realize, through the analyst's explanations and his own astute observations, that he was talking about his hot, erect penis. His preoccupation with certain superheroes—Spider Man, The Thing, The Flame, and Plastic Man—was based on his fascination with his penis. Defenses having been interpreted, once more drive derivatives appeared more clearly. Jim recognized his sexual feelings.

Jim's diminished fear of his own sexual feelings and father's changing attitude toward his son enabled Jim to become less fearful of his father and talk to him more, to ask him for a skateboard. The analyst was able to reconstruct and to relate present fears of father to similar earlier fears of his father and sexuality—fears that had occurred during the oedipal period.

Now Jim could deal with his oedipal competition with his father, but not as yet with his sexual feelings toward mother.

Again displacement became an important resistance and defense as Jim talked of other boys touching their penises. When the analyst pointed out this resistance, Jim talked more about his bodily sensations. Again, resistances and defenses were interpreted. This time he was attributing his erections to pinworms and anal squeezing rather than to the *ideas* that actually caused the erections.

Jim kept away from these ideas for a while and concentrated on the act and related sensations. But soon he was telling his sexual fantasies—a ropelike thing goes up in the penis into the balls and pulls the sperm out—and discussing his parents' mating. The analyst treated with skepticism Jim's denial that they slept alone in a room of their own on vacation, and soon Jim was talking about his mother wanting to take him into her bed and "huddle" with him when his father was away. The interpretation of the projection involved didn't lead to further clarification immediately, but in a few weeks Jim came back to the "huddling."

When Jim talked of the possibility that men hurt women, the analyst suggested that Jim was talking of "other ideas" to "cover up what you would like ladies to do to you." The interpretation had an astonishing effect. Jim told of a sexual fantasy of being immersed in quicksand, a fantasy associated with mother and danger. The analyst didn't interpret the resistances that followed because Jim knew of his fears. He waited patiently for five sessions until Jim told another version of the fantasy—a woman (associated with mother) bites off a man's penis and is punished for it. This in turn was connected, through a dream, with Jim's fear of rattlesnakes. The analyst interpreted his fear of being bitten by them as a punishment for thinking of ladies (mother). The rattlesnake phobia of the oedipal stage could now be reconstructed.

Not surprisingly, Jim's strong resistance emerged and he wanted to stop the treatment at this point. Things seemed to be getting too hot to handle. But he persisted, and soon more fantasies about mother and patient being in bed together appeared; the mother squeezed Jim.

The oedipal configuration became even clearer as Jim talked of a song in which the father leaves and kills himself because mother had an affair with her stepson. Jim recognized his own wish to get rid of father and have mother for himself. After this Jim avoided giving in to his mother's actual advances.

As Jim entered prepuberty, masturbatory fantasies and acts were discussed more than ever, and Jim again wished to leave treatment, be independent, and avoid sexual feelings toward mother and father. Interpretation led to Jim's remaining in treatment and discussing the negative oedipal aspects of his feelings as well as his interest in girls. He teased the analyst more and more, expressing both antagonism and attraction, which he could discuss with the analyst.

The analyst was able to do a reasonable amount of reconstruction. He reconstructed Jim's conflicts during his oedipal period, in particular his fear of rattlesnakes. Jim feared punishment for his wishes to possess his mother and get rid of his father. He felt he should be bitten for these desires, including his wishes to be huddled, hugged, and squeezed by mother.

Jim had a remarkable capacity for insight. He could see connections between defense and drives warded off when the analyst pointed these out. Later he made his own connections as a reflection of his recognizing cause and effect. The fact that he was a bright boy was not sufficient explanation for his capacity for insight. Tactful interpretation was necessary to enable him to use his limited logical capacity. As Jim entered prepuberty, with its beginning formal logic, he acquired greater maturational capacities on which interest in the past and present could be built. It was in prepuberty that the reconstruction mentioned above became effective. It was then that he could talk about termination with an eye to the future.

Conflicts were not resolved all at once. They appeared repeatedly in different forms. Hence resistances, defenses, and drives were recognized and interpreted again and again, constituting a repetitive working through.

Not that everything went smoothly all the time. In analysis the unconscious forces that resist insight and recovery can be potent indeed, and the analyst's own unconscious needs will, at one point or another, almost always facilitate the patient's resistance. Sometimes, conventional analytic technique will serve to slow things.

As a result of the interpretive work, a change in the balance of defenses occurred. Repression diminished remarkably. Jim soon became more aware of this antagonism to his father and later recognized his sexual feelings toward his mother. He stopped attributing his huddling solely to his mother's desire for this activity (i.e., projecting his wishes for his mother to his mother). He no longer attributed sexual feelings to other boys, but owned up to his own wishes. Displacement of fears from parents to the rattler who would bite him and thus punish him for his illicit sexual desires ceased, but displacement came to be used adaptively in his new object seeking; his feelings toward his mother transferred to girls his age.

As these defenses altered, Jim became more able to tolerate hostility, affection, narcissistic hurt, and anxiety (which diminished). The greater tolerance also reflected a superego change; Jim did not experience the severe guilt he had early transformed into symptom formation.

Not only did Jim's symptoms disappear, but he also made developmental advances. At the start of the analysis, this 10-year-old's temper tantrums, difficulty maintaining friendships, and trouble sitting still in school and completing his work signified that he was not firmly established in latency. Latency-age children are able to maintain a proper balance between sublimated activity and the use of isolation and reaction formation on the one hand, and less controlled outbursts of drive-dominated behavior on the other; Jim leaned too much toward the latter.

As the treatment proceeded, Jim became a latency child. Midway through analysis his symptoms had largely disappeared. He had more friends and was doing well in school and regressing less at home. Sexual interests and activity were present but did not dominate the picture. Simultaneously, bodily changes revealed that Jim was entering prepuberty. He started the growth spurt and grew dark hair on his arms and legs. Jim's psychological reaction to prepuberty was to seek more independence and to avoid consciousness of incestuous involvement. Regression was minimal. Soon he was ready to enter the terminal stage of treatment.

The termination issue was initially introduced defensively by Jim and discussed periodically during the second year of analysis. A mutually agreed-upon date was established 3 months before termination. The rationale for termination was the resolution of Jim's symptoms concomitant with the analytic work on his castration anxiety and construction of his oedipal phase. The positive feelings toward the analyst and the father became more readily apparent at the time of termination. A range of feelings and issues was expressed and worked through during this period, including the expression of sadness.

Eventually the analysis ended with Jim's preadolescent status firmly established, achieving appropriate developmental level, which is a prime criterion for termination.

REFERENCES

Bornstein, B. (1949). The analysis of a phobic child. Some problems of theory and technique in child analysis. *Psychoanalytic Study of the Child* 3/4:181–226. New York: International Universities Press.

Colarusso, C. (1991). Analysis of a neurotic boy. In *Psychoanalytic Case Studies*, ed. G. P. Sholevar, pp. 199–238. New York: International Universities Press.

Fenichel, O. (1945). *The Psychoanalytic Theory of Neurosis*. New York: W. W. Norton.

Freud, A. (1965). *Normality and Pathology in Childhood*. New York: International Universities Press.

Freud, S. (1912). The dynamics of transference. *Standard Edition* 12.

_____ (1923). The ego and the id. *Standard Edition* 19.

_____ (1926). Inhibitions, symptoms, and anxiety. *Standard Edition* 20:77–175.

_____ (1937). Analysis terminable and interminable. *Standard Edition* 23.

Glenn, J. (1991). Discussion of analysis of a neurotic boy. In *Psychoanalytic Case Studies*, ed. G. P. Sholevar, pp. 239–254. New York: International Universities Press.

Hellman, I. (1985). *The Analysis of Defense*, ed. J. Sandler and A. Freud, p. 11. New York: International Universities Press.

Moore, B., and Fine, B. (1990). *Psychoanalytic Terms and Concepts*. New York: American Psychoanalytic Association.

Morgenstern, S. (1991). Course on Resistance, Philadelphia Association for Psychoanalysis, Fall 1991.

Pearson, G. (1968). *A Handbook of Child Psychoanalysis*. New York: Basic Books.

Rangell, L. (1983). Defense and resistance in psychoanalysis and life. *Journal of the American Psychoanalytic Association* 31:147–171.

Sandler, J., and Freud, A. (1985). *The Analysis of Defense: The Ego and the Mechanisms of Defense Revisited*. New York: International Universities Press.

Schafer, R. (1973). The idea of resistance. *International Journal of Psycho-Analysis* 54:259–285.

Sholevar, G. P. (1991). Introduction to analysis of a neurotic boy. In *Psychoanalytic Case Studies*, ed. G. P. Sholevar, pp. 193–197. New York: International Universities Press.

Stone, L. (1973). On resistance to the psychoanalytic process: some thoughts on its nature and motivations. *Contemporary Science* 2:42–73.

8

Interpretation

Bertram A. Ruttenberg, M.D.

Introduction and Review of Classical Concepts

The jewel in the crown of psychoanalytic therapy is the process of interpretation. In dictionary terms, the act of interpretation is to give an explanation, an understanding of another's words or deeds (Random House 1967), or to expound on the meaning of something (Oxford 1971). The American Psychoanalytic Association's glossary of psychoanalytic terms and concepts (Moore and Fine 1990) considers interpretation to be

> the central therapeutic activity of the analyst during treatment, a process whereby the analyst expresses in words what he or she comes to understand about the patient's mental life. This understanding is based not only on what the patient brings to the analysis in the form of distorted memories, fantasies and other manifestations of psychic conflict but based also upon observation of the way the patient distorts the relationship with the analyst. [pp. 103–104]

This chapter will review the basic psychoanalytic concepts and techniques of interpretation, and how they have been extended and adapted to analytic work with young children, both neurotic and otherwise disabled but with serious emotional disturbance involving repression and other neurotic defenses that hinder emotional growth and habilitation, who would respond to psychoanalytically oriented psychotherapy with interpretation.

Arthur P. Noyes (1953), a pioneer in the adaptation of psychoanalytic concepts and technique to psychotherapy, wrote, with characteristic lucidity,

[Interpretation] is the process whereby the therapist helps the patient to understand the meaning of his mental phenomena and behavior—usually mental phenomena of the existence of which he is not even aware. In order that the patient may acquire an understanding insight into his difficulties and thereby improve his adjustment, and reconstruct his personality to a desirable extent, there are many phases of his mental life of which he should have an understanding knowledge—an emotional, not merely an intellectual, knowledge. [p. 573]

The impartment of such an understanding, however, is one of the most difficult tasks of psychotherapy and requires great skill and tact and discreet timing. The acquiring of an insightful understanding by the patient is a slow process and must not be hurried—a premature interpretation mobilizes anxiety and antagonizes the patient. [p. 574]

Dr. Noyes describes how the patient must be brought to a state of readiness by preparatory interpretations of his defenses in order to be able to tolerate the painful revelations. The patient's defenses need to be respected. "Whenever the patient cannot see the obvious it is because he needs his blindness" (p. 574).

Otto Fenichel (1941) was the first to systematize the steps, rules, process, and signs of effectiveness of interpretations. In many ways his succinct presentation has not been surpassed, although more recently Ralph Greenson (1967) wrote in detail on this subject and included many clinical examples. In the following summary I draw freely from these two sources.

Fenichel describes a preparatory period in which connection between events, surface feelings, and manifest behaviors are made, connections that make the patient curious (you are behaving as if you . . ., or, like you did in the past when . . ., or just the way you complained your father did to you), and gets the patient intrigued with the process. General avoidance of knowing should be pointed out in a way that will support, not tear down, the ego defenses: "You are concerned that . . . ," "afraid you might . . . ," rather than "you want to. . . ."

After demonstrating the patient's oscillating dynamic between defense and expressed derivative (surface manifestation of an underlying conflict), the process of interpretation can begin according to the following rules:

1. Start at the surface with the least repressed material, that which is most available to the ego.
2. The subject matter of the session is determined by the patient's verbal or behavioral associations.
3. Interpretation of resistance and defense precedes interpretation of content (ego before id).

4. Avoid interpretations that are either too superficial or too deep. The former may be seized on to avoid going further; the latter may be too threatening and overwhelming to the ego, the agency with which the therapist has to deal.
5. Because of the economic tendency toward overdetermination, given behavior having more than one meaning (cf. Waelder [1936], Principle of Multiple Function), one must focus on the most important instinctual conflict at that moment, meeting the patient where he is, affectively and developmentally, and interpreting in his idiom (which may not be verbal).
6. The dosage of interpretation should be such as to cause as little psychic pain as possible. One would not want to leave the patient defenseless.
7. One must aim toward the integration of the interpretive understanding with the total picture, and with the here and now.
8. Interpretation of symbolic behavior or dream material, in the form of standard symbol intellectualizations, can harm the progress of treatment, even though accurate, inasmuch as they may not be where the patient is affectively at the moment. The analyst should do not interpret until considerable associative material (verbal or behavioral) has been obtained.

The interpretive process involves confronting the experiencing ego with something it has heretofore warded off or denied. It may be something that is uncharacteristic of the person, or conspicuously absent.

The attention of the experiencing and reality-testing part of the ego is called to this behavior or attitude; the analyst emphasizes that it is the patient's own activity or idea that he or she is *actively* generating, that there are reasons and motives for this activity, and that there are connections to other behaviors.

The validation of the interpretation can be surmised by the fact that the interpretation is accepted and rings true with affective as well as intellectual relaxation of tension, and new flexibility of attitude through the therapeutic rapport and trust. In identification with the therapist, and pushed by his intrigue with the process, the patient self-observes and comes to see the discrepancy between what he has experienced in the past and the present reality. Having drawn the past into the present, the patient brings out more associative material, less-distorted derivatives, and gradually the origins and motives for his behavior pattern or fear become clear.

Working through is the process whereby the basic steps of recognition, confrontation, clarification, and finally interpretation (which Greenson [1967, p. 39] calls "the ultimate and decisive instrument" which . . . "assigns meaning to a phenomenon") are repeated again and again, examining behavior and attitudes from every aspect at different times and in different connections. Each interleaving interpretation and overcoming of resistance to allow further awareness of warded-off unconscious content brings the patient to a higher level of understanding and cohesion. Working through is a long-term process, the antithesis of *abreaction*, which is a discharge of psychic energy or affect, an immediate response with little permanent effect. Working through, by contrast, integrates the warded off components into the total personality, and adds to emotional maturity and ego strength.

Oremland (1991) has added a perspective to the concept and technique of interpretation that stresses the connection between the more verbal process engaged in the analytic psychotherapy of adults and adolescents, and the much more diversified and activating interpretative approach used with children. Oremland looks on the process of interpretation in the analysis of adults as an interactive intervention on the part of the therapist, which adds an experiential factor above and beyond the assignment of meaning and motivation to the patient's behavior. The interventions support healthy defenses and reality testing. By adding meaning to what is being experienced in the therapeutic session, interpretation becomes the most supportive and least regression-inducing of the therapeutic interventions. The therapeutic interaction itself becomes the object of the analysis. Because most information about the meanings and motivation of transference enactment in the therapeutic session comes from the therapist's empathetic experiencing and countertransference awareness of the patient, Oremland feels that inferences about the transference are the most valid and the interaction between patient and psychotherapist is, for the purposes of therapy, the true and immediate "here and now."

INTERPRETATION IN THE PSYCHOANALYTICALLY ORIENTED PSYCHOTHERAPY OF THE CHILD

Theoretical Issues

In considering the use of interpretation in the therapy of young children, a number of complicating issues come to the fore that highlight the differences between the treatment situation with children and that with adults.

First of all the young child is brought for help when his or her disturbance produces concern, discomfort, and disruption to the family, or upon the recommendation of others (teacher, pediatrician, the court, etc.). The child is dependent on his caretakers and may be the targeted member of the family through whom family conflicts are acted out. The child, in turn, may be acting out the subtle and unconscious agenda of a parent. Thus the child often enters therapy unmotivated, resistive, and scared. On the other hand, when the child does seek help and when there is no responsive awareness and action on the part of his caretakers, the child has no recourse but to either withdraw or act out until enough pain and embarrassment is caused to push the family into seeking help for the child. When the child senses parental ambivalence about therapy, conflicts in the treatment situation over loyalty and over betrayal of family secrets are set up, which inhibit openness and full revelation. Thus it is essential that the child feel support and approval from his caretakers for his therapeutic work so that he will feel free to go on with it.

I have stated above that interpretation of the transference is the sine qua non in the psychoanalytic psychotherapy of adults. With adults and adolescents, what is transferred to the therapeutic situation from the past as contrasted with the present can be made clear. With young children, however, only partial transferences are possible. There is a present reality that the child comes from and returns to after therapy, which is current, ongoing, and on which he or she is dependent, which splits the focus and indeed may be a major contributor to current reactions.

The psychoanalytically based psychotherapy of adults is largely a talking cure, though the astute analyst is also picking up body language, affective expression, and behavioral style and patterns on which to base his interpretations.

With children the avenues through which the therapist can gain insight and understanding and, in turn, provide clarification and communication of meaning, are varied and ever-changing. They are also closely tied to the developmental profile and phase specificity at the moment in each area of functioning and for each mode of clinical assessment, elicitation of response, and interpretive intervention. In simple terms, to make a connection and impart an understanding one has to engage the child where he is developmentally, and using the mode and metaphor that will have meaning for the child.

It follows that since infancy and early childhood is a time of rapid dynamic interplay and maturational change, the psychoanalyst-psychotherapist must be intimately and exquisitely familiar with all aspects of infant and child development and the dynamics of parent–child dyads and triads in order to understand which adaptive behavior and defenses are normal at any given age and which are pathological, and what mental processes are going on to produce what is being observed.

Only with this basic information is it possible to understand what is happening within a child or within the family constellation, and to be able to then therapeutically prepare the child for an effective interpretation that is mutative—that is, one that brings together a number of small understandings of connections between id, ego, and superego so that it reactivates arrested development and/or removes a painful symptom or disturbing behavior. There are many general and specific descriptive and developmental schedules and schemata that can serve as guides to the therapist, some behavioral-descriptive and others more analytically and dynamically oriented and examining a specific line such as object relations or narcissism. Several example follow.

Arnold Gesell and collaborators have provided, since 1940, the classic, detailed running descriptions of the development of normal children, culminating in Gesell and Amatruda's "Developmental Diagnosis" (Gesell and Amatruda 1974).

Anna Freud, in *The Ego and the Mechanisms of Defense* (1946), provided the therapist with a dynamic description and delineation of the defense mechanisms upon which so much of our interpretation of ego defenses depends. Also, her *Normality and Pathology in Childhood* (1965), using object relationships as a prototype, provides developmental lines with sequential steps that help orient the therapist as to the normality versus pathology of the behavior and changes that he observes, and its developmental phase specificity.

Erik H. Erikson's *Childhood and Society* (1950) brought cultural anthropology to bear on the understanding of psychoanalytic development. In Chapter 7 of that volume he delineated the eight stages of man, contrasting at each stage the developmentally healthy state versus the failed counterpart.

Rene Spitz (1965) has provided a detailed study of the development of object relationships in the first year of life.

Margaret Mahler and associates (1975) describe the slow psychological birth of the human infant, with a detailed scheme of how the infant first separates from its symbiotic relationship with its mother, and the four subphases of differentiation towards individuation.

Call and colleagues (1979), in their "Psychiatric Intervention with Infants," describe the many factors to be taken into consideration when psychiatrically assessing and treating an infant in his family. They provide a month-by-month listing of the expectable manifestations that concern parents yet which are normal and, indeed, signs of psychological health. They also include a detailed month-by-month descriptive list of signs of psychological and psychophysiological disturbance from birth to 3 years, including a valuable summary of Winnicott's methods of approaching the assessment and treatment of infants.

Three recent conceptual perspectives on infant and child development, based on clinically oriented direct developmental observations, have been presented by Greenspan, Temeles, and Stern.

The work of Greenspan, culminating in his most recent book *Infancy and Early Childhood* (1992), looks at infant and child disorders from the point of view of regulatory function and the adaptation to experience, and the ability or failure of the multiple systems in the organism to integrate. In his scheme there are six developmental levels of the ability to organize and integrate experience and respond to it. Their individual profiles point the way to specific therapeutic intervention and interpretation. His descriptive developmental schedules are presented in terms of attachment and adaptive and affective responses.

Margaret Temeles (1986) has put forth a "developmental line for narcissism," which complements Anna Freud's object relations theories and focuses on the acquiring and depleting of narcissistic supplies and the attendant vicissitudes of self-esteem, which is often the subject of interpretation—how one feels about oneself, and how that has shaped one's behavior.

Finally, the scheme of D. Stern (1985) brings yet another perspective, that of the child development observer and researcher with psychoanalytic antecedents. He argues that infants are prewired, as it were, to relate and differentiate themselves almost from birth, going through ever more complex modes of relating and communicating, not displacing but overlayering and continuing throughout life.

Developmental and emotional disorders present themselves in a myriad of qualitative aspects, and I have found that my ability to understand and communicate interpretively has been extended considerably by having this variety of conceptual and descriptive perspectives through which to view the child and to express one's formulations. Often a perspective that illuminates and makes sense out of what one child and his family is presenting does not seem to work for another. Similarly, trying to interpret in terms of one way of looking at things may get across to one child but not to a second.

Clinical Issues and Technique of Interpretation

Sandler and associates (1980), reporting their discussions with Anna Freud on the technique of child psychoanalysis, stressed the more active role that the child analyst must play through the preparatory processes of reality orientation, clarification, confrontation, and reassurance. Anna Freud emphasized the importance of gaining parental approval and support for therapy.

The reality of the child's dependence on the availability of parental care, and his need for parents as real objects, limits and blurs the development of a full transference neurosis within the treatment situation which is the core basis for interpretation in the psychoanalysis of adults. In fact the child's early thoughts and fantasies about the therapist and therapy may not be transference projections at all but an age-appropriate fantasy about meeting a stranger or doctor—which will, however, give some introduction to the child's fantasy content and style. Preinterpretive explanation and reassurance to the child about initial fears and anxieties carries the child until he is in a position to retrospectively contrast what he brought to therapy with what he found it to be in reality. The therapist can elicit this by asking, "What did you think it would be like?" At that point, making interpretive connections can begin.

What may be transferred to the therapeutic situation includes (1) the child's habitual modes of relating, and (2) the fears and expectations from current relationships with the child's family (which I call *lateral transference*) rather than from the past, which are responsible for the child's reluctance to reveal what is going on—issues of loyalty or fear. This inner conflict may become so severe as to educe the presenting symptom:

An 8-year-old girl with elective mutism was brought for treatment. Casual dollhouse play, then puppet play, revealed her perception of a family about to break up, with terrible battles between her parents that had to be kept hidden because father, a public figure, was up for election and had actually exclaimed to his wife in front of the child (as I learned later from the mother), "You can't leave me! At least not till after the election!" An interpretation connecting the girl's reluctance to speak at all in school for fear of revealing family secrets, coupled with the reassurance that what she said and played out in therapy would be our secret, removed her mutism and allowed her to begin dealing with other preoedipal and oedipal conflicts brought on by long-term family problems.

Other elements that may be transferred to the therapeutic situation are (3) past experiences (derivatives of the repressed experience), and (4) the development of a transference neurosis—only partial and blurred by the availability of the real parents.

Anna Freud (Sandler et al. 1980) described the following reactions to interpretations:

1. Immediate or delayed response in which the child may verify or deny the interpretation,
2. Increased or decreased anxiety and accompanying resistance. Increased anxiety may be due to the ineptness of the interpretation by virtue of its being poorly phrased, badly timed, and out of phase. Increased anxiety may be the child's now-habitual way of responding to an inquiry:

Eight-year-old J., referred for school refusal, sat in the corner of a couch, looking worried and anxious, and, in a barely audible voice, responded with a whining sound or "I don't know" to seemingly innocuous questions about his school, his family and pets, his interests, and how he was feeling. He leaned against his mother for comfort and looked to her for some answers, yet he did not respond any better to her encouragement or rephrasing of the questions. He was not oppositional or defiant. He was not physically afraid of me, for when the general questioning and the supportive noting of worried affect were put aside, he could be engaged in a game of catch with a soft sponge ball, at which point he would get up and eventually throw hard and competitively with some excitement and laughter, only to return to his worried affect and uncommunicativeness if asked a question. His teacher, whom he adored, and his school principal had reported this same response to questions about his feelings. My noting this contrast and interpreting through wondering if there were something on his mind that he found too scary to bring up, brought a reduction in his anxiety but no further information at that time, yet enabling a return to school as long as mother was in the school building. (We will return to this case later as an example of involving the parent in the interpretation and response.)

3. The child may react positively by bringing up more connecting material. Passive acceptance without further productivity is in itself a defense.

INTERPRETATION OF RESISTANCE AND DENIAL

4. Resistance to interpretations may show in many ways. The child may react by changing his play, by "clamming up," or by no longer reporting dreams. The child may run to the bathroom frequently or stay there for a prolonged period. The child may panic or angrily shout to drown out your interpretation, hit out or spit, run out of the room, or, having left, refuse to come back. These negative reactions are usually the ego's responses to feeling that its defenses are about to be overwhelmed, and the therapist would do well to back off at

that moment, with the comment acknowledging that what was said
had distressed the child.

In my experience there are situations when the defensive reactions of
denial and counterattack are so chronic and automatic that the therapist
has to address the child's defenses in the child's metaphor and manner
of defensive attack by means of an interpretive counterattack, so to
speak:

D. was a thin, pale 9-year-old brought by his adoptive father and new adoptive
stepmother, because of increasingly severe tantrums in school, which involved
throwing desks and chairs, breaking down into infantile crying and screaming
fits (over claimed inability to do the class- and homework) in front of peers
without apparent shame, threatening to kill himself, wishing to die and making
some suicidal gestures, and wanting to run away. He complained he was no
good and that everyone hated him. Hospital studies implicated depression and
learning disorder. Though he responded with improved behavior to guided
structuring at home, one-on-one support teaching, psychotherapy, and chemotherapy for attention-deficit disorder with hyperactivity and depression, his
aggressive outbursts continued.
     D. had been given up for adoption reluctantly by his young, college-student
mother, who, disowned by her family, could not support him. His adoptive
mother claims she refused to let herself get attached to the child for fear of the
pain of the loss, should he be reclaimed. When the adoptive parents separated
when D. was 7 years of age, D. went with adoptive mother, who, because of
D.'s difficult behavior, shipped him to his adoptive father. Despite the demands
of his executive job responsibilities D.'s adoptive father was sincerely committed
to caring for and working with D. D., however, always wanted to go back to his
adoptive mother, painting a rosy picture of what life was like there and of his
attachment to his dog, which he had to leave behind because no pets were
allowed in his father's apartment house.
     Father established a new relationship with a fine woman with two early
adolescent children of her own, who took on the task of being a mother to D.
and helping in his rehabilitation. She pulled up her own professional roots and
moved in with her children, married D.'s adoptive father, and formally became
his second adoptive mother. He rejected his new mother, accelerated his
wanting to go back to his prior mother, and despite her direct assertions to the
contrary, kept insisting she wanted him back. This denial persisted, as did his
ever-increasing testing the limits of his new mother's patience. Father could not
be firm because of his own experience with an abusive father. Father was
supported in setting limits, and many preparatory interpretations were made
concerning denial and D.'s own feelings of worthlessness associated with
having been given up twice. There seemed to be no way his new mother could
gain his trust. He attempted to provoke me to reject him by his destructive

behavior in the playroom, requiring physical restraint as he did at home; and yet he left little tantalizing signs that he really wanted to be accepted. He would relax when taken physically in hand. After he had attacked his stepsiblings, a conjoint session including the parents was held in which he screamed out his hatred for his adoptive stepmother and adoptive father and the sibs, and his wanting to leave home. I summed up the reality of his biological mother's inability to care for him and her happiness at learning he is with people who love him and care for him, and reinterpreting his denial of the situation of his first adoptive mother's rejection and how his feeling of unworthiness and lack of confidence keep him from learning (thorough testing had not revealed an organically based learning disorder or attention deficit). This was met by warding off, via a crescendo of yelling and aggressiveness, which I signaled father to contain. At that point I decided to meet him at his level, reflecting his aggressive mode and yelling threatening verbal metaphors, and to administer the "shock treatment" to his now-maladaptive ego defense—the mutative interpretation that would sum up and produce change. I grabbed his shoulders, yelled "Shut up and listen!" I added, "You're jealous!" He screamed; he cursed and tried to run from the room and I signaled father to exert his authority. He broke down in tears as I, enlarging the interpretation, said that he felt no good because two mothers had already turned him away and he'd rather die than believe it, and that despite how loving and dedicated his new mother has been, he could not accept this because to accept it he would have to accept the reality of his two previous rejections. He was jealous because his stepsiblings had never been given away by their mother, and living with them was a constant reminder, whether he was aware of it or not, of the difference.

A lot of pathetic weeping followed, but he stayed and allowed himself to be held. This interpretation overcame the major resistance to further treatment. After a few sessions, he re-repressed his pain over his losses. But indications that a nonverbal working through was going on were reflected by these signs. Relationships at home and cooperation in school gradually improved, and by the next summer he was able to say he did not want to return to the same summer camp program because he had acted so badly and the kids would remember. He now cared about his image. Unfortunately, further working through in the face of early puberty and other stresses presented by middle school was severely limited by third-party payment restrictions, and the gains did not hold but required further intervention on an inpatient level.

Many of the preparatory interpretations alluded to in the above example reflected the techniques discussed by Anna Freud in Sandler and associates 1980, where she talked of the preparatory work of clarification and confrontation with reality—in my example, forceful, to meet and match the forcefulness of his defense, followed immediately by the mutative interpretation of his jealousy, which in itself was his own contradiction of his denial. With all of this in the treatment situation, which at the moment included his parents as auxiliary therapists, he experienced ego support through the limit setting and momentary physical restraint; acceptance, not rejection; supportive empathy, not anger (mostly through nonverbal means: the firm restraint, then the holding and comforting). His initial trauma of loss had been at a preverbal level, and, as we found, verbal assurances and interpretation on my part that were relatively affectless did not meet him at that level. It took the affect-laden two-word phrases and the nonverbal accompaniment to reach him. To have interpreted the derivatives, his death wishes for his siblings (which were also turned on himself as wishes to die) at this point, would have been premature and counterproductive.

Anna Freud recommends that initial interpretations need to be of defense, and the relating of defense to what is defended against is made in stages. She notes that this preparatory explanation to the child of the reality of his situation is especially needed when the child has a physical handicap or when one or both parents are seriously disturbed. This relieves the child of blaming self for the situation.

INTERPRETATION OF THE DEFENSE AGAINST ANXIETY

We see this problem existing in divorce situations or when a sibling is hurt, has elective surgery, or dies. One clarifies and relieves anxiety by noting and correcting the child's self-blame by explaining the reality of the situation. The sibling rivalry or oedipal death wish is not approached for a long time, if at all, and then only through an ego-supportive interpretation acknowledging the ego defense: "You are afraid you might have wished that . . .," and so forth.

A 12-year-old boy developed severe anxiety when his younger brother was scheduled for an overnight hospitalization for a tonsillectomy. History given by the parents indicated that he had been an only child when his brother was born at age 4, and had actually tried to harm the baby, after first acting like the infant did not exist. The patient was of course *not* confronted with this information, but was just asked casually how he felt when he first saw his new baby brother. He remembered only how puny and helpless the infant seemed. He had no conscious memory of his earlier attitudes. He now treated his brother with the bemused toleration afforded a kid brother. He expressed fear that something would happen to his brother—he had heard of anesthesia deaths and uncontrolled bleeding from even minor operations. He had nightmares, then could not sleep. After going over, step by step, the realities of his brother's operation and the negligible chance of danger, which he accepted intellectually, anxiety decreased but sleep problems persisted. Keeping in mind his mother's description of his early but unremembered hostility to his infant brother, I asked him to draw his family. In the drawing he placed his brother between him and his mother. I asked him casually how old he was when his brother was born and mused that it must have been rough on him and quite a change to have all the attention shifted to the new baby after having it all to himself. He said he thought he was glad. I said I was surprised, for most 4-year-olds would not have been very happy, and even, down deep inside, might have wished the baby would go away. It would only be natural for a 4-year-old to feel that way. And did he remember that when he was 4 years old, he thought that wishing something was like doing it and that it could happen just because he wished it— sometimes even though he didn't *really* want it to. He was relieved, and the sleep problem ended.

Let us analyze what happened in this interpretation:

This recognition of the unconscious anxiety-producing hostile wish and my generalizing and diluting it by attributing it to "most kids" *at that age* made it more acceptable and normal and implied that his reaction was a carryover from his original death wish *without my having to say it in so many words*. His ego knew that I knew. My observation about the 4-year-old equating wishes with deeds also implied that at 12 he knew better, and that perhaps by identifying the anxiety as belonging to the 4-year-old in him and exposing it to reality he could take hold of himself with the reality of the 12-year-old and didn't have to be anxious or guilty anymore. All of this was implicit, not explicit, in the interpretation and thus more palatable. Thus interpretations are like negotiations: You try to save face. You don't have to rub the patient's nose in it and extract a confession; it's enough that you know the ego gets the message. You are in effect working with the unconscious; sometimes you let the sleeping dogs lie—not asleep, but not unleashed, either.

DISPLACEMENT AND EXTERNALIZATION OF CONFLICT AND "YOU ARE NOT ALONE IN THIS"

There are many aids that can facilitate the interpretation and allow a degree of displacement and externalization of the warded-off impulse that is producing the neurotic derivatives and symptoms. A dollhouse with family and animal dolls and puppets; hammering and punching toys; and toy trucks and cars are used in this way and allow both affective discharge and playing out the conflict in a displaced and projective way.

R. is a sweet $9\frac{1}{2}$-year-old girl with two older sisters in a home where father explodes with anger in the mornings. Father has verbally abused the mother, who in turn has little self esteem and is phobic, anxious, and depressed, some of which antedated her relationship with her husband. R. is considered a good girl in school, but hypersensitive, with a tendency to give up, crying easily, and feeling she cannot do the work. She would get headaches and get sick. The initial clinical impression was that this was neither attention deficit disorder nor a specific learning disorder, an impression confirmed by thorough testing. The first two sessions were exploratory; she didn't want to come ("There's nothing wrong with me. I just get a little worried."), but she came—passively. In the third session she described a roller coaster ride. The girls were screaming; the boys were roaring. "What did you do?" I asked. "I was roaring" (a pun on her name). At this first hint of aggression I tossed her some animal biting puppets. She became transformed, and her puppet attacked my old lady puppet with total intensity and tenacity—"I hate the old lady!" R. tore her head off and tore the limbs off the little boy doll . . . "till there's nothing left of you." This intense angry affect was limited to the puppet and doll play and was nowhere else in evidence. (During testing she had characterized a plant in the psychologist's office as a man-eating plant.) At that point I could only comment on how angry the gotcha! bird puppet was, and wonder why, which of course she didn't know. I wondered if she knew anyone who got angry like that? Sometimes her daddy—but she immediately dropped the subject. A weak, musing observation that girls are afraid to roar like boys and show their anger but that she had said she could roar was not picked up. The aid (puppet play) allowed the anger to come out in a strictly circumscribed way. She and I know it is there; the why and the extent will have to wait for future sessions. Any interpretation of cannibalistic fantasies is a long time off, if ever, in her case.

In the next session, the puppets were people, not animals, and the Queen beat up the King: swift blows and vicious biting off of heads. Again this did not spill over beyond the puppet play. My offhand interpretive comment, "Sort of like your father and mother, but this time Mom wins," again brought no reply, but again the impact of the interpretation could be seen in the change in play content in the following session.

Other interpretive techniques involve

1. Supportively referring to another child: "I know a child about your age who . . ." or "When I was your age I remember . . ." (this was described above).
2. Pointing out the conflict by saying "Part of you would like to . . . but the other part would be unhappy if . . ." or by bringing out the contrast between the big boy versus the little boy or baby.

3. Having the child tell a story about a picture on which not only the child's impulse but also the feared disapproval can be projected or displaced from the self onto the figure in the picture. For example, "That little boy is thinking about doing bad things and his daddy will be angry." Using the same picture, the therapist can also make an indirect interpretation by talking about the same child. Here, as in any interpretation, the degree of directness and depth should take into consideration the load of stress already on the child's ego.

PLAYING OUT THE CONFLICT— REVERSAL OF ROLES

4. Playing out the conflict, letting the child assign the roles to both the therapist and himself and providing grist for the mill of interpretation.
5. A favorite technique of Berta Bornstein (1961, personal communication and supervisory instruction) was to reverse the roles, with the therapist becoming the child patient and the child becoming the therapist-doctor. Here, acting the child, the therapist has a chance to put into words what he understands the child's fears and fantasies to be, and the child can act out and reflect the therapist as perceived or fantasied by the child. Here interpretation of the "here and now," the child's current anxieties which he or she may be denying, can come out.

It was Fred Allen (1942), a pioneer in the child guidance movement, who stated that the value of interpretation is in its association with the primary value of the immediate experience with the therapist. The therapeutic impact arises from the experience itself—"helping the child to be what he can be in the here and now, and assisting him to move toward responsible and creative uses of the self, which has emerged out of the past" (p. 129).

Here he is in accord with the later ideas of Oremland (1991), who is thinking more in terms of a "here and now" transference experience within the therapeutic situation and its consequent interpretation. In my opinion, exclusive focus on the here and now leaves out other rich material arising and presenting itself for interpretation. It should form only part of the total therapeutic approach. However, in any event, the child's manifest content must be accepted as having significance in its own right, not merely as a derivative or screen for deeper conflicts.

R. is a beautiful nearly 13-year-old, the second of six siblings, flanked by three sisters; the two youngest children are boys. She was brought by her parents, a youthful handsome couple in their mid-thirties. Father is a police lieutenant. R. was brought because of an episode of extreme panic and following a physical attack on her sister by some neighborhood teenagers.

Six months prior to this anxiety attack, R. had begun expressing fears of the devil harming her, and she developed obsessive-compulsive rituals to ward off the devil. At age 4, after recurrent bladder infection R. was hospitalized for 10 days during which a blockage in her urethra was surgically removed. Mother was allowed to stay with her. R. had always been very religious, concerned with Christian ideals, with helping people, yet somewhat dependent and immature.

Psychological testing showed average intelligence, neurotic-level conflicts, and no severe ego disturbance or psychotic/delusional tendencies but rather neurotic conflicts about violence and aggression expressed in obsessive-compulsive tendencies and intense anxiety. Parents report that she always was a very sensitive child and was quite jealous of attention given her siblings, and never was comfortable being left alone. She avoided bathing and would leave the bathroom door open when she would bathe.

On the first visit, R. insisted father come with her. She kept close to him and seemed a bit seductive. She described fears of Freddy Krueger (a sadistic character seen on television), of the devil, and of her own thoughts. She thinks someone will die and is compelled to do something (her rituals) so it won't happen. "If it isn't just right, I have to do it again and again."

My first comment was to commiserate about how much time this must take from homework and play. "Yes, even with homework, if I cross it out, I have to do it over three times." She feared the devil would stab her. "I'm afraid I want to go to him, and if I don't do something (ritual), I'll go to him."

I asked, "Is it intriguing, a temptation?"

She answered, "That's a thought!" and reported a dream in which the devil had sent someone to get her, a girl in her classroom, a girl who flunked; she's a showoff.

"Sexy?" I asked.

She laughed nervously. "She's pretty, she acts like she's 15, and flirts with the boys."

"Are you scared at the way she is behaving?" I asked.

She replied, "She's too fast. It's scary."

"Yours is a scary time of life," I mused.

"I tell myself not to do what she does. I'm getting a funny feeling in the pit of my stomach."

"Anxiety," I said. I asked her for three wishes.

"Peace in the world; me to go to heaven where the good people are; and more people should follow Jesus and God," she said. "The devil is pushing me to do what God wouldn't want me to do."

At the third weekly visit she and father, who brought her, looked like a young couple. She was no longer concerned about her skirt being pulled down primly when she sat. She reported going to a slumber party with her friends and her sister. She got thoughts about the devil and that if she didn't swallow five times the devil would get into the house and get her sister. At the fourth visit, rituals were all based on odd, not even, numbers. Although her anxiety had decreased by the fourth visit, problems with studying, and near flunking, increased. The teacher makes them keep their hands on top of the desk, she informed me, and I noted that she still kept her hands hidden in her long sleeves.

There were other spontaneous fantasies she had to undo by ritual. She didn't take the textbook out of her desk in the right position. If she didn't correct it, Mary would get bloody. She had to say "bloody Mary" 100 times. The parallel to confession and doing Hail Marys was called to her attention, and she felt it was like doing penance but she was puzzled as to why.

In a conference with the parents after R.'s fourth session, I explained to them that R. was feeling the hormonal pressures of puberty and emerging adolescence, stirring up thoughts and impulses that she finds overwhelming, and has to put out of herself as the devil. She turns to religion, ritual, and her mother at night for control. Mom needs to see that she is fully informed about her body, sex and reproduction, and help her set limits. They can expect testing of these limits, defiance of rules, and increased assertiveness and wanting to run with the crowd of girls that she now sees as the devil's agents. I suggested that they support her involvement with an excellent school counselor on a regular basis. She resisted coming to the next session. A weird dream in which the devil held her hands behind her back and covered her mouth drove her to seek sanctuary in her mother's bed. I interpreted that she sensed there were thoughts that she felt she had best keep secret. I noted that she was now biting her lip and her nails and cracking her knuckles. The parents unfortunately had translated my caveat into a stern system of time limits as when to be at home, and loss of privileges—grounding—at any violation, or bad report at school.

As these conflicts translated into the typical conflict of generations with her parents, her anxieties decreased, and by the sixth session she came in smiling and without the oversized jacket that had hidden her hands. She described how she had been grumpy, screaming at her sisters, and had given everyone a rough time. "Speak of the devil!" I commented. She got the point, laughed, and said she had apologized to everyone. I looked up to find her staring at me, and I asked, "Are you wondering what else I know about you?" She blushed.

In the few sessions left (managed care had limited it to ten; the family supported several more), through the use of Thematic Apperception Test cards, issues about relationships, love, hurting and helping others came out, as did the reality of her average intelligence and her preparing for a helping profession. She was passing all her courses, and anxiety was no longer a major concern. She sublimated through sports activities. Devil fantasies and warding-off rituals had all but disappeared.

In her next-to-last session I summed up her challenging and self-assertive behavior and said a bit sadly, "You know you've been getting wilder and wilder all the time. Maybe this devil you feared was in you was really a part of your thoughts and impulses you couldn't accept as coming from you. You are beginning to recognize and hopefully control and take responsibility for them; your parents are trying to help with their restrictions." She was angry because her parents wouldn't let her go with a group of peers (ages 14 and 15) to the seashore for a weekend. I agreed with them and told her I felt she couldn't do that until she could demonstrate that she had the devil in her under control, and she is still struggling with it, although it doesn't scare or panic her anymore. In her final session she reported that her goal is now to attend community college.

"Not with C's and D's," I countered. She knows she can do better. She reported a good working relationship with her counselor, who seemed to be a big sister/mother type without the hindrance of the emotionally charged oedipal and counteroedipal factors involved in her ongoing relationship with her parents. Relations with her parents improved in the face of, perhaps because of, the firm limits they were setting.

Comment: After the history interview with R.'s parents, and the first interview with R., it was clear that this was neither a case of obsessive-compulsive disorder, nor an ego disorder moving toward psychosis. R. was a deeply religious child faced with pubertal awakening of sexual impulse and oedipal fantasies, which she had to split off and attribute to the devil, and devise elaborate rituals to protect herself and her family. The external controls provided through her religious beliefs were no longer sufficient. The problem for the therapist is how to give her and her family an understanding of what is going on in a way that can be accepted and made use of by the child and her family, in a way that respects and supports their defenses. Here issues of quantity, timing, and metaphor are of utmost importance.

This is the *art* of interpretation. In the twelve sessions covering a 6-month span, there was no way that her increasing testing of her mother and passing period of seductiveness with her father could be worked through in terms of her oedipal wishes, nor could her anxiety in the bathtub, in bed at night, or her hiding her hands in long sleeves be worked out in terms of masturbatory impulses or actions.

Seeking safety from the devil in mother's bed was a way of seeking external control and assuring herself that mother was O.K., and of protecting her mother from her own unconscious wishes to displace her. Indeed, as she became a more normal, assertive adolescent, her anxiety diminished under the controls she had provoked from her family, primarily her mother; and the visits from the devil and her neutralizing rituals disappeared. In my interpretive explanation to R.'s parents I used R.'s metaphor of the devil to call to their attention the adolescent awakening that was going on and frightening her, and suggested how they could discuss these issues with her so as to signify their acceptance of these changes in her. I predicted, before the fact, her shift to a more normal, albeit more rebellious, early adolescent and supported them in setting limits. With R. the interpretations involved first how this was interfering with her school work, then her temptation and intrigue with the devil. Her response was a dream in which she is scared by her implied interest in being like a girl who flirts and is too fast. I watched developmental changes take place and largely kept silent regarding mutative interpretation, but I suggested that I knew there were secrets I would not push her for, respecting her defenses. Then, commenting on her behavior, I equated it with the devil ("Speak of the devil!"). The mutative interpretation was the final one, that the devil she feared was in her, part of her, and her responsibility to control (not in those words, of course). In essence, that interpretation was my parting charge to her.

INTERPRETATION TO THE PRESCHOOL CHILD— THEORETICAL AND CLINICAL ISSUES

Therapy with the young preschool child is more likely to involve predominantly preoedipal issues related to loss of love, trust, insecurity, and being helpless in the face of physical or psychological assault. Diagnosis of neurosis in the *young* preschool child is blurred. Neurotic formation is infantile and incomplete, and conflicts are expressed as disturbances of affects and in bodily function and regulation; and in developmental arrest, or regression from developmental levels already attained (loss of speech, loss of toilet training, return to mouthing and wanting a nursing bottle or breast). Pure infantile neuroses as pathological disorders involving oedipal conflicts requiring analysis are rare. They are more likely to be an intermix of oedipal and preoedipal traumas, losses, or other deprivations, requiring long periods of working through for each level of interpretation.

The neurosis itself is usually an incomplete entity in which the disorder may be better characterized as areas of neurotic defenses responding to a stressful environment and to inner adaptive dysfunction or deficit, which conspire to lower self-esteem and deplete healthy narcissistic supplies.

These origins and issues extend the problem and the nature of the intervention far beyond that of dealing with the classic structural ego, id, and superego interaction.

This analytic partial case history will not only illustrate key interpretations and the process of working through over time, but also will show a parallel clarification and working through process in the mother, which led to not only an improved relationship between her and her young daughter but to maturational changes in the mother as well.

M. was referred by her analytically oriented pediatrician at $3\frac{1}{3}$ years of age for severe behavior problems. Her parents elaborated: "She doesn't relate well to other kids nor initiate play with them. When others are having fun, M. is sullen. She is moody and nasty, stiff and inflexible." They added that M. is controlling, gets upset if mother leaves the room, yet pulls away if picked up and cuddled. M. is very hostile to her only sibling, a brother 22 months younger. She noted the genital difference right away.

Her parents made a handsome couple. Father, age 31, an academic, was very intellectual, orderly, and self-controlled. He presented himself as immersed in work and self-confident. He tended to explain and defend his daughter's behavior.

Mother, 29, a willowy, arty brunette with hair pulled back severely into a ponytail, spoke with intensity of how she felt threatened, even attacked, by her daughter M. She was self-deprecating, afraid of her own aggressive impulses, and felt guilty for her preference for her son, a husky blond blue-eyed boy, outgoing and friendly to everyone.

Both parents agreed that the paternal grandparents are closed-minded, rigid, country club types. The grandmother dominates the grandfather, which father resents. The paternal grandmother interferes, pampering M. and rejecting her brother, which mother resents. There are no problems with the maternal grandparents.

A description of the medical background is pertinent. Pregnancy was planned in the sixth year of marriage. It was a breech birth without complications. M. was fussy and became hypertonic by 7 months. Motor landmarks were normal, M. talked in sentences at 2 years. At 2 years 6 months, she was fearful and shy and fought toilet training. At 2 years 9 months, M. developed cystitis and pyelitis with much abdominal pain.

A month later, because of a constricted urethra she was dilatated in the urologist's office, without anesthesia. Mother described M. on a GYN table in stirrups, terrified. Relief was not sustained; symptoms returned. She was hospitalized a month later for 4 days, and urethrotomy was performed under general anesthesia. She would not look at her mother the next day when she visited. Dysuria with cystitis and vaginitis developed a month later, this time treated with antibiotics, vaginal suppositories, and subsequent catheterization by the office nurse. In her doll play at home she would catheterize her dolls. Behavioral problems with tantrums, nastiness, and withdrawal followed, leading to her referral for psychotherapy, 6 months after cystitis had begun.

In her first visit, M. at first refused to separate from her mother but soon forgot that her mother was there. Her hand puppets were biting horns, fingers, noses, and ears. One doll has a hole between her legs, the other doesn't. M. noticed the bull's penis and pumped up the cows udder with it. I noted to myself, but not yet to her, that her cystoscopies and retrograde pyelographies involved catheterization and filling her bladder with fluid, and that the theme of her play was castration and invasion in an oral-sadistic mode, in which she identified with the aggressor.

She was very bright and conversational as she played and said, "You know, they catheterized me in the hospital. They hurt me." She totally ignored my request for more details. I should have known better than to have asked. She had her hand puppet bite my nose and fingers. "My puppet won't really hurt. I only eat food, nothing else" (a denial of cannibalistic urges?). She announced that her brother is a boy, her father a great big man, while she and her mother are girls. Though I saw her as having regressed to oral-sadistic and urethral preoccupations after premature stimulation of phallic-vaginal preoccupation secondary to her traumatization, I accepted her statements of memory of the trauma and her reassurance that her puppet won't really hurt, it was just play. I made no interpretation. I didn't have to; her own push for help was carrying the therapy, and as it turned out, there were other key issues.

In her second visit, mother remained downstairs with younger brother. M. noted, "I can make old sick cars and trains better because I'm a man." She was astraddle, and walking a large truck between her legs. In response to my question, "Can't a woman do it?" she said, "I don't know how or why, but only he can." Several times she threw away or hit a lady doll. ("I don't like her.") A crocodile destroys the furniture looking for his mommy. Phallic squirting play followed.

The next session found M. even more reluctant to separate from her mother. She was looking for a puppet with teeth and found a wolf puppet. It bites the arm off a he-baby, who then turns into a wolf. After running over babies with a truck (all identification with the aggressor) she announced, "I have a baby, he's a boy."

Her next two sessions (4 and 5) changed the theme to one of activity over passivity, attacking the aggressor rather than identifying with him. She runs over the wolf. Bites the wolf's snout. "*I'm* eating the wolf." "Don't cry! Be brave!" She puts a peg in her mouth. "Its a drinking bottle—it's a nail." I thought (to myself, of course) that she was exploring the dual function of a penis to squirt and to penetrate. She pulls the wolf's jaws apart: "So wide!" Again I interpreted to myself that she was reproducing the situation when she was in the stirrups, converting helplessness into being the active one, the aggressor.

By the sixth and seventh sessions new themes are appearing—loss and death, first by a denial that people (grandparents) die. The Try-to-be-brave-while-they-are-biting theme continued. I suggested that maybe this was how she was trying to feel when she was catheterized. I noted that her paintings were yellow, like her urine from the catheter.

In her play, after the wolf ate all the babies, grandma rescued them and hid all the babies inside. Then the restorative theme of mother, father, and little girl together was played out.

After an August vacation, mother complained that M. was horrible to her brother. She can't stand M.'s obnoxious aggressive behavior, it embarrasses her before her neighbors.

In the second month of therapy (September) the biting, castrating play and the theme of male–female differences continued with all sorts of variations (e.g., girls can't be doctors, they can't give injections). New themes appeared. M. put a ball of clay under her dress and delivered her own baby, which she called "bad" and promptly threw in the wastebasket. I interpreted, "Bad babies get thrown away, they get abandoned," and that when she was in the hospital she must have felt bad and discarded. Her response to the interpretation was to start real metaphoric role playing. She said to me, "You be the little girl. I be the mommy." This was an opportunity to interpret via putting the words in the little girl's mouth. She had already rammed the snake in my (the little girl's, and perhaps by overdetermination the doctor's) mouth, an upward displacement of what had happened to her, and reversing and taking the active role. She said (as mommy), "Good bye, little girl."

I asked anxiously, "Are you leaving me?"

"Yes!" she said, sternly.

"At the doctor's?" I asked.

"Yes!" she hissed.

"What will happen to me?"

"You will die!"

"Don't leave me, am I a bad girl?"

"Yes!"

In the third month (October) the abandonment theme continued, but it was now about being discarded into the hospital, having been promised no pain and no needles, and feeling betrayed because she was penetrated and hurt. Though the hospital was on fire, she must stay! At Halloween she did not want to wear a mask (anesthesia).

By December, inasmuch as M. repeated some of this in her play at home I was able to tell mother that M. is portraying (mother's) hostility to her under the guise of worry and concern.

Mother blurted out, "M. brings out the monster in me!" I also interpreted that M. acts out mother's hidden impulses for her and represents the part of mother that she would like to deny and discard. Mother confesses that it is all she can do to control her impulse to do physical violence to M. In fact, when M. was much younger, mother handled her quite roughly and angrily and now finds herself being cruel and brutal to her again.

In November mother noticed the first signs of self-control in M. She is more feminine.

At the end of January M. played the Jewish Sabbath ritual of covering her head, blessing and lighting the candles, and presenting the ritual bread to the head of the household to bless and cut, and then said to me, "Imagine you're the daddy. Lie down here, I won't eat you. I'll lie down too." This oedipal play must have frightened her because she immediately said, "I hate you!" She filled all the holes of the knockout bench with clay "so you couldn't hammer in the pegs" and filled the wolf's mouth with clay so he couldn't talk or bite. I felt she was telling me to back off from the interpretations, and a period followed of further repetitive working through of current themes.

In February M. began portraying more graphically what had happened to her in the hospital and interleaved oedipal themes. The knockout bench became a surgical cart. The little girl gets a "deep needle" and is wheeled to the operating room. Daddy says he will be back, but he doesn't come. He is at home hugging Mommy. She angrily jabs the needles into the doctor's eyes (fortunately a designated hand puppet, not me). I interpreted to M. her defensive regression to an oral-aggressive defense by attack, biting back, like the wolf. That was all she could think of doing. She gave a diabolical laugh and said it looked like they were going to eat me up. "I'm the lion but the lion is friendly now." Meanwhile, M.'s mother informed me that she is working out her hatred for M. messing up her life in her own therapy, which she had begun in response to what had been stirred up in her by M.'s therapy.

In March M. played the nurse who shoved the ball-point pen between the legs of the little bendable dolls.

"They went away and left me all alone." M. took the role of the efficient but firm nurse who took care of her in the hospital. I commented that the nurse was a bit like her father. April saw a gradual shift from playing it out to talking it out, and a concomitant shift from phallic castration to phallic oedipal themes. The wolf now bites and hisses. There is an increased interest in daddy. She orders me to be the daddy and lie down on the couch. (My office is one-half standard desk, chair, and couch, and the other half a playroom area.) She giggles. She returns to the catheterization themes. The hospital cart becomes the irrigation cart. Mother reports that she hides and denies her abdominal pain at home, for fear of being taken in for yet another catheterization. In her play therapy, M. cannot sustain the oedipal themes. She destroys the clay wedding ring and goes back to oral- and phallic-sadistic themes of biting and penetrating. I interpret; she is angry that I know her secret (oedipal). She brings in a policeman, a superego theme. Mother reports that playing out the hospital scene goes on at home, and her nastiness during the Purim celebration was unbearable to her mother. Perhaps M.'s nastiness was the outward manifestation of inner anxieties and somatic memories stirred up by the symbolism of Purim, which is a Jewish festival commemorating the biblical story of Queen Esther and her uncle Mordechai and their triumph over Haman, the persecutor of the Jews. Esther and Mordechai triumph through Esther's intercession with the king, who did not know that she was a Jewess.

This story is traditionally reenacted by the children in the congregation, and a carnival is held. *Hamentashen*, triangular filled pastries representing Haman's three-cornered hat, are eaten.

The triumph of the good girl over the persecutor through the king's intervention (king = oedipal father/therapist, a role M. often assigned to me) seemed to make Purim themes symbolically pertinent to the themes being enacted in her therapy at the time. In her play in therapy M. takes the mother's role: "Little girl, stop being messy and clean up."

In the ensuing months the above themes recurred over and over again, each time examining yet another facet and with an increasing sense of control and verbalization of more and more of the whole episode, but also with periods of regression—it is impossible to detail the steps in this presentation. Mother, now more empathetic and sensitive to her daughter's conflict over letting loose, and identifying with it, stated that, figuratively, she would like to see M. "get into the mud and enjoy being loose." Keeping to her metaphor I suggest that rather than M. doing it for her, they should do it together. As if sensing an unspoken permission, M. goes through a quick period of anal themes and farting and making a mess and playing out forcing the girl to be sitting on the potty, and on to being coy and interested in her dress. More and more she puts the puppets aside and acts the seductive feminine role. This alternates with themes of being the nurse assisting the doctor examining the girl and saying severely, "She has to be crushed!" Entwined was the little girl's masochistic wish to be hurt. Themes equivalent to rape emerge by July. "I don't want to be a girl," after one year of therapy (sixty sessions). But she then bounds back by making a clay object that sticks out and remarks that it has curves and boys don't have curves. It is a remarkably true rendition of a mons veneris and the vulval folds. She then impales it with a pen. I interpret that she sees value in being a girl. She can be just as big there but different. Yet there is also danger in being a girl; you can be hurt as she was, and mommy and daddy couldn't protect her.

This is a very skeletal account of the first year of a 4-year psychoanalysis that took 110 sessions. Themes were repeated and elaborated again and again. She repeated and sustained oedipal play, transferring to me and assigning me the role of father she would lie down with. In the end of the third year she played out the Jewish Sabbath ritual again. She identified the challah, the Sabbath bread provided by the mother, which the father then ceremonially cuts with the knife, with herself as the *kallah* (bride) under the canopy. I could now make the integrative mutative interpretation in which her operation was indeed in her mind, but also her defloration as her father's bride. Somewhere she had mixed up the doctor with her father. That's why she felt she was a bad girl and why she felt she was left by her mother and father and why she felt her mother was so angry at her. (Indeed her mother was, but for her own reasons.)

She was reassured that most girls have nice thoughts about their fathers and even before kindergarten would like to marry their daddies, and that it's O.K. to think that then. Afterwards they learn that they have to wait till they grow up and can have their own man and their own babies. So she was not bad, she was normal, and because she also had that trouble with her peeing and the doctors had to do all those hurtful things, and Mom and Dad were not allowed to stay with her, she thought she was being abandoned because she was bad. So now she is all mixed up about men and what they do to ladies and whether she would like it or not and whether she would rather be a boy or girl. Because she is scared and felt she was abandoned she is also very angry and we're going to have to work some more on all her mixed-up thoughts and feelings now that we know and she knows her secrets, some of which she didn't even know before. We spent the fourth year of her analysis working on her issues of trust, her sadomasochistic conflicts, her angry feelings, and her oedipal conflicts. In that time her I.Q. steadily rose from high average through bright normal to superior levels. Her school performance became steady and without impulsive and tantrumlike episodes. She became a leader, had lots of friends, and was able to sustain good relationships. She tolerated the birth of a sister late in 1973.

However, by the fall of 1975, a year after the analysis ended, her mother was still not sure that M. loved her, but pointed to distancing individuating behavior that many midlatency children have. M. still retained scars of her traumatic experience and some mood swings with depression were evident (still feeling somewhat "apart," as she says wryly when her parents reassure her that she is "a part" of the family). She is still at risk, but the family is now poised to seek help should disturbance arise.

Mother was able to see, in her parallel self-examination in response to what emerged from her daughter during the last years of her daughter's analysis, that she had decided to have a baby (M.) for the wrong reasons: because peers were having babies and her sister did. Somehow she resented M. from the beginning, a resentment that M. picked up even before her traumatic experience. Mother, during the last year of M.'s analysis, had figuratively and literally begun to let her hair down and began to enjoy the whistles of the construction workers, something that would have offended her before. She felt that she was no longer so hyper and uptight.

Father, who during the analysis was upset by this invasion of his rigidly constricted sense of the logic and order of things, made a career change and is happy with it.

Comment: I have tried to give you a taste of the immensely complicated and overdetermined mental and emotional processes that take place in a traumatic neuroses superimposed on a possible (prematurely stimulated) oedipally based infantile neurosis, a process greatly influenced by parental conflicts. What comes from the child opens up vistas in the parent, and visa versa. I have tried to show again how premature interpretation is of no avail, and how the process of working through must examine and reexamine the conflicts from every facet, but that with each return and with each interpretation one sees both new material and a somewhat more integrated review of old material, and some small increase in developmental maturity manifested in the way the conflict is understood and adapted to. The process is long and tedious, but in the end (if one can say there is an end) it is gratifying.

INTERPRETATION THROUGH AFFECTOMOTOR INTERACTION

The younger the child, the more likely it is that the therapy will be related to the activity of the child and interpreted through the affecto-motor interaction and play with the therapist (though the therapist may need to verbalize as a vehicle to carry the affecto-motor message). Infants with enteroceptive and proprioceptive (core and rind) disorders (of eating, bowel retention, sleep and motor discharge disorders) fall in this group.

Although exceptional 2- and 3-year-old children may be surprisingly verbal, even to the point of having the capacity for symbolism and abstraction, it is their nonverbal play that carries the bulk of the affect-loaded information needed for interpretation. One must guard against interpreting too high (*not too deep*), that is, oedipally, when the affect, despite the form and manifest content, is preoedipal, infantile, and involves loss of the protective envelope.

G., at age 3 years 4 months, was driving with his mother when their car was rear-ended by a tractor trailer truck at 50 mph and pushed toward a car that had stopped suddenly and that she had slowed for. Both had been securely belted, G. in his safety seat. Though the car was totaled, neither was physically hurt, but because the mother was wearing a neck collar from a previous whiplash, injury rescue workers carried her off on a plank stretcher, and despite her entreaties to take her child out of the car seat and let him ride with her, he was left with the police and saw her being carried off. This extremely bright, very verbal and motorically active child became quite hyper when returned home and reunited with his mother. He immediately began playing the incident out, smashing his tricycle into the wall or down the steps, yelling, "I'm in an accident," and defensively displacing the affect and splitting it off, telling his brother, "My friend had an accident. A truck hit him and they had to take his mother out on a board and in an ambulance. I'm not scared, but he was and worried about his mother."

Three days later he was brought for assessment and treatment because of nightmares; persistent complaints of pain in his right foot; a need to have his mother nearby; a loss of bowel control, which had been attained 3 or 4 months earlier; and general whiny, anxious behavior.

In the first session he played at an 18–24-month level, filling and dumping "by accident," but also being in charge, pushing the truck and being the doctor. I said to the child how good it must feel to be in charge and be able to make things happen the way *he* wants. In subsequent sessions, or at home between sessions, concerns over loss were expressed in such questions as, "Why do people get old, sick, and die?" (there had been recent losses, including a cat) and by playing out being in charge, the boss, the doctor. Sleep problems were interpreted in terms of his fear of going to sleep and waking up to find his mother gone. With the reassurance that she would be there, he was able to fall asleep if his mother were in the room, but anxiety about separation ("Hold me," "I need you") persisted. Interpretations were about his worry that he can't ever be sure that Mom will be able to protect him.

In our play he constructed a Tinkertoy crane, and we moved dump trucks and moving vans. We emphasized *his* role and *his* strength. Big boy versus baby themes appeared, and we talked about how it felt good to be big and strong like Daddy—but yet it also felt good and safe to be Mommy's baby.

He continued to "poop" in a diaper. I noted that his grandmother used the word "accident" to designate what he was doing. I suggested that this was an accident that he could control—and not be helpless. He continued to have periods of phobic anxiety associated with driving, during which he clutched his penis and wanted to be sure everyone was buckled in and that they weren't going near the expressway. There had been a previous auto accident when he was 1½, in which both his mother and older brother were hurt. Could it be that some of the intense anxiety went back to that time he could hardly remember to tell about, but that he could remember the feelings, although he was just a baby then? These interpretations were made both to G. and to his parents, who used this knowledge to give him supportive reassurance.

He went from controlling the truck to deploying his body as a whole, as a diving, jumping, attacking, karatelike unit. ("You're running and smashing like *you* are the truck.") He had to check to see that Mommy was O.K. in the waiting room. He began to build and put things together and at home to tape chairs to tables—to fix things that belong together. His anxiety and night fears took on a controlling and manipulating quality rather than one of seeking protection. Anal preoccupation with smells and oppositional testing out followed. A summer vacation and wanting to run with his peers motivated his pooping in the pot and being proud of it. He did many things with his father that fostered his identification with Daddy's manly ways. Preoccupation with gender differences paralleled these interests.

At present G. has started in a class with 4½-year-olds. Though he is 9–12 months younger than most, he holds his own academically and in play. At home he still wants to be close to his mother, but the developmental quality of his behavior has changed in the past 2 weeks. Mother's presence at sleep time is needed for only 10 minutes or less. He announces he wants to be married to Mommy and suggests his father sleep downstairs, which of course is countered with a gentle explanation that Mommy is Daddy's wife. When he grows up like Daddy he can get his own wife; meanwhile Daddy and Mommy take care of him and help him grow up.

When he regresses, it is to a more anal manipulative state—his mother says he no longer feels like a tiny, clingy baby. Indeed, at times he has exceeded the anal levels and is cocky and assertive. The taping together of things seems to be a protection against breaking off (castration) and splitting apart of things that belong together.

Comment: The above clinical vignette took place over a 4-month period in which this very bright and verbal child reacted to a trauma that shattered his belief in the all-protective mother, called up and worked through affect from a previous trauma at age 1½ years—a trauma "unspeakable" in Winnicott's terms, which caused loss of bowel training and a regression to a more infantile need for mother to allay his anxiety. The trauma and the defense against the regression, with emphasis on the big boy theme, led to a somewhat premature oedipal preoccupation.

The developmental estimations and interpretations that I shared with G.'s parents supported and directed their understanding responses to their child, and he may yet be able to resolve his oedipal conflicts smoothly. (A week after this was written his mother reported that at dinner G. announced that he wanted his high chair put away and saved, so that when he grows up and marries and gets a wife he can use it for his sonny boy!) Though I interpreted his insecurity and loss of trust and his feelings of helplessness and need to be in control, I felt no need, and found no opening, to interpret his oedipal wishes beyond noting his wish to be like (not replace or displace) his father. His regression to anal behavior after *he* suggested that father be displaced was the warning signal that such interpretation or picking up of his statement would be premature and overwhelming. Just because a child says it, acts it out, or dreams it does not mean he is ready to hear it from the therapist. One must watch carefully to see how he defends against his own statement or acting out. If regressive defenses appear, his ego is demonstrating it would not be able to handle such an interpretation.

SETTING THE AFFECTOMOTOR TONE

Because infants under 2 years of age have fantasies not yet attached to word production, but are rich in affects, we look for memories expressed affectively and somatically (Call et al. 1979). Even with older children and adults, memories of traumatic events that occurred in the preverbal period of development (under age 1½ to 2) do not come back as word memories but in affecto-somatic form, and have to be reconstructed into word pictures.

In working with infants, one interprets and reassures by facial expression, calm voice, by the holding attitude, by calmly enduring infantile rage and not replying in kind, so that trust and security can be established. This is a kind of nonverbal interpretation by affecto-motor body language that says, "I will not allow you to hurt yourself or drive me away, or take control" (all of which is reassuring to the child's budding ego). Supportive interpretations to the parents, such as, "It must be upsetting when your child doesn't respond," and "I can tell you are blaming yourself, when it wasn't really your fault" or "Most parents would get angry if their child did that," make them feel understood and accepted.

I was asked to see the 5-month-old grandchild of an acquaintance of mine whose daughter had married an Englishman and settled in England. She was coming for a visit and was devastated by the diagnosis of infantile autism made by her

English pediatrician. The infant was sluggish from birth, sucked poorly, and did not give the usual rooting and molding responses. The mother, who felt lonely and depressed during her pregnancy and had anticipatory doubts about her mothering abilities, had her suspicions of being a bad mother verified by her infant's lack of response (which in a later review of the birth records seem to have resulted from the use of long-acting barbiturates as part of mother's predelivery preparation). The mother became depressed, tense, anxious, and fearful of dropping or otherwise harming her infant. When the 2–3-month social smile failed to materialize, the pediatrician, noting how uptight the mother had become, began blaming her for the infant's autistic condition.

At 5 months this infant would not respond to his mother with a smile, cuddling, or eye contact and would feed only in a perfunctory, affectless way.

Mother was continually in tears, and also angry and frustrated. Her self-esteem as a mother was nil. My object was to assess the infant's capabilities and deficits, and the mother's, looking for her strengths and how to elicit them. Further, in the short time (1 week) we had I would try to bring them into a synchronous engagement in the process of my assessment, clarification, and nonverbal interpretive behavior as I demonstrated engagement and attunement, and elicited interactive involvement with her baby.

I asked the mother to play with her baby the way she would at home. She held the baby tensely, and the baby stiffened in response to her attempts to have him smile, coo, or even look at her. I noted the mother's tension, and gently suggested that babies are very sensitive to their mother's state of tension or relaxation and respond in kind.

I reached out for the infant as we sat on the floor; the mother surrendered him with relief. After swaying with the babe in arms from side to side in the cadence of *her* breathing (hers, because it was her rhythms he would be returned to), and picking up the rhythms in the cadence of my voice, almost hypnotic, I began asking mother about her childhood, her initial daydreams of motherhood, about her courtship and her marriage.

As we continued talking I would pick up the baby's sounds and echo them in pitch and rhythm, and comment on the baby's movements as to what the baby can do, touching or moving the part of the baby being remarked about.

I guessed that the latter part of her pregnancy and her early months with the baby must have been frightening and lonely, so far from home, and away for the first time, in a cold damp country in winter, with a different life-style and with a busy husband trying to establish himself. Although in Britain it is common practice that the baby care is left to the mother and the governess, in this instance it was all left to her.

I asked about her baby's behavior in his first 4 months, and how she felt when . . . or what she did when this or that happened. I was able to say, "That is just what Dr. Spock would have recommended," or that you did just what Dr. Brazelton did to get the baby interested. In other words, "Mother, you had the right instincts, you did the right thing." Her mood lightened, and when I laid the baby on the floor and, on my knees, leaned over until our heads nearly touched—back and forth—the baby became alert, gurgled, and began kicking his arms and legs. I vocalized and shook my head to the rhythm of the flailing arms and legs. With repeated approach and withdrawal, the baby smiled a flicker and vocalized in a rising pitch. Mother was encouraged ("Now you do it") to take my place over her child, and was responded to in kind.

I swept up the baby, held him cradled in my left arm in a bottle-feeding position, semidanced around, reached out and drew mother in with my right arm and close to her baby, and we swirled around as a unit. "Take hold of your baby," I said; we were both laughing by then. I pulled back: "Keep going!" She became giddy, and I motioned her to sit down, and rock the baby. I hummed a lullaby as they wound down to the slowing cadence of the lullaby. The baby slept and the mother relaxed, almost dozing herself. "See, you're not uptight and your baby is not stiff." Go home and play with your baby, talk to your baby, be where your baby is at."

In the next session (and last—she had to return to England), I said, "Show me what you've been doing." There was at first a tentativeness and fear that she might not do well before the critical eye of the master. I verbalized this to her and suggested that the overcritical eye was her own (her superego, but I didn't call it that), which she felt was coming from her husband, his countrymen, and her pediatrician (projection, but I didn't call it that). She has been too hard on herself: "Look how well you are doing!" I paraphrased a country folk song: "Have fun with your baby. Make love to your baby!" She held her child with a self-assurance that had not been present in the first session, and a lively affective interchange was going on. She had met her baby at its level and picked up the baby's cues.

I told her to insist that her husband take part like we had done here; he might even find it fun and relaxing.

She wrote that the baby had continued to respond, and sparkles now. She feels better about herself, they have become a threesome, and incidentally she changed her pediatrician. The new one is warm and empathetic, with children of her own.

Comment: What on earth does this impromptu unorthodoxy have to do with analytically oriented psychotherapy and interpretation? Well, we did have a goal: to assess the child and the mother's capabilities. I guessed, later verified, that the infant's original sluggishness was not organic but iatrogenic, but it was enough to crystallize the mother's self-doubts and loneliness into a self-defeating attitude, with anxiety, and depression heightened by her need to defend against underlying anger and resentment, a vicious cycle. The positive capability for normal function was there in both mother and child, and we proceeded to elicit, engage, exchange, and integrate it. But interpretation? Yes; interpretation is to give an understanding. The nonverbal interpretation to the infant through my picking up on his movements and vocalizations and my meeting and responding at his level was that there was someone out there who could "read" him—who was emotionally attuned to him—and as that someone became "someones" and included his mother, he sensed a growing assuredness and hence a feeling of security. It was also the relaxed firmness and lack of uneasiness in the way he felt he was being held that transmitted a message, "I'm O.K., you're O.K."

With the mother—and remember our basic principle that with young children it's the family dyad or triad that must be treated—I could verbally interpret her lack of self-esteem and her heavy-handed self-criticism, and clarify for her how the vicious cycle had been set up and demonstrate to her how the conflict could be resolved, and go on to work it through with her and her baby. What made it happen so fast? Perhaps because we *had* to do it in a limited time, and mother was seduced into doing it. Q.E.D.

Note: This vignette took place years ago. At present there are also "how to" books that I might present to the family, such as Stanley and Nancy Thorndike Greenspan's *The Essential Partnership* (1989).

TRIADIC INTERPRETATIONS: INCLUDING THE PARENT/CARETAKER IN THE TRIAD

A young mother brought her 1¾-year-old son, S., with the complaint that ever since he learned to walk at 1 year, she can't control him. He is stubborn, willful, and he will bang his head on the floor or wall to get his way. I observed them in the first session. Little S. made a shambles of the playroom, picking up and dumping everything in his path, ignoring his mother's efforts to get him to play with or put back the play materials. He would look at her and deliberately do what she had said no or "Don't touch" to, including the hot globe of a desk lamp. If she persisted, he began banging his head, which clearly upset her. "I can't stand it when he does that, so he wins every time."

The second session was an interaction between S. and myself, which mother observed through a small window. This time the playroom was bare, just table, chairs, and carpeted floor. S. looked around, looked at me, whined, and began to make head-banging gestures. I remained impassive. When the head-banging threats ceased, I asked him if he would like to play with a toy. He could talk in simple phrases, and he said O.K. I opened a cabinet door. He began to pull them out and dump, I stopped him, put them back, closed the door, and said, "Choose one—one at a time." He chose one. I closed the door. When he had mastered it and lost interest, I asked, "Would you like another?" He nodded. I said, "O.K., put this one back first." He whined, began the gesture toward head banging. I said, "Put it back," he did, and he chose another. The interpretation, made behaviorally, was, "I'm the boss here." Having established that, we went on to have some fun, reciprocal play, catch, roughhousing and with good affective interchange. He wanted to come again.

Afterwards, discussing this with his mother, I remarked that somehow he got a different message from me than from her about who is in charge, and that in order to feel secure a little child should feel that his parents are all-powerful.

Mother began to cry and described how she has always had a problem with males. Even her dogs. She couldn't get them to obey her, so she took them to a trainer who looked at them and said "Sit!" and they sat! When she asked why they didn't do that for her he said, "Lady, they know I mean it." She went on to tell me that she had seven older brothers who always bossed her around, and that she never felt she could prevail with any man. That's why she separated from her husband; she felt like nothing. I reassured her that she was indeed stronger and more responsible then her child, and that his victories only made him feel insecure and unhappy. Because of the deep-seated nature of her problem, she was referred for analysis.

Comment: The interpretation to the little boy was nonverbal. To the mother the message was that there must be some reason why you can't control your child . . . and that he needs your control. What she then brought up verified the interpretation.

In the case of a somewhat older child, one interprets and works through by playing out the traumatic situation (hospitalization with procedures, auto accidents; see the cases of M. and G. above).

A vignette of the case of J. has already been cited earlier in the chapter to illustrate an interpretation that brought a reduction in anxiety but not of clamming up, and brought an ability to return to school under certain conditions.

We now carry the case further to illustrate that interpreting in the presence of the parent may also be valuable even with a school-aged child who is capable of talking but overwhelmed with anxiety, inasmuch as the interpretation may overcome parental denial and guilt (usually unconscious), and may reveal a key piece of information enabling further interpretation to the child.

J. had improved enough so that mother no longer had to be on the school premises, or even at home (across the street) within telephone reach, and she could go back to work. However, he remained unabashedly tearful, impulsively gave up in class if he did not understand a problem immediately, or quitting a peer game—for example, softball, if he missed a catch. He would make himself look foolish by tripping and falling and responded to everything academic with "I can't" or "I don't know." He would complain of headaches and stomachaches. Thorough neurological and psychological testing for organically based learning disability came up with nothing. With one-on-one tutoring he did well in his academics.

In therapy sessions he would retreat to the corner of a chair, fearful and cringing, if asked about school or his fears. He was afraid of the subject, not of me, for if we played catch he could get active and throw hard and competitively and laugh. He could be this way also with his father. He enjoyed their outings.

When I invited his mother into a session, and the subject of school came up via her questions to him, he would revert to this anxious state and cling to her. I pointed out to both of them that he also was nervously clutching and fingering his neck as he whined, and could it be that there was something associated with school, or another other situation in which he was helpless and mother was not in a position to protect him, a situation that he can't remember because it's too scary, too overwhelming to deal with; yet his body does so with worry, anxiety, and stomachaches? We already know that when he was little (15–18 months) and in the hospital for ear problems and finally a tonsillectomy, they wouldn't let Mom stay in the room with him even though he was panicked. We also know that at 18 months he was knocked out by an object thrown by his 3-year-old brother and developed partial seizures, then at age 3 a big one, and that with medicine the seizures went away. In neurology clinic at age 3, they had to tie him down to draw a blood sample and again sent Mom out of the room. And seizures haven't come back even though they took his medicine away a year ago. Maybe he's afraid that he could get the shakes again, another thing he can't control. J.'s response was to burrow in closer to his mother.

The following week, J.'s mother reported that he was introduced by his kindly male principal to his new teacher-to-be for the fall term. He stated to his mother, "I like her, she's not mean." He also had had a great time camping out with his father and brother, and was very assertive and physically active. J. sat still with his worried look but admitted he had had fun. Mother had recalled that in kindergarten he came home crying, "Mrs. P. yelled at me," and did not want to return to school. Teacher told mother that this was her teaching style—she raised her voice at all the kids. J. was terribly sensitive, and afraid of her.

Then mother and father started looking back, that night, and both recalled an incident that had happened when he was in first grade and the school anxiety had escalated. A grandmotherly neighbor often baby-sat with J. She was raising her grandson Charley, of J.'s age, whose maiden aunt, K. K., visited frequently and was fiercely overprotective of Charley. "I'd *kill* for Charley." One afternoon J. came home hysterical. "K. K. choked me." There were red marks on his neck. K. K. told mother she pulled Charley off J., but mother found out that although K. K. would allow her nephew to beat up a peer, she would knock the child to the ground if the child would fight back at Charley.

At this point I made the mutative interpretation: "It was all a matter of being powerless, and having no control over what was happening to him—strapped down in the hospital—ear tubes, tonsils out. Look, you're holding your throat again!" I continued: "Later they studied you or your seizures, and you were afraid of the needle and you cried and cried, fought and fought, but it didn't do any good. They tied you down and sent your mother out of the room. Even she couldn't protect you! It really was scary. Again you were helpless, and that's also what this is all about. You must have felt like you couldn't even control your own body; when you got the seizures you even made in your pants and couldn't help it." Mother interjected that he had told her last night that he was afraid that if he had another attack, it would kill him.

"When K. K. choked you, Mom wasn't there—though she went right over when you told her. In school there was a mean teacher and Mom wasn't there to protect you. That's when you stopped playing with other kids your age."

I said that we must all work out our feelings about this. J. must be angry about being left, though he *now* knows Mom was helpless, too. It is always scary to find out that Mom and Dad aren't Supermom and Superdad after all. We've all had to find that out. We are working on those feelings and how they spilled over to school—Mom wasn't there if he needed her. Once he found out that Mom would take off and be there, he felt a little better. He also knew where she would be if he needed her, even when she is at work. But really he's a big boy and doesn't need her now like he did when he was a baby and in the hospital or in kindergarten; he can speak for himself. J. sat impassively but not cringing. Mother was in tears, blaming herself: "It was like child abuse." I reassured her that these were situations not in her control. What we need is to get J. and his family talking about how each felt so we could work out his difficulty in trusting his caretakers and his peers.

J. went on to do better academically and finished out the school year. He invited nine boys from school to his "best birthday I ever had," but again got upset when a bigger boy kicked him. Mother expressed disappointment that he was acting like a 2-year-old. He squirts kids with a squirt gun, then says, "I'm not allowed to get wet." I suggested that he was doing to boys what Charley did to him. Perhaps he thought, "If I grow up . . . I won't need Mom to protect me— I'll lose Mom!"

He began to be preoccupied with birthdays, deaths, and anniversaries: "Pop-Pop's birthday is in 2 days." (And you're acting strange and getting headaches and chewing your fingers again.) "Paw Paw (Who is he?), my great grandfather, he died." J. could not tell me how long ago he died (about 1½ years ago), or where, or what he died of. I told him I was told that everyone else loved Paw Paw too. They cried and got their feelings out while he couldn't . . . just like he couldn't when his dog had to be put away. His dog had to be sacrificed after he had bitten J. on the back. Perhaps he is afraid to cry—it hurts too much— he will feel overwhelmed by his feelings—and I am sure that he is worrying about what could happen to him.

The next session he looked scared and unhappy. Again the repeated "I don't know." "*You do* know but don't want to deal with it," I replied. This time he could tell me he was worried about his great-grandmother. I told him that his crying about the little things so easily took the place of crying about Paw Paw, whom he loved so much and was helpless to keep from dying. And now, he was told, his great grandma was very, very sick. He would feel better if he could talk about it.

J. began to talk to his mother, venting his anger at Paw Paw: "He died and left me!" At the time, he chose not to go to the funeral and though he was the closest, never cried although his parents and his brother did. "Am I going to die too and go to heaven?" Now that great grandma is dying, J. requested to see her. Mother said, "I realize I made a mistake in trying to protect him, so I am taking him to see her." They have been reassuring him that it's O.K. to cry. His father is taciturn and macho and not verbal or emotional. Somewhere J. learned it was bad to cry. Meanwhile he had a good, very physically active week at the beach. He and father were buddies. He became assertive, did not throw a tantrum when frustrated, and began to show discomfort at mother hugging or tickling him. He saw his great grandmother, who died shortly after his visit. He was able to mourn yet did not cry at the viewing. He still is working through his feelings about her death and the other deaths. Over the summer he has joined the scouts and is actively engaged with his peers. He is very actively involved with father and brother. They had a successful family reunion; he was competitive, and won a lot of prizes. He wants to march in the parade and was looking forward to school. He is pleased with himself, and the school is pleased with him; he has taken off academically. J. still sets himself up to be picked on, however. He occasionally reverts to whining at home and wants to sleep near his mother, who now refuses until he can tell her why. He can now say "I'm scared." I reassure her that he probably doesn't know why he is scared. Perhaps he's afraid he could lose her too and wants to make sure she is O.K. In any event I praised her taking things in hand and providing structure. She is aware, as is J., that there is yet more to work through.

This is a taste of the large amount of tedious and persistently repetitive supportive clarifications and interpretation that goes on in working through.

The themes are preoedipal: loss and helplessness. There is some hint of oedipal themes but these are more tied to the theme of baby versus big boy; his oedipal conflicts, I predict, will not be a problem.

At one time in analytic work there existed a rule with some child analytic teachers whereby analysts were to let the child know that "you don't tell your parents; you save it for the analyst." Parents were discouraged from getting involved and listening to their child's concerns. That was wrong, a position perhaps fed by the omnipotent self-importance that some felt then, or at least behaved as if they felt. J.'s case described above had to be done on a once-a-week basis. Having the mother as an intermediary therapist, and father cooperating with a strong, supportive relationship that involved a lot of physical activity and affective exchange, and doing things together rather than doing much talking, helped make a successful result possible. Remember that S., Freud's original child analytic case, though not so freewheeling, was through the father's exchange with Dr. Freud. It would be nice, of course, if we had the luxury of five sessions per week, but it is the basic method that counts, and interpretation and working through are at its core.

Where the trauma occurred in the pre-language years, interpretative play and interpretation can take place in front of the parent, and the interpreter-therapist can give voice to the infant's original concerns, saying what the infant could not say. Sometimes, in turn, the parent has associations for the nonverbal infant or the child who was not verbal at the time of the trauma. On the premise that she was the verbal member of the dyad, I have regularly had the mother free-associate while watching through a one-way mirror a therapy session with a nonverbal autistic child, bringing back repressed memories on the parents' part (See the case of L., below).

In work with nonspeaking autistic children as well as with other very young children, one frequently interprets to the caretaker–child dyad (usually the mother–child dyad). Keep in mind that an interpretation is an explanation, and that one of the purposes of interpretation is to elicit further information clarification. Given that the mother was the verbal part of the autistic dyad, and indeed is the articulate part of any normal dyad at the stage when the child has only preverberal affecto-sensory motor memories, it makes sense to interpret to both mother and child in the hope that the precipitants of Winnicott's "the unthinkable (or unspeakable) anxiety" (Davis and Wallbridge 1981, p. 46) of the child can be put into words by the mother. This is traumatic stress material that is rarely if ever presented in the initial developmental history given by the parents, in whom a self protective "say it isn't so" denial is operating. (See also the case of A., below.)

L., a 7-year-old autistic girl, was on a developmental plateau after having established an infantile, nonverbal relationship with me and her chief child-care worker. She was born at term, but precipitously, She was a ruminator who did not hesitate to back you off with projectile vomiting if she felt you were invading her space. Because a skilled infant observer noted that she used a corner of the playroom as if it were a crib and stayed within that limited space, and because, while playing peekaboo with her and varying the position of the napkin first covering my eyes and then just my nose and mouth, I noted that her eyes widened in fear when I shifted to the latter, I asked her mother to come in and observe the next play session through a one-way window, telling her to recapture for me anything it brought to mind from the past. Mother emerged from the observation booth visibly shaken. She had wanted to put this behind her. L. was fine when brought home—alert, even precociously reaching out and responsive. However, at the age of 1 month she developed a bad respiratory infection, which kept coming back despite the use of antibiotics. A pediatrician told her that L. suffered from a lack of gamma globulin and that she would have to be protected from germs or she might die. Mother frantically, and over the protests of her husband and L.'s older sister, set up a germ-free nursery. She forbade anyone but herself from entering, and she wore a surgical mask when entering to care for her daughter. She did handle her and pick her up, but as I interpreted to mother later, the baby saw no mouth movements to associate to the human voice. Mother said, "When I watched, I was reminded of that—how it must have looked to her when I wore the mask. L. pulled herself up early and would move along the edge of the crib and cry for me. Finally, by about 7 or 8 months, she lost her spark—gave up—her legs became rubbery and she wouldn't stand up anymore. Then she refused the bottle from me, so I had to prop it up for her." (Later on she was able to associate L.'s unusual finger movements in front of her own face to the way L. would curve her arm around a cribside post and her fingers under the propped-up bottle, after I had remarked to mother that these finger movements had the same rhythm as an infant sucking.)

I noted that this uncovering had caused L.'s mother much pain, but I was sure that she had done what she felt had to be done to save her daughter's life. I suggested that we both keep thinking about it and meet again the following week. I felt that any probing on my part would have been taken as accusatory (the question of dosage and timing of interpretation). I hoped that when she returned, *she* would make the interpretation.

She greeted me on her next visit with "I'll bet I know what you're going to ask: Why did I let it happen?" I nodded and asked, "Have you figured it out? It must have been something specially frightening to overcome your basic maternal instincts, for I *know* you're a good mother. I see how well you've raised your older daughter."

She said, "My mother has never liked me or my kids as much as my sisters. She came in one day while L. was congested and snapped, 'She sounds just like your brother did just before he died of pneumonia' (age 3). I got frantic and called the doctor."

I retorted, "And stayed so frantic you could not act on your gut feeling and get another opinion. You were marching to another drummer from your past."

When her older daughter was born, the woman in the next bed had cried when they did not bring her baby; they finally broke the news to the woman that her baby had died. After L. was born, the baby was not brought to her mother, and no one could convince her that L. had not died. (She was born precipitously on the way to the hospital and considered contaminated, and was kept isolated until they left the hospital.) I exclaimed at the many circumstances that had conspired to shape her fears, but the real clincher seemed to be missing. I paused, then asked, "Could it be that she herself had not been too happy about a new sib coming, and felt when he died that somehow it had been her fault? Kids at 4 and 5 feel wishing is like doing, though we grownups know better."

These types of interpretive interventions are important because the associative response of the parent to what she witnesses between her child and the therapist brings back affectively loaded memories that she has been trying to forget (deny). Her more informed state and integrated information about herself and her child allows mother another chance to work through old conflicts, which have shaped her responses to her child, leading to better understanding of her child, her relationship to her child, and a supportive relationship to both her child and the efforts of the therapist. Indeed, L.'s anxiety decreased, as did her mother's guilt, and their relationship improved. She later could understand why her autistic daughter could be so devilishly destructive of her best furniture pieces and selectively trash her mother's clothes, leaving those of her now grown sister's, side by side, intact. She could understand her daughter's anger at her inadvertent rejection in terms of what she herself had felt at the hands of her own mother. When our program had to send L. to another program (L. having long exceeded the age limits), her mother was bitter and unforgiving, and I in turn had to understand her anger as a transference of her own identified feelings of rejection, which I interpreted—but to no avail, the mother not having been in a therapeutic alliance for herself with me.

RECONSTRUCTION AND INTERPRETATION

Even when the very young child had developed speech and had related and communicated before the trauma, the "unspeakable" event can be so overloaded with affect that it cannot be put into words by the child and has to be slowly played out and reconstructed in nonverbal ways. Here too, interpretations shared with the parent can elicit needed information.

A. was referred at age 4 with the diagnosis of autism and atypicality confirmed by first-class psychological testing. Both parents have superior intelligence. Both family backgrounds were free of nervous or mental disorder; mother was enuretic into latency. Pregnancy and perinatal period were normal. A.'s social and motor milestones were accelerated. He was very cuddly. He was breastfed for 23 months. He gave it up abruptly at that time. By 14 months he was using four-to-five-word sentences and phrases and had a vocabulary of more than one hundred words. From 17–24 months A. had a series of negative experiences in baby-sitting and day-care situations culminating at 24 months in a private home day care setting in which he suddenly developed panicky crying, banging on doors and windows, not wanting to be closed in, and refusal to return to the day care setting. He lost his recently achieved toilet training. An anxiety-driven hyperactivity began. He ran in circles, flapping his hands then twisting and wringing them as he held them over his head. Later he began twisting crayons and paint brushes in the same manner. He stopped talking. By the times I saw him at age 4, he had begun to jargon and talk in phrases with slurred or infantile articulation. He had been entered in a series of special preschool programs in which he was described as perseverating, keeping to himself, and tuned out most of the time. Cognitive and social development was very slow. He became fascinated with lawnmowers and vacuum cleaners. He would perseveratively open and close doors. A.'s mother was present in the first sessions as an observer and interpreter of his slurred speech. She would bring his 3-month-old stepsister and nurse her. My first interpretation was that A. was telling me via his doll play that he is jealous of his nursing baby sister, which mother dismissed with "He doesn't even notice," at which point a wooden block came flying from A.'s direction and hit his sister on the back of the head. I said to mother, and for A.'s ears as well, that he not only understand what I was saying, but also that maybe I understand how he feels.

The advanced degree of his premorbid development (fully relating and talking) and the signs of his attachment to his mother suggested that something other than an autistic process was responsible for his condition. I shared this with his mother and stepfather, who reiterated the history of negative day-care experiences in which A. could name the teachers he didn't like, and culminating in his being shut in a room where mother found him with a load in his pants, banging on the door and window. Also, F., the mentally ill adult son of M., the proprietress, had been wandering around; a few days before, A.'s mother had come into the playroom and F. was there wrapped in a sheet. Mother now recalled that a few other mothers were pulling their children out at that time.

In subsequent sessions A. perseveratively painted unrecognizable scribbles, mostly in red paint, and gave them the names of barnyard animals and birds (chickens, ducks, etc.). He stared at these and would jump and flap and twiddle the paint brush. This went on for weeks, during which time he became both more dependent on his mother and more demanding of her time. He began to use the toilet and have a bowel movement just when mother was nursing his sister, and demand that she wipe him. "I don't want Mommy to hold L." (his sister). I told him that he wanted to be the baby, the only baby. In the midst of one of his scrawl drawings of animals there appeared a life-sized erect penis. When he gave it a nonsense name, in response to my asking "What is this?" I said, "It looks like a big man's penis." Since he made no response, I had no further questions or comments. I had a growing suspicion that a traumatic sexual abuse had occurred at age 2, but decided it was premature to raise the interpretive question at this time. He did begin to be concerned with the tackiness of the paints on his fingers. Compulsive handwashing began. His hand and finger twisting and wringing changed, taking on the quality of one trying to get something sticky off his fingers. At home he began to masturbate and also stick the four fingers of one hand into his mouth. He developed facial tics. Mother remembered that he used to love to play with finger paints, but this stopped abruptly just before she had withdrawn him from the nursery school, when he began to bang frantically on doors and windows, and his sudden violent reaction to anything messy or tacky on his fingers began.

At this point mother reported that a magazine article on child sexual abuse had set her thinking. The possibility that F., the proprietress's mentally ill son, had been sexually abusing A. had been gnawing at her mind but she had tried to suppress it because it had been too awful to think about and she felt guilty for not removing him sooner.

Mother asked A. if he remembered M.'s house. She reported that his response was to get up from the lunch table and open the back door. He began to cry and to look down at and clutch his genitals. Later she drove him by M.'s house. He stared, said nothing but wanted to cling to his mother. I suggested that she not press him with questions, and wait to see what he would bring out.

At the next session he painted his hands red and went through the hand wringing and washing. The following session he pointed toward the back of my house and said "M— —'s house" and was afraid to come upstairs to the playroom (above a detached garage). He opened a service closet door that he had a explored on previous occasions. He pulled out an upright vacuum cleaner and began manipulating the curved handle the way he had been manipulating paint brushes and rods, then sliding his hands up and down the curved section as if masturbating. Mother, who had been observing, asked, "Are you at M.'s house? Did F. do anything to you?" His response was to hop up and down frenetically and chant about milk and a baby cow in bed with its mommy, and climbed all over his mother as if pressing for her acceptance. He regressed to smearing his feces at home and calling himself "bad boy." Several sessions later he found a set of 14-inch round, tapered table legs in a cabinet drawer, began rubbing one against his cheek and mouthed it sideways, then put the tapered end into his mouth and began sucking. When I put the legs back in the drawer, he was driven to repeat and perseverate in the activity. In subsequent sessions A. went back to the vacuum cleaner and this time put his mouth around the end of the handle and sucked.

My only interpretation to A. was that something terrible had happened to him at M.'s house that he can't seem to put into words but is trying to show us. He referred to himself as "bad" and "bad boy" and to his baby sister's loaded diaper as "dirty" and "bad."(Remember that mother found him in a room crying with a load in his pants, a week before the "last straw" event at M.'s.) He was reassured that he was not bad, but the grown-up person who made him do it was the bad one. He periodically would go to the couch and pull his mother's coat over him like a sheet or blanket. He shoved a woodwind instrument down his throat till he gagged.

For A.'s mother and stepfather I reconstructed the probability that he was sexually molested by F. through oral insertion, being led to manipulate F.'s penis and probably F. having manipulated A.'s penis as well. Speech stopped because his area of traumatization was his mouth. The hand motions act out his manipulation as well as tactile involvement with the sticky ejaculate and handwashing. Mother tracked down a few other families who had pulled their children out at that time. None wanted to talk about it but implied that things had gone on, and one said on parting, "If you go to court I'll back you up."

From then on issues turned from learning and interpreting the meaning of his behaviors (I am telescoping 4 years of three-weekly, then twice-weekly, analytic therapy into this summary) to the reparative work of turning A.'s passivity and helplessness into activity—having some control over his situation.

Though he was eager to come to each session, he wanted to leave early. I interpreted to both that when he was at M.'s he had to wait till Mommy came, often a little late, and he was locked in a room more than once. Now he wants to be able to say when he can go home, and it was important for him to feel he could be in charge and his request should be honored. His water play involved not only handwashing compulsion but exquisite control of the stream of water from the spout. He insisted on being the one who turned it on and off. I had to resist the temptation to shut it off as it began overflowing. In turn I put him in charge of mopping up, not as a punishment but as part of the job. Each session he would produce a tremendous b.m., at first calling mother to wipe him but then, at my insistence, doing it himself. He should be the boss of his body (I was tossing in a little developmental stimulation as a secondary gain, because he had been toilet trained and then had regressed after the sexual trauma). At home and in therapy he had to be the one to open and close the doors and turn the light switches off and on, and would panic and tantrum if someone else got there first. Interpretations centered around his need to be the boss, to be in control, because he had been so helpless and powerless. He took over my desk and chair and periodically became the doctor; I took his role, using it as a way to verbalize for him what I felt he was struggling to communicate. Meanwhile, he was making cognitive progress with a developmental therapist who was focusing on learning and mastery issues and who found out that if he were allowed to work out his own solutions to tasks presented him, he would learn faster. The progress paralleled his progress in therapy.

A. took charge of watering my waiting-room plants, choosing the watering can with the long spout.

Once he looked in the mirror, put his four fingers in his mouth, and shook his head from side to side as he manipulated his fingers. I interpreted that he was moving his head so as to avoid something being put in his mouth. He said, "I cleaned it—feels ugly."

"What with?" I asked.

"With my fingers." He began to rub his fingers.

"As if you're getting something sticky off them," I said. (The reader will remember that I had made this observation to myself a few months before but did not feel he was ready for the interpretation at that time.) He looked scared and was quite depressed that night.

In subsequent sessions he charged at me with a snake and picked up a rubber knife and said, "Cut it! Cut it!" He made explicit drawings of an erect phallus, complete with glans and scrotum.

He began to put his fingers in his mouth and stared with a faraway look. I wondered if he were thinking of F. "Yes." He looked out the window to the back of my house. He was afraid I would take his pants off. He said, "He took off my pants." "Did he touch you?" I asked. He pointed to his buttocks and then to his genitals. He began to laugh wildly.

At home he told his mother he didn't like the food at Mrs. M.'s. Big, hard. It hurted. It got soft. Because he frequently sought candy from me and also ate Play Doh, I asked what the food tasted like, candy or Play Doh; then I reversed it. Play Doh or candy? He said Play Doh (Play Doh is salty). He was able to say later "F——is bad." "He hurt my face." He pointed to his temporomandibular joint, which hurts if one's mouth is opened excessively wide.

By the Christmas season at home, his controlling the lights and his running back and forth and finger manipulation continued but slowly diminished. However, he became more openly aggressive in the sessions.

Issues of anger became paramount. He began hitting mother, and conflicts about yet another pregnancy and new baby complicated the therapy. Strict limits had to be set at home.

He began physically attacking me as if I were F., while his cognitive functioning in special classrooms increased, as did his I.Q. by testing.

His repetitive activities at home and school were ameliorated to some extent by the addition of clomipramine to the therapeutic regimen, and the frantic need to be in control of the doors and light switches diminished. His infantile speech became more mature, but he found a lot of pleasure in manipulating words, asking questions (Why? What do you mean?) and making clang associations. He began acting silly and provocatively "crazy" to the point where the school psychiatrist was wondering about schizophrenia and urged antipsychotic chemotherapy, which I resisted. A. said, "Its fun to act crazy," a denial of his panicky frenetic state from ages 2 to 4 (I told him, "Just like you were after F. did that, but now you can turn it on and off. You're the boss of it.") This behavior in school diminished and ceased after a year.

As to transference, A. never completely gave up equating me with F. despite interpretations, physically attacking me. After a long plateau because of a bad back, which limited my ability to set physical limits, and for other considerations, he was transferred to a female psychotherapist with whom other issues came up and therapeutic progress resumed.

Comment: This partial case history illustrates the role of reconstruction as part of the preliminary work enabling clarification and interpretation. This case, which categorically fit *DSM-III-R*'s description of autism, was really a posttraumatic stress disorder that arrested and regressed development at a very crucial period in normal development. This case illustrated the role of the process of reconstruction and interpretation, and how interpretation to the adult caretaker can elicit information crucial to the understanding of the genesis of an acute disturbance. Also, in the young child we see how traumatic a state of helplessness can be and how, given the proper interpretation, waiting until the child can accept it without being overwhelmed—even waiting as long as I did may have been barely enough time—one can, through interpretations, work through the therapeutic task of establishing activity over passivity and give the child a measure of security in having control, first of his environment (a healthier defense) and then over himself (a developmental maturation). This also illustrates the possibility that at a certain point a second therapist may have to complete the job.

INTERPRETATION TO THE HANDICAPPED CHILD: ADDRESSING ISLANDS OF NEUROTIC DEFENSE

Since the parent was and is a part of the dyadic or triadic relationship with the very young child, it is helpful to have parents involved in the therapeutic process. This is especially true when providing therapy for young developmentally disabled, minimally brain-damaged, or otherwise handicapped children. Almost without exception there is a secondary emotional disorder with neurotic defenses (denial, reaction formation, etc.), anxieties, and lowered self-esteem. These children feel rejected, derided, unloved, and unworthy, and react to the world with mistrust.

Minimal brain dysfunction interferes with play and cognition via poor memory, distractibility, poor motor coordination, and poor impulse control, thus contributing to low self-esteem and poor self-image, as well as poor family and social interaction.

Interpretation therefore must not only clarify reality but support and assure continued ego control, and encourage his mastering of experience by changing passivity into taking action.

In general, dealing with the handicapped child's neurotic defenses through clarifying interpretation of poor self-image opens up the way for the child to be motivated to make full use of his special education and remedial training.

While most autism and pervasive developmental disabilities have a neurological basis, they too have secondary emotional components, anxieties, and self-image problems that benefit from psychotherapeutic intervention.

THE LIMITING IMPACT OF THE THIRD PARTY PAYMENT AND MANAGED CARE SYSTEMS ON INTERPRETATION AND WORKING THROUGH

Finally, a word about the impact of managed care on the psychoanalytically oriented therapy of the young child. In my descriptions of the use of interpretation as the key element in the therapeutic process, I have outlined a process by which the therapist elicits, listens, and observes what the child is saying, feeling, and doing, and vis-à-vis his detailed knowledge about human development, assigns meaning and understanding to what he observes and then imparts to the child his understanding in a way that can overcome or bypass resistance, not overwhelm the child's defenses and cause anxiety and further resistance. This is accomplished through a series of clarifications, making connections and integrating interpretations. One must at the same time develop a therapeutic alliance not only with the child but also with his caretakers, on whom the child is dependent in the here and now. Furthermore, in order to make real changes this process must be repeated over and over again in the course of working through. This is a slow and long-term process, which is less and less often supported by third-party insurance payments—especially the managed health care plans that are directing the insurance programs for big companies.

In many instances, knowing there are only a limited number of sessions to do the job, one has to obtain the background history, come to an understanding of the problem, and make an introductory or even a mutative interpretation—or at least one that intrigues the patient into a therapeutic alliance—often making intuitive (really one's own unconscious scanning) assumptions by virtue of one's years of experience and clinical feel, assumptions that usually turn out to be correct or at least close. For example:

A large 13-year-old boy, looking perhaps 18, was referred by the school for academic failure, disruptive behavior, alcoholism, and suicidal threats escalating over the past 1½ years. At home he refused to help out. His father had died almost 2 years before. I dwelt on his depressed and angry affect and asked a few questions about his father's death. I interpreted that he missed his father and what they used to do together, was hurt and angry about his loss of his father, and that he hadn't really finished mourning his death, and that drinking and disruptive school behavior and flunking was a way to punish his father as if to say "See what happens when you leave me—come back and get me in line." He knows father can't, so I proposed, "Why don't I take over for awhile via therapy? First of all, here's a pill for your depression and mood swings. It will take the edge off the pain and sadness enough for us to be able to work on your problem. You can't drink alcohol with this pill, or you'll feel like someone shot you through the head. You have a lot of talking and crying to do about your father— it's O.K. to cry—you can do it in here. It's O.K. to help your mother. She needs it; she has a bad heart. I guess you've been told you're the man of the house now." He nodded yes. "Well—in a way you are, but it's not like taking his place. No one could do that. But I'm sure he'd like to see you help out. I'll call the school principal and see if we can get you back in, but you've got to promise to get down to work."

This "crunching" of interpretations defused his oedipal conflicts, encouraged his mourning, noted and accepted his anger and hurt at his father's leaving, suggested he was trying to punish his father by hurting himself, and allied me as a father substitute in working things out with the school—all in the first session. He did stop drinking. He called to bring his sister in to meet me; she needed help too. He was accepted back at school. We did some further work on his feelings, but I could only get to see him twice monthly, then monthly. This was not psychoanalysis but what I like to call "psychoanalytically oriented intervention"—more spare and lean than psychoanalytically oriented psychotherapy, which has the luxury (if it sounds cynical, I am) of weekly or twice-weekly sessions. His improvement held up for a year. Obviously, without building a solid structure by working through, his new ego strengths were shaky, not fully his own but partially, through transference identification and incorporation.

Too often, unfortunately, this will be the patched-on "cure" of the future until the insurance companies and whatever national health care plan that, hopefully, replaces the present system come to their senses and realize that a *thorough* job of psychotherapy is cost effective, reducing recidivism and the secondary, much more expensive, problem of substance abuse and associated criminality.

Meanwhile the psychoanalytic principles of defining, clarifying, and interpreting the problem and intriguing the patient into the therapeutic alliance can be used in dealing with the managed care reviewers. They too are human beings, by and large intelligent, compassionate, and interested. I try to make them a part of the therapeutic alliance, clarify and explain to them generally without revealing family or personal details. I get the name of the reviewer and request the same reviewer for allotment of further time. I find that they become involved, sometimes in spite of themselves, and often offer more in frequency and number of sessions than I ask for: "Don't you want to talk things over with his mother more often? I think it's helped." By treating them with respect, and giving them the experience of following cases through to completion (they may have otherwise have put an arbitrary limit on the number of sessions, saying "too bad but that's the rules"), one develops a therapeutic ally. As an ally they too want to see this kid get better, and they feel they have had a personal stake in the patient's recovery. Another example that psychoanalytic principles of human nature apply to us all!

REFERENCES

Allen, F. H. (1942). *Psychotherapy with Children*. New York: W. W. Norton.
Call, J. D., Reiser, D. E., and Gislason, I. L. (1979). Psychiatric intervention with infants. In *Basic Handbook of Child Psychiatry*, vol. 3, ed. J. Noshpitz and S. Harrison, pp. 457–483. New York: Basic Books.

Davis, M., and Wallbridge, D. (1981). *Boundary and Space: An Introduction to the Work of D. W. Winnicott*. London: Karnac.

Erikson, E. H. (1950). *Childhood and Society*. New York: W. W. Norton.

Fenichel, O. (1941). *Problems of Psychoanalytic Technique*. Albany, NY: Psychoanalytic Quarterly.

Freud, A. (1946). *The Ego and Mechanisms of Defense*. New York: International Universities Press.

———— (1965). *Normality and Pathology in Childhood*. New York: International Universities Press.

Gesell, A., and Amatruda, C. S. (1974). *Developmental Diagnosis*. 3rd ed. Ed. H. Knobloch and B. Pasmanick. Hagerstown, MD: Harper & Row.

Greenson, R. (1967). *The Technique and Practice of Psychoanalysis*. New York: International Universities Press.

Greenspan, S. (1992). *Infancy and Early Childhood: The Practice of Clinical Assessment and Intervention*. Madison, CT: International Universities Press.

Greenspan, S., and Greenspan, N. T. (1989). *The Essential Partnership*. New York: Viking Penguin.

Mahler, M., Pine, F., and Bergman, A. (1975). *The Psychological Birth of the Human Infant–Symbiosis and Individuation*. New York: Basic Books.

Moore, B., and Fine, B., eds. (1990). *Psychoanalytic Terms and Concepts*. New York: The American Psychoanalytic Association and Yale University Press.

Noyes, A. P. (1953). *Modern Clinical Psychiatry*. 4th ed. Philadelphia: Sanders.

Oremland, J. D. (1991). *Interpretation and Interaction Psychoanalyses on Psychotherapy*. Hillsdale, NJ: Analytic Press.

Oxford English Dictionary (1971). New York: Oxford University Press.

Random House Dictionary of the English Language (1967). New York: Random House.

Sandler, S., Kennedy, H., and Tyson, R. (1980). *The Technique of Child Psychoanalysis–Discussions with Anna Freud*. Cambridge, MA: Harvard University Press.

Spitz, R. (1965). *The First Year of Life*. New York: International Universities Press.

Stern, D. (1985). *The Interpersonal World of the Infant*. New York: Basic Books.

Temeles, M. (1986). A developmental line for narcissism. Paper presented at the Vulnerable Child Seminar at the Midwinter Meeting of the American Psychoanalytic Association, New York City, December 18.

Waelder, R. (1936). The principle of multiple function–observations on overdetermination. *Psychoanalytic Quarterly* 5:45–62.

9

Countertransference

Robert C. Prall, M.D.

Countertransference reactions are ubiquitous in psychotherapeutic and psychoanalytic treatment of children and adults in both inpatient and outpatient settings. The more disturbed the patient, the more prone the therapist and staff to respond with countertransference reactions that may adversely affect the outcome of treatment. Thus, an understanding of the potential for countertransference and identification of the common areas of difficulty can assist in training and supervision and in the process of self-examination by the therapist in the course of everyday work with disturbed patients.

DEFINITION AND REVIEW OF THE LITERATURE

There are many divergent uses of the term *countertransference* in the literature. Some authors use the term in the broadest sense to include any reactions of the therapist to the patient, while others apply it strictly to the therapist's unconscious reactions to the patient's unconscious transference manifestations.

Countertransference in Work with Adults

Freud in 1910 spoke of countertransference for the first time. Speaking of the analyst, he stated, "We have become aware of the 'counter-transference,' which arises in him as a result of the patient's influence on his unconscious feelings, and we are almost inclined to insist that he shall recognize this counter-transference in himself and overcome it."

He added, " . . . no psycho-analyst goes further than his own complexes and internal resistances permit; . . ." (pp. 144–145).

In 1915, in "Observations of Transference Love," Freud dealt with the problem of the female patient's love for the male analyst and the analyst's reactions to this problem. "For the doctor the phenomenon signifies a valuable piece of enlightenment and a useful warning against any tendency to a counter-transference which may be present in his own mind. He must recognize that the patient's falling in love is induced by the analytic situation and is not to be attributed to the charms of his own person . . ." (pp. 160–161). He indicated that the treatment must be carried out in abstinence, and that "we ought not to give up the neutrality towards the patient, which we have acquired through keeping the counter-transference in check" (p. 164). He stated further, "It is therefore plain to him that he must not derive any personal advantage from it [the patient's love for the analyst]" (p. 169). "Those who are still youngish and not yet bound by strong ties may in particular find it a hard task" (p. 169). "The psycho-analyst knows that he is working with highly explosive forces and that he needs to proceed with as much caution and conscientiousness as a chemist" (p. 170).

Reich (1960) stated, "Counter-transference is found to represent not only an interfering agent, but an essential catalytic one needed to achieve the therapeutic goals of psycho-analysis" (p. 389). Reich further indicated that countertransference responses, either libidinous or aggressive, or defenses against them ". . . or identifications and ego attitudes connected with a specific past conflict in the analyst" may cause anxiety, inappropriate emotion, lack of understanding, or boredom in the analyst (p. 389). Reich also indicated that it is a misconception to equate countertransference with the analyst's total response to the patient, that is, all conscious reactions, responses, and behavior. She clarified that "the delicate process of trial identification is fraught with many hazards, and its failure manifests itself as countertransference. . . . [The analyst] may return love with love, hate with hate, failing to identify and to detach himself again." Or "he may get stuck in some of these trial identifications because they please him too much: he becomes unwilling and unable to relinquish them . . . the analyst remains identified with the patient (or the latter's object). He behaves and feels like the patient, which will render him blind to the patient's defences" (p. 391). She concluded, "we should be alert to our own feelings, stop to investigate them and analyse what is going on. For the analyst's awareness of his undue emotional response warns him of an obstacle that interferes with his competent functioning, and ought to be removed. *"The counter-transference as such is not helpful, but the readiness to acknowledge its existence and the ability to overcome it is"* (p. 392).

Kernberg (1965) differentiated between two concepts of countertransference, the classical approach and the totalistic one. The classical approach is that delineated by Freud originally, and espoused by others, which relegates the concept of countertransference to the analyst's unconscious reactions to the patient's transference. The totalistic approach includes the total emotional reactions of the analyst to the patient, both conscious and unconscious. This approach uses a broader definition of countertransference and advocates more active use of it. In describing this approach, Kernberg pointed out one of its positions. "When the analyst feels that his emotional reaction is an important technical instrument for understanding and helping the patient, the analyst feels freer to face his positive and negative emotions evoked in the transference situation, has less need to block these reactions, and can utilize them for his analytic work" (p. 40).

Kernberg also described a continuum of countertransference reactions to patients from those experienced with neurotic patients on one end to those with severe disorders, including psychoses, on the other.

> When dealing with borderline or severely regressed patients, as contrasted to those presenting symptomatic neuroses and many character disorders, the therapist tends to experience rather soon in the treatment intensive emotional reactions having more to do with the patient's premature, intense and chaotic transference, and with the therapist's capacity to withstand psychological stress and anxiety, than with any particular, specific problem of the therapist's past. [p. 43]

He added that countertransference thus becomes an important diagnostic tool. In his discussion of countertransference reactions to borderline or psychotic patients, Kernberg stated that the most serious countertransference disturbances in handling the pregenital aggression are those involving the severe, archaic aggression in the patient, "expressed typically by the therapist's emotional reaction to the patients who always seem to have to bite the hand that feeds them" (p. 49). He added, "In dealing with severely regressed patients, dedicated therapists of all levels of experience live through phases of almost masochistic submission to some of the patient's aggression, disproportionate doubts in their own capacity, and exaggerated fears of criticism by third parties" (p. 50). He added two important points. First, "Willingness to review a certain case with a consultant or colleague, as contrasted with secrecy about one's work, is a good indication of concern" (p. 52). Second, "The therapist's lack of experience or of technical or theoretical knowledge has to be differentiated from his countertransference reaction. This is not easy because these two factors influence each other" (p. 53).

In Winnicott's paper (1949), "Hate in the Countertransference," he made cogent observations concerning the therapist's reactions to severely disturbed (psychotic) patients. He stated that "the countertransference needs to be understood by the psychiatrist. . . . However much he loves his patients he cannot avoid hating them and fearing them, and the better he knows this the less will hate and fear be the motives determining what he does to his patients" (p. 195).

He classified countertransference phenomena as (1) countertransference feelings based on relationships and identifications that are repressed, which require more analysis for the therapist; (2) identifications and tendencies belonging to an analyst's personal experience and development, which provide a positive setting for analysis; (3) the truly objective countertransference, the analyst's love and hate in reaction to the patient's actual personality and behavior, based on objective observation.

Winnicott stated further that with psychotic and antisocial patients, one must be aware of the countertransference to sort out the objective reactions to the patient, including hate.

He pointed out that just as a mother has to tolerate hating her baby without doing anything about it,

> the analyst must find himself in a position comparable to that of the mother of a new-born baby. When deeply regressed the patient cannot identify with the analyst or appreciate his point of view any more than the fetus or newly born infant can sympathize with the mother. . . . A psychotic patient in analysis cannot be expected to tolerate his hate of the analyst unless the analyst can hate him. . . . An analyst has to display all the patience and tolerance and reliability of a mother devoted to her infant; has to recognize the patient's wishes as needs; has to put aside other interests in order to be available and to be punctual and objective; and has to seem to want to give what is really only given because of the patient's needs. [pp. 202–203]

It is important to keep in mind that every action or reaction of the therapist is not based on countertransference. As Anna Freud (1954) pointed out in discussing the wide variety of approaches that analysts make to similar cases, "they are determined, of course, not by the material, but by the trends of interest, intentions, shades of evaluation, which are peculiar to every individual analyst. I do not suggest that they should be looked for among the phenomena of countertransference" (p. 359).

Others in the literature indicate that countertransference reactions are more common with more severely disturbed patients. Kohut (1971) noted the countertransference phenomenon of boredom in working with the mirror transference in treatment of the narcissistic personalities, whereas Kernberg (1980) attributed the boredom to the patient functioning as if he or she were self-sufficient. Adler (1986), in his discussion of Kohut's and Kernberg's approaches to therapy of the narcissistic personality disorders, stated that "the narcissistic personality disorder patient's defensive style and/or 'fragmentation' present countertransference difficulties that make treatment seem stalemated under the best of circumstances" (p. 433).

Countertransference in Child Therapy

In a panel on the differences between child and adult analysis (Casuso 1965), Marianne Kris stated in her discussion, "While it is very tempting to use parameters on the rationale that the special conditions of the young age of the patient require it, the rationale is usually a poor one and what actually takes place is that the analyst projects onto the child an uneasiness of his own" (p. 161). In the same panel, Anthony subscribed to the view that countertransference in child analysis is one of the great obstacles in the way. In addition, Bonnard pointed out that countertransference problems are often occasioned by seeing a child in a room where the analyst worries about cherished objects. Rangell indicated that the child analyst should resist the tendency to become the proud parent and to unconsciously hold on to the patient through subsequent development so as to enjoy the success of the analysis.

In inpatient settings for children, the countertransferences are extremely complicated because of the large number of workers from various disciplines who must relate to the child patient in a consistent fashion for therapy to succeed. Ekstein and associates' (1959) frank discussion of the failure in residential treatment of a symbiotic psychotic child owing to massive countertransference problems among the staff is of considerable significance in this connection.

Szurek and Berlin (1973) and their colleagues at the Langley Porter Neuropsychiatric Institute described a number of major countertransference problems in the work with psychotic children. Among other papers in that collection, Christ (1973) gave a candid discussion of the countertransference difficulties he encountered as a trainee in regard to the sexually provocative behavior of a nearly mute 14-year-old girl.

Yandell (1973), in the same volume, explored countertransference problems related to the expression of sexual drives in psychotic children, presenting six cases illustrating tension-filled instances in which the therapeutic problems related to the expression of sexual drives in the child. As with Christ's case, the work with these children highlighted the frequency with which young trainees are faced with sexual countertransference problems.

Christ (1973) pointed out the great difficulty in working with psychotic children. "I am finding that the willingness to work for long periods of time with uncertainty and apparent absence of confirmatory data from a patient is requisite for the therapist working with the nonverbal schizophrenic child" (p. 495). He also commented on the silence in the literature on countertransference problems at that time. More recently there has been an increase in the attention to the subject in the literature.

In a similar setting, Prall (1959) and his colleagues at the Eastern Pennsylvania Psychiatric Institute, in their many years of psychotherapeutic work with psychotic children, uncovered findings similar to those of Szurek and Berlin. Many of these findings were presented in a series of workshops at the American Orthopsychiatric Association on the research into the treatment of childhood psychosis. It became clear that the work conducted in various centers showed many common denominators in terms of the etiology and treatment of childhood psychosis as well as awareness of the tendency to countertransference problems in this type of work.

Prall (1960), in the introduction to the panel on "Training in Orthopsychiatry," described many of the countertransference tendencies encountered with mental health trainees. He pointed out that the choice of a mental health profession is motivated by inner needs, personality patterns, and personal satisfactions derived from the work. It is our obligation to train personnel (1) to be helpful to patients, (2) to do no harm, (3) to be as objective as possible in observations and reporting what transpires, (4) to be aware of and keep one's own needs under control, (5) to be noncritical and nonjudgmental and to keep one's own value judgments to oneself in order to help the patient develop his or her own values, (6) to maintain therapeutic optimism and avoid therapeutic nihilism no matter how difficult the treatment may become, and (7) to avoid acting out one's own emotional needs with patients or vicariously through patients. Most significant, (8) one must keep narcissism and omnipotent rescue fantasies under control so that one may tolerate the slow and usually laborious process of helping people to develop and mature emotionally. These are among the most important countertransference factors that contribute to the phenomena of "burn-out" and job dissatisfaction, particularly in inpatient work with seriously disturbed children and adolescents.

COUNTERTRANSFERENCE DIFFICULTIES IN WORK WITH PARENTS

An important area of potential countertransference conflicts lies in the work with parents, as pointed out by Prall and Stennis (1964), who stated, "Difficulties in work with parents result from the therapist's guilt, fear, or anxiety about his relationships with them. Avoidance of the parents, postponing interviews, undercharging them, or showing antagonism often result from the therapist's unresolved guilt toward his own parents, displaced onto the family of his patient" (p. 9). This may lead to problems in being sufficiently firm and direct with the child's family.

The Preparatory Period of Work with the Parents

Young or inexperienced therapists may find it difficult to stand up to powerful, controlling, or dominant parents who attempt to control and manipulate the therapeutic situation, for example, by trying to bargain about fees or attempting to rearrange the appointment times to their convenience.

Another countertransference pitfall for young and inexperienced therapists is the problem of establishing their role of authority with the parents at the beginning of treatment. The tendency to capitulate to parental demands in order to curry parents' favor can lead to interferences with the treatment situation. It may prove particularly distressing to the young therapist when the parents demand to know how much experience one has had with this type of case and what the therapist's experience has been with successful treatment of such children, when the young therapist may never have treated such a child before. It is not uncommon for parents to attempt to manipulate the therapist into helping them cheat on insurance claims. For example, if there is a new insurance plan that requires a 6-month waiting period before payments may be made, the parents may ask one to use a false date for the beginning of therapy so that they may collect the third party payments.

This is not only highly ill advised, in that it allows the parents to manipulate, it is also dishonest and illegal. Because one must sign insurance forms attesting to their veracity, one should never give false information. It is also essential in all of one's dealings with parents and children to remain scrupulously honest in all one does and says at all times. Allowing oneself to be corrupted can only serve to undermine one's veracity and authority and gives the parents a sense of being able to blackmail or otherwise cajole the therapist into doing what they wish.

Another pitfall to be avoided in this connection occurs when a family offers to make a large payment in advance for treatment. Such an arrangement would compromise the therapist's objectivity and independence, since it would give the family the feeling that they own the therapist and could therefore make excessive demands on him or her. One should politely refuse such an offer and point out that reimbursement can only be accepted for services rendered. Accepting an advance payment would cause great difficulty if the family were not cooperative and one wished to terminate the treatment relationship.

There are some parents who will soon become threatened by the child's positive attachment to the therapist, particularly those mothers who have an unresolved symbiotic attachment to their child. It is necessary to recognize and avoid countertransference reactions to such a response and to promptly help the parents with their fears of "losing their child." One must explain that it is necessary for successful therapy for children to become attached to the therapist temporarily, but that it is our aim in treatment to use the therapeutic relationship to help the child overcome the problems of which the parents have complained and that it is not our intention to try to take the child away from them but rather to help the child get along better with them.

Occasionally parents may forbid the therapist to discuss certain topics with their child such as family secrets, skeletons in the family closets, a miscarriage, parental divorce, previous marriages, the child's adoption, religion, or sexuality. In the preparatory period of work with the parents before seeing the child, it is imperative to establish the ground rules for therapy, which must include the parents' willingness for one to discuss *any and all areas* of the child's life, thoughts, fantasies, and feelings that may emerge in therapy, including taboo areas that the parents may fear. If one states that it will not be possible to treat the child with such limitations, most parents will relent. If they do not, it is most likely that the case would not proceed in a satisfactory manner and one should refuse to begin treatment. If the therapist has countertransference difficulties with regard to fear of the parents, it will be difficult to handle such delicate issues.

The Informative Alliance with the Parents

Because children usually are not capable of telling about their past histories or their current environmental situations, it is essential to maintain what Mahler referred to as the "informative alliance." Kramer and Prall (1971), in their description of Mahler's child analysis training program at the Philadelphia Psychoanalytic Institute, reviewed her conceptualization of the working alliance with the parents.

> We do *not* substitute the information gathered from the informative alliance for that derived from the therapeutic alliance with the child. The material from the parent . . . serves as background information, a kind of corollary stream of information which confirms and clarifies our understanding of the child's material and the forces in his reality environment. . . . We do not make use of the content from the informative alliance in such a way as to rob the child's ego of its autonomy in the analysis. [p. 493]

Confidentiality

Other preparatory steps should include helping the parents to respect the confidentiality between child and therapist. If this is not adequately handled, many parents will insistently implore the therapist for details of what their child is saying and doing in therapy. Often countertransference issues regarding parents make it difficult for some therapists to hold the line on confidentiality, and they submit to pressure from the parents to reveal the child's material. Doing so can rapidly undermine the therapeutic alliance and the child's trust in the therapist, and should be avoided.

At other times parents, or other relatives, may telephone the therapist with some piece of family news (e.g., a pending separation, divorce, or illness in the family) and indicate that the therapist should not tell the child that they have called. This, again, is countertherapeutic and must not be agreed to. In the preparatory phase, it is necessary to cover such situations with the family and explain that we must be completely honest with the child at all times and not keep secrets. If such a call occurs, one should advise the caller to inform the child about the call and what was reported and to obtain the calling person's agreement that it will be necessary to deal with the child's reaction to the news when it comes up in therapy.

It also happens that parents will request the therapist to be the bearer of bad news to the child because they, themselves, are afraid of the child's affective displays and are reluctant to deal with difficult issues. This is also contraindicated, although it might be possible to invite the parent to join in the therapy session for a few minutes at the beginning of an appointment to discuss the difficult issue with the child in the therapist's presence. The therapist can then deal with the child's emotional reactions in treatment.

Family Background Issues

Other potential countertransference issues may arise in the course of the therapist's attempting to obtain the family background history. Some parents are reluctant to reveal their personal histories and information about their family history including mental illness, alcoholism, or drug addictions in the family. It is imperative to be firm in presenting the need for truthfulness on the parents' part if one is to be able to help their child, since family patterns of personality types and various disease entities—for example, manic-depressive illnesses—are most important to our understanding of the child's diagnosis and treatment planning. The unconscious identifications between parents and their children can shed considerable light on the child's psychopathology. Thus, one must obtain detailed information concerning the parents' perceptions, ambitions, fantasies, feelings, and aspirations for their child as well as the parents' attitudes about the child's conception. One should not be afraid to pursue these issues in spite of parental reluctance.

Countertransference Problems with Parents during Child Therapy

Overidentification with "the hurt little child" in its struggle with the "bad parents" can only lead to major countertransference problems with the family and often results in parental negative transference and broken treatment relationships. One should remember that the parents are real people who have had serious trouble coping with their offspring whom they have entrusted to our care, and one should avoid criticizing them. Instead, one should maintain an empathic attitude toward the parents at all times. One tends to encounter negative reactions to parents more frequently with those therapists who are not parents themselves and have not suffered the pangs of parenting children through difficult times. Negative attitudes toward the child's parents also occur more frequently with those therapists who have had severe struggles and negative relationships with their own parents.

An additional parental countertransference pitfall lies in unconscious rescue fantasies and a tendency to compete with the parent for the child's affection, or to set out to show that one can be a "better parent" than the child's own parents. This serves to heighten the child's loyalty conflict between the therapist and the parents and results in therapeutic difficulties.

When such a situation arises, a child may show evidence of the heightened loyalty conflict in the waiting room by clinging to the mother and refusing to come into the playroom or protesting about not liking the therapist. Then, once in the playroom, the attitude quickly changes and becomes positive. Often such a child may not want to leave at the end of the session. Inexperienced therapists sometimes become anxious and find this difficult to handle. One should interpret the loyalty conflict by saying to the child, "It seems to me that you have very mixed feelings about being here: not wanting to come into the playroom, and then not wanting to leave when the time is over. I think this has to do with your not being sure whether you like this place at all or whether you prefer to be with Mother instead." One may also deal with the loyalty conflict by saying, "It seems to me that you want Mother to be sure that you don't like this place and that you want to be with her instead."

Mahler (1960) also cautioned against expressing negative attitudes to a child about the parents. The child may say all manner of negative things about the parents, and one can make a confrontation such as, "You are certainly feeling very angry about the way your parents treat you, and I can understand why." But one should avoid saying, "Yes, they really are terrible people," since, no matter how cruel or abusive the parents may be, if one criticizes them, the negative transference increases, and the child will invariably come to their defense and say, "Don't *you* say that about *my* parents!"

On the other hand, siding with the parents against the "bad" child and admonishing about the bad behavior that has annoyed the parents will hinder the development of the positive transference and the therapeutic alliance essential to treatment. Injudicious use of the informative alliance material from the parents can make the child's ego feel attacked rather than supported by the therapist. (See Kramer and Prall [1971].) Thus one should avoid reciting the bad things that the parents have reported, which would make the child feel that you are on the parents' side rather than on his or hers. Of course, one must not ignore the parents' complaints, but the child must be helped to deal with them in an ego-syntonic fashion rather than being overwhelmed by a list of parental complaints, which can only serve as a further narcissistic injury and lead to negative transference and increased resistance.

Countertransference and Fees

Parents, as part of their difficulty in caring for their child, may fail to pay the fees for therapy. Thus it is important for the therapist to remain apprised of the timeliness of payments for treatment as therapy progresses. If the payments fall behind, this is very often due to parental negative transference and signals the need to meet with the parents and discuss their feelings about the child's progress, or lack of it, and to clarify their feelings behind the delay in payments. Unless payments are kept current, countertransference difficulties may ensue. One soon becomes tired of waiting endlessly for reimbursement for the work done, and resentment may build up toward the parents. There is a real danger that the parents may stop the child's treatment, much to the detriment of the child, if such a situation is not cleared up promptly.

Sometimes there are legitimate financial difficulties, such as loss of the parents' employment. If treatment is essential for the child and one is dedicated to helping the youngster, it may be possible to offer to reduce the fees temporarily until new employment is secured. Often parents will agree to this and offer to pay the balance later when they can afford to do so. Sometimes it may be possible for the grandparents or others in the family to help out by supporting the child's therapy if they have the resources. One should not abruptly break off treatment with a child in the midst of dealing with the many issues involved in solving the riddles of the psychopathology.

Intrusive Parents

A very troubling source of countertransference difficulties lies in dealing with intrusive parents. There are those parents who will endeavor to intrude on the child's appointment times. This occurs especially when there is a major negative transference to the therapist on the part of a parent. The critical parent may criticize the therapist's handling of various issues in front of the child or attempt to give instructions on how one should treat the child or what to tell the child. This is, of course, very detrimental to the child's therapy and should be dealt with firmly by insisting that these matters be dealt with in separate appointments with the parent at the earliest opportunity.

Some parents are very inquisitive about what is going on in therapy and will quiz their child insistently after each visit. One may overhear a mother in the waiting room asking her child, "What did you tell the doctor?" Or she may ask, "Did you tell the doctor that you were a bad girl in school today?" It is imperative to help such a parent to stop this kind of interrogation, since it will interfere with therapy if the child feels that its mother wants to know everything he or she tells the therapist.

By contrast, another problem that often evokes countertransference difficulties may occur when a parent develops a strong positive transference to the therapist and attempts to enter into a therapeutic relationship with the therapist, thus shutting out the child. This may manifest itself by parents insisting on phoning the therapist at all hours on the slightest pretext, or whenever they are anxious. Such situations may need to be handled by referring such a parent to a colleague for therapy after discussing with the parent the need for additional help.

One of the most annoying behaviors of parents is their forgetting appointments or showing up at the wrong time or on the wrong day. Severe transference and countertransference difficulties may occur when two child patients and their parents appear in the waiting room at the same time. These difficult situations can provoke anxiety and distress for the therapist who must send away one patient without his or her being seen. One technique for dealing with these situations is to have a firm policy of charging for missed appointments that occur without sufficient notice or without legitimate reasons. It is best to have this policy in writing, in a treatment-plan form signed by the parents, so that they cannot say that they were unaware of the policy. To help avert such situations it is helpful to write out the appointment schedule for parents, thereby reducing the likelihood of confusion.

Countertransference Reactions to Parents' Separation and Divorce

When one has been treating a child for some time and the parents decide on separation and divorce, this may occasion considerable countertransference reactions for the therapist. All too often the therapist may have stronger positive feelings for the parent who has been more supportive of the treatment. Likewise, negative countertransference reactions may occur toward the other parent. This may lead the therapist to tend to side with one or the other parent. If one receives a subpoena to appear for a deposition or in court to testify in favor of one of the parents in a custody dispute, this can only serve to interfere with the child's treatment. Having to choose between the parents heightens the child's loyalty conflicts and places the therapy in great jeopardy.

To illustrate this type of situation, a case in which the author had treated two of the children in the family, beginning several years earlier, will highlight the dilemmas one may encounter.

Allen, the middle sibling of three, with a half-brother, Jack, 4 years older, and a newborn sister, Heather, 5 years younger, was referred for therapy at age 5 while in kindergarten. He was depressed and moody and said that everyone hated him and that he was no good and should be dead. He was overweight and had very poor peer relationships. In school he had behavior problems and was not adjusting well to the school situation. At home he was very jealous of his new sister and was difficult to manage.

During the therapy with Allen, which lasted for 3 years, I had formed positive relationships with both parents, who were supportive of treatment and interested in their children's welfare. I attended several school conferences with both parents and the school staff, during which we worked out special programs for Allen. A close working relationship was maintained between me, the parents, and the school throughout the therapy.

In therapy, Allen complained that his older brother, Jack, was lucky because he had two daddies and got two presents on birthdays. Allen had felt shortchanged all of his life. His sister's birth had made things worse, and his rivalry with Heather was quite striking. We were able to make slow but steady progress in treatment. By the end of the third year of the once-a-week therapy, Allen was in much better spirits, doing well in school and getting along better with peers and at home. Treatment was terminated when Allen was 8 years old, with rather good improvement.

Soon afterward the parents called to say that Heather was having difficulties. She was then 3 years old and had begun to have nightmares, a severe sleep disturbance, and separation anxiety along with some day wetting and regular bed-wetting after having been dry earlier. She was no longer willing to stay in the Mother's Day Out at their church and clung to her mother almost constantly. At night she would come into the parents' room and insist on staying all night. She would sleep on the floor near the bed.

Heather had known me since she was a baby, having often accompanied Allen to my office. When I saw her for evaluation there was no separation anxiety noted. I made the diagnosis of Separation Anxiety Disorder and began once-weekly therapy. In treatment she revealed that her mother and father were arguing a lot, which was upsetting her. Although they were well off, there was trouble about money. It seemed from what Heather said that Daddy was mad at Mommy because she spent too much money.

In the informative-alliance visits with the parents it came out that they were having rather serious marital problems and that Heather was reacting adversely to them. At that point Allen also began to show signs of becoming upset, and he asked to see me. It soon became apparent that the parents' marital relationship was deteriorating, and it was not long until the parents told me that they were planning a separation.

Both children showed intense loyalty conflict struggles, since they were quite attached to both of their parents. Allen had started to gain more weight and told me about the kids at school teasing him and calling him "Lard Ass," which upset him considerably. Heather's sleep disturbance worsened and her separation anxiety became more pronounced as the family situation disintegrated.

Shortly afterward the parents decided to file for divorce, and both children seemed to react badly, with much distress. They told me that they wanted their parents to get back together because they loved both of them.

The issue of custody of the children became a bone of contention between the parents, and they each asked me to support their respective side in the custody battle. I steadfastly refused to take sides and indicated that doing so would make it impossible to help the children with their emotional reactions to the divorce, with which they both needed much help. Taking sides would result in major transference problems since the children loved both parents and were suffering marked loyalty conflicts. I could not side with one parent and still be an objective, unbiased person for them.

When both attorneys involved called to try to persuade me to support their respective clients, I refused but offered to serve as mediator to help both sides attempt to resolve the conflict. Thus we met together with the parents and attorneys at my office, and I was able to help them work out a joint custody plan that seemed to be in the best interests of the children. Although I do not generally recommend such a plan, it was agreed that the children would spend equal time with each parent, rotating between the two homes which were close together in the same school district. Because the family had recently moved from one house to the other and still owned both homes, the kids had lived in both houses and had friends in each neighborhood. This made it easier for them to make this kind of adjustment.

This plan has worked out rather well for the children, who still see me occasionally. The parents still call for help with their questions from time to time. The mother has remarried and has a new baby, and the father is engaged to be married. I have met with the new fiancée who will become their stepmother, and I will continue to be available to help her and the rest of the family as needed.

Maintaining one's neutrality in family disputes is essential. If negative countertransference feelings toward one parent lead the therapist to become involved in giving legal testimony for one of the parents, this invariably interferes with therapy. In supervision I have heard of disastrous outcomes for treatment when a therapist has gone to court to advocate for one parent of a child in treatment. For therapy to continue, it is absolutely essential to maintain one's neutrality.

Exceptions to this guideline occur when one learns of physical or sexual abuse, where the law requires that one report such evidence to the authorities. This will often have severe repercussions for the child's therapy.

Countertransference Problems in Therapy with Children

Bleiberg (1987) stated, "Perhaps the greatest obstacles therapists contend with during the initial phase of treatment stem from countertransference. Typical countertransference reactions described in the literature include: dread of the sessions and irritation; feeling of being fooled by patients with related wishes to show them who is 'really in charge'; feelings of worthlessness, helplessness, and defeat; verbal and nonverbal rejection of patients; boredom or indifference" (p. 446).

Kramer and Prall (1971), reporting on Mahler's principles of child analytic technique, indicated "the need to avoid playing 'God', and to refrain from moralizing or judging" (p. 495). Some therapists tend to inflict their own moral standards and judgments on child patients rather than allowing them to develop their own. Because we work with children from many religious and ethnic backgrounds, it is imperative that the therapist become familiar with the various religious tenets and principles in order not to contradict the child's beliefs. Children are often very curious about one's religious beliefs, and it is our responsibility to keep our beliefs to ourselves and draw out the child's beliefs. I remember one little 5-year-old boy who, at election time, asked me," Are you Jewish or Republican?" This led to some interesting revelations concerning the parents' dinner-table political discussions.

Needless to say, one should also keep one's political and religious beliefs to oneself when working with patients. If one has strong political leanings, all well and good, but one should avoid placing bumper stickers on one's car, since curious children invariably figure out which car in the parking lot belongs to the therapist. It is essential to avoid countertransference reactions to the child's religious, political, and ethnic proclivities.

Prall and Dealy (1965) described therapist's countertransference reactions in the therapy of patients with childhood psychosis. They describe the following areas of difficulty in learning to treat these more disturbed children, which commonly lead to countertransference reactions that are worthy of examination.

Problems in Communication and Countertransference

One of the most difficult areas for beginning child analysts and therapists is to learn to understand the nature of children's communications. It is not uncommon in work with disturbed children for the patient to spend several sessions with little or no verbal communication. One must become familiar with the child's various modes of communication including play, motility, and affective expressions.

Mahler (1960)[1] and Kramer and Prall (1971) noted that it is also necessary to talk to the child in the child's own age-appropriate language and using the child's own words rather than adult language.

Communication and Countertransference: The Nonverbal Child

Disturbed children's communication can cause difficulty for the beginning therapist who is not fully cognizant of age-appropriate means of children's communication. The adult analyst and the psychiatrist trained in medical school and in adult psychiatry may tend to expect children to be verbal and to sit still and discuss their complaints and feelings as do the adults with whom they have worked. The disturbed child or adolescent is often quiet, passive-aggressive, or mute. This may result in negative countertransference reactions and efforts to coerce the patient into talking about things that are troublesome. If the trainee is worried about what to tell the supervisor, and there is no verbal material from a child to report, frustration and anger may result in increased efforts to get the child to talk, with a resultant increase in the child's resistance. A vicious cycle thus begins, and an impasse may be reached in treatment.

This type of countertransference reaction is quite prevalent with electively mute children who refuse to talk in treatment and can be quite challenging cases to treat. As with severely passive-aggressive children and adolescents, such youngsters can be very provocative in their withholding of verbal material and can tax the patience of an inexperienced therapist. With the nonverbal or withholding child, it is imperative to de-emphasize efforts to enforce verbal communication and to develop skills in understanding nonverbal communication and the language of play, drawing, clay modeling, and body language. Gestures, affective facial expression, posture, motility, artistic productions, and symbolic puppet or dollhouse play often offer the only access to the child's thought life and can convey a wealth of information if understood by the therapist. Without such understanding, negative counter-

---

1. The material attributed to Dr. Mahler is from the seminars on child analysis that she taught at the Philadelphia Psychoanalytic Institute from 1950 to the 1980s, as well as from her visits to the Eastern Pennsylvania Psychiatric Institute Children's Service where she served as consultant on the treatment of childhood psychosis.

transference reactions may result and will be manifest in the therapist's annoyance toward the child, dread of seeing the patient, boredom, sleepiness, lateness, or missing and canceling sessions. The narcissistic injury inflicted on the less experienced therapist by this type of child can be quite pronounced.

By way of illustration of such a difficult case, a severely autistic 6-year-old boy, the middle of three siblings with a relatively normal brother and sister, was so regressed and chronically self-destructive that he was hospitalized at the Institute Children's Service, where research in treatment of childhood psychosis was being undertaken. Jami had been withdrawn from birth, had bonded poorly, and had shown autistic symptoms from very early in infancy. At the time of admission he showed a marked delay in speech, toilet training, cognitive development, and all areas of ego control and socialization. He was preoccupied with spinning and twirling objects and himself and made little or no eye contact. His capacity for object relationships was severely impaired. He was largely nonverbal, very regressed in all areas of functioning, and constantly agitated. There was little evidence of ego control over his aggressive impulses, as he would frequently bite and spit at the staff. His severe organismic distress took the form of psychotic temper tantrums during which he would throw himself down and smash his face on the floor. Jami's disturbed motor behavior included repeated efforts at self-destruction and obliteration. He would continually withdraw from human contact through such maneuvers as climbing into the toilet and trying to flush himself down, hiding under rugs, and at other times climbing under beds or into bureau drawers trying to shut himself in. When we attempted to hold him or stop him from these self-destructive acts, he would scream violently and have psychotic temper tantrums of severe intensity and interminable duration. He showed signs of massive anxiety at human approach and, likewise, at separation from people, such as at bedtime when he refused to go to sleep. Owing to his language delay he was unable to verbalize his fears, which were pervasive and of marked intensity, but he gave nonverbal clues as to the nature of his persistent fears. His behavior pointed toward severe self-punishing spurious superego development, as he would frequently dash around hitting his head, shouting,"Bad boy, Jami!"

He showed evidence of faulty definition of his body boundaries in his feeling his way around the walls of the unit and seeming totally lost most of the time. The severe degree of oral fixation was noted in his spitting, biting, sucking, and mouthing anything in sight. When regressed and lying along the edge of the floor, he would pick mop strings from under the baseboards and eat them. While outdoors, he would eat dirt and sand, and anything he found in the playground would go into his mouth. At meals he had very strange and irregular eating habits, alternately refusing to eat and at other times gorging himself. He also showed a marked intolerance for change and resisted moving from one activity or area to another. It was most difficult to get him to go outside, and when he did, it was equally hard to get him to come in again. His

frightfully distressing and disturbing behavior tended to promote strong negative countertransference reactions among the entire staff of the unit, who found
it exceedingly difficult to console him or to perform any simple bodily care such
as bathing, teeth-brushing, toileting, dressing, and undressing.

The author began intensive therapy with Jami, who was in treatment during
a prolonged hospitalization in the inpatient unit. From the outset there was
obvious fear of physical contact, which was usually warded off by his screaming
and hiding. At first, whenever I entered the ward he would scream and hide
behind one of the worker's skirts and refuse to go with me to the playroom. For
many weeks I continued to visit him and spent the time on the ward.

Over the years of supervision of trainees, it often became apparent to
me that this type of withdrawal could lead to strong negative countertransference reactions characterized by injured narcissism, feelings of
rejection, and inadequacy, and all types of rationalizations would be the
result. The young trainees would say that the patient "was not ready for
therapy," or that they were the wrong choice of therapist. A male
therapist might say, "Perhaps a woman therapist is indicated," and vice
versa. It became clear to us that the work with autistic children required
a high degree of persistence and maturity that was not always available
with new child psychiatry trainees (see Christ 1973).

One should not embark upon this type of work without a thorough
knowledge of nonverbal communication and a real commitment to
persevering and persisting against all types of resistance. We usually did
not assign seriously disturbed children to the part-time residents in
adult psychiatry who rotated through the unit for training in child
psychiatry, since they did not have the level of sophistication required
for this difficult work nor was their time on the unit sufficiently long to
permit therapeutic change to occur with these very disturbed children.
Such assignments would mean frequent changes of therapist, which is
positively contraindicated in the therapy of psychotic children.

With Jami, I persisted in my visits to the ward and used every trick in my
armamentarium to get close enough to him to begin some meaningful interaction. I finally got some glimmer of a response from him by imitating one of his
obsessive forms of behavior. Jami had daily spent hours frantically building
higher and higher block towers and knocking them down. While lying on the
floor near him, I built a large block tower and kicked it over. A little smile
flickered across his face, so I built another tower quite close to his leg and
eventually he kicked it over. This began a series of building and destroying
games that finally allowed him to begin to relate to me insofar as I was able to
enter the autistic world where he dwelt.

In our years of work with autistic children we learned that it is necessary to
empathically tune in on the children's idiosyncratic preoccupations and attempt

to insinuate ourselves into their autistic orbit. Eventually, through this method, Jami was able to allow himself to go with me to the playroom, but he continued to resist any attempts at physical contact. If I offered him candy, he would withdraw and attempt to climb out of the window. One day, quite by accident, contact was finally permitted. A large, empty cardboard box was inadvertently left in the playroom, and Jami promptly climbed under it and hid from me. I climbed under the box with him and, in this dark, womblike environment, Jami climbed on my lap and allowed me to hold him, rock him and sing to him for the first time as he sucked voraciously on his thumb. It became apparent to me that he had been attempting to regress into a prenatal intrauterine position by his self-obliterative, hiding, and withdrawing forms of behavior. In addition, his strenuous defenses against physical contact seemed to represent a fear of the ambivalently feared and wished-for symbiotic reengulfment by the mother. The readiness with which he sought contact in the dark box spoke to the wish for closeness that was so stoutly defended against in the light.

We kept the box in the playroom for weeks, and it became his refuge to which he began to look forward. Eventually he began to take my hand and pull me to the playroom to this cozy, dark environment. Finally, when the box had deteriorated so that it was no longer useful, he permitted the physical contact in the open. At this point he began to sing back to me the songs I had made up that included his name.

A quasi-symbiotic attachment was gradually formed between us, which enabled Jami to slowly emerge from the autistic position he had assumed. Mahler (1968) pointed out that emergence from the autistic shell was invariably accompanied by painful affects and marked anxiety. When she consulted with me about Jami on one of her visits to the unit, she observed that he seemed to have been enabled to come out of his autistic orbit through the development of the attachment to me, which was, albeit, highly ambivalent. This ambivalence was shown in many ways; for instance, while sitting on my lap, he would suck and kiss my arm and then suddenly bite it without warning.

After many months of treatment, Jami's nonverbal expressions of his intense fears allowed understanding of what he was attempting to communicate. Late one night while making rounds on Jami's ward, I found the night-duty child care workers in the nurses' station attempting to ignore Jami's screams from the bathroom down the hall.

They had all reached a point of despair in trying to console him and had withdrawn from attempting to help him. It was clear that their negative countertransference reactions were based on frustration of their rescue fantasies as they talked of having the best intentions about helping the boy, but he had rejected all their efforts and they had left him in the bathroom in frustration and anger at his lack of response to their efforts.

When I entered the bathroom, Jami was sitting on the toilet screaming in great distress. He clawed at and inserted his fingers in his anus and pulled violently on his nose, his fingers, and his penis. Understanding his nonverbal communication, I sat on the floor near him and said that I understood what he was trying to tell us, namely, that he had to make b.m., but was afraid that making b.m. was like part of him coming off such as his nose, his fingers, or his penis. I added that his b.m. was not a part of his body but the leftover waste from the food he had eaten, and that it was not the same as his fingers, his nose, or his penis. These were all permanent parts of his body that would never come off, and that the b.m. was supposed to come out. I said that everybody made b.m. including me and all of the nurses and workers, his brother, sister, and mommy and daddy and even the president of the United States.

With this, Jami stopped his screaming, relaxed, and had a large bowel movement. By pointing to the toilet paper and to his bottom he nonverbally asked me to wipe his bottom, which I did. He then climbed down from the toilet and crawled onto my lap and, exhausted, promptly fell asleep. I carried him to his bed, where he slept peacefully the rest of the night.

The obsession with building and destroying block towers could now be understood in terms of his preoccupation with bodily dismemberment, disintegration, and castration fears. When this was interpreted, it enabled Jami to gradually begin to overcome his fears. His anxiety slowly decreased, and toilet training was soon completed.

Only through an understanding of the child's nonverbal communications and the therapist's awareness of what the child is attempting to communicate can one avoid the all-too-frequent countertransference reaction of frustration that accompanies failure to comprehend the bizarre, idiosyncratic behavior. Such failure to understand leads to the therapist's feelings of helplessness, hopelessness, withdrawing libido, becoming bored or sleepy, and to therapeutic stalemates.

Countertransference Difficulties with Affective Responses

A frequent area of countertransference difficulties lies in the therapist's inability to tolerate various types of powerful affective responses. With more severe disorders of childhood and adolescence (as well as adulthood), there is often a failure of modulation of the affective expressions, and the raw, unfiltered affects can prove rather overwhelming to the uninitiated. Some therapists become uncomfortable with patients' anxiety and attempt to use reassurance by telling them not to worry. Others find it difficult to tolerate depressive affects of sadness and grief and try to cheer up the patient rather than allowing the expression of the affect and exploring its origin. Some therapists cannot cope with the intense aggression frequently encountered with disturbed children and adolescents. This type of countertransference reaction leads to failure to set realistic limits and the tendency to attempt to please the child at all costs so as not to promote an angry reaction. This permits the patient to control the therapist and the therapeutic situation, to the detriment of treatment. Patients' intense sexual impulses and preoccupations are also difficult for many therapists to accept and frequently lead to major countertransference problems.

The therapist's capacity for empathic understanding of painful affects and tolerance for *all* the affects encountered are essential tools in therapeutic work. The ability to tolerate anxiety, hostility, grief, longing, and sexuality without experiencing anxiety, counterhostility, despair, guilt, or sexual arousal is an absolute requirement for the successful therapist of disturbed children and adolescents.

Countertransference and the Aggressive Child

By contrast with the nonverbal or mute, regressed child, some children and adolescents may become extremely aggressive, destructive, hyperactive, or noisy. It is imperative to deal therapeutically with the aggression, since aggression directed toward the therapist is a common phenomenon in therapy with disturbed children, and negative countertransference feelings can readily be stirred up.

Returning to the example of Jami, the aggression he had formerly directed mainly to himself in banging his face on the floor and hitting his head gradually subsided as he began to turn the aggression against me. He would be sitting calmly on my lap with his back to me (his favorite position because it involved no eye contact, which he continued to find difficult to tolerate), when suddenly he would violently smash his head against my sternum. Sometimes his head would hit a shirt button, which I found very painful.

This realistically hurt and made me angry. Recognizing my negative feelings, I told him so. I said, "That hurt very much when you did that, and I did not like it. I know you have all kinds of mixed feelings about me, enjoying our time together and liking to sit on my lap and having me sing to you, while at the same time you are very scared of getting close to anyone and afraid of how scared it makes you feel to come out of hiding and let yourself make friends with anyone. I don't mind your being scared and angry, but I don't like you to hurt me or yourself. We must find other ways to show it when you are angry."

The therapist has a right to feel angry when physically hurt by the patient. Ignoring the pain and saying nothing is quite unrealistic and does not help the patient control the direct expression of aggression (see Winnicott [1949]).

If the child's aggression gets out of control, as Berlin (1973) clearly pointed out in his descriptions of therapy with childhood psychotics, it is essential to use protective, nonpunitive physical restraint to avoid the child's hurting himself or the therapist. One must not be afraid to lend one's external ego control when the child's ego loses control of the aggressive id impulses.

One particularly annoying and disabling behavior of a seriously disturbed child toward one of the child psychiatry trainees occurred on the Institute inpatient unit when he would repeatedly grab and smash the therapist's eyeglasses. Behavior such as spitting in the therapist's face and soiling during therapy can, understandably, produce negative countertransference reactions that require a great deal of patience, forbearance, and self-examination.

Countertransference and Limit Setting

A frequently noted problem area with some therapists is the inability to set firm and consistent limits and a tendency to give in to the child's attempts to wheedle, cajole, and manipulate. Particularly with the more seriously disturbed adolescent or child whose demands and temper tantrums can have tremendous force, one must have the courage and superego strength to withstand these onslaughts and to "hold the line." If one is afraid of the child's aggression, giving in to avoid angry reactions that make the therapist anxious may allow the child to control the therapeutic situation. Such capitulations do not promote ego growth that requires sufficient, well-timed frustration to permit the child to develop frustration tolerance. It is essential for the child or adolescent therapist to possess a firm superego and the capacity to set limits. Giving in to children's demands or allowing them to get out of control and destroy things or hurt the therapist will not promote personality growth and will result in treatment failures (see Bixler [1964]).

I recall a child analytic candidate who saw a very aggressive little girl for evaluation and allowed the child to stomp on and break all the dollhouse furniture she had played with. Because this was not handled promptly, the child refused to return for further visits. In discussing this episode, Mahler pointed out that realistic limits are essential for the support of the child's ego. She added that one should neither allow oneself to be bribed by a child nor should one try to bribe the patient. She indicated that there is no place in our work for coercion, exhortation, or threats, which are to be avoided (see Kramer and Prall [1971]).

Similarly, allowing oneself to be manipulated into answering the child's demands or persistent questions is also not conducive to the therapeutic process. Withholding personal information is as important as setting limits on destructive behavior, since the child cannot be expected to develop frustration tolerance if one gives in and fulfills all the child's wishes. In addition, supplying personal information undermines the efforts to get at the child's fantasies, theories, and feelings about the therapist. Such questioning is often an effort to deflect attention away from the child and put the spotlight on the therapist, which serves as a resistance that should be interpreted. One can often turn a question around and ask the child what his or her thoughts and feelings are about the subject under discussion.

Faulty superego formation and ego control over the impulses is invariably involved with seriously disturbed youngsters. Consistent limits and not allowing oneself to be manipulated by the child's powerful affective outbursts foster ego growth and development of the superego by means of identification with, and incorporation of, the therapist's ego and superego strengths. We must continually serve as external ego and superego to the immature child who lacks sufficient ego and superego control over the impulses. When the child's aggression begins to get out of control, one must side with the strengths of the ego and state, "I will not let you hurt yourself, or me, or break anything in the playroom because that would only make you feel worse, not better, and we are here to help you gain control of the wildness in you that makes you so unhappy."

Another approach that proves therapeutic when a child's wildness gets out of control is to state, "We must work together to strengthen your inner police force to help it control the wild side of you that wants to break things. You can be the sheriff and I'll be the deputy, and we will work together to get your Mr. Wild Guy under control." This type of control of the aggression often leads to games of "good guys and bad guys" or "cops and robbers" where one can be on the child's side against imaginary bad people to catch them and give them "time out" in jail. Time out is a concept with which most disturbed children are familiar from experience in school or at home, and the taking control of their wild side leads to active mastery of the aggression, as contrasted with passively and masochistically submitting to its sway and being punished at home or in school for their destructive behavior.

Firm but kind and consistent limit setting offers the child a new model for identification different from the frantic, harsh, punishing, and rejecting parental images that have been internalized, and which must be replaced if the child is to improve in treatment.

Countertransference and the Child's Wish to Leave the Therapy Room

Very often in supervision, therapists have told me about taking their patients outside to play. They indicate that the child insisted on going outside and they were powerless to say no. This is particularly nontherapeutic and should be avoided at all costs. Once outside the therapy room, a child may run around inside the building, bang on other people's doors, and make a lot of noise. If they get outside, they may run all the way around the building, climb trees, or run out into the street, and there is a real danger of the child being hurt.

I am reminded of one male therapist who took a latency-aged boy patient outdoors, only to have him climb a tree. Triumphantly, in a show of phallic exhibitionistic prowess, he urinated from high up in the tree! It was obvious from the subsequent material that this youngster was defending against his severe castration fears.

It is virtually impossible to have a real therapeutic interchange in wide open spaces, and one ends up chasing the youngster rather than attempting to understand. Children use such distancing techniques as a defense against dealing with their conflictual feelings, and this should not be reinforced by complying with their wishes to go outside. It is far better to hold the line and insist on staying in the therapy room. If necessary, with a really rebellious child, I move my chair in front of the door to avert a hasty escape by such children. One can interpret the child's wish to escape from dealing with painful feelings and state that our job is to try to understand what makes him or her unhappy and upset.

Sometimes, when confronted by my refusal to allow them to escape, such children may begin to scream at the top of their voice, "Help! I am being kept prisoner! I'm being tortured! Somebody save me!" Needless to say, unless the therapist has his or her countertransference feelings under control, it would be quite easy to give in and allow the child to leave the room. However, this does not promote ego growth. Instead, one should remain calm and continue to refuse to let the child leave the room. Under such circumstances, I would whisper, "I think you are very scared of thinking about what brought you to this place and you are really wanting to avoid dealing with the things that worry you so much." The whispering often calms youngsters; they will stop screaming to listen and this may break the tension. The therapist's calmness and firmness under fire is the most therapeutic tool with which to combat such behavior. Losing one's cool and talking loudly to the child only serves to exacerbate the situation.

Curiosity about the Therapist

Invariably, child patients are very curious about the therapist, just as with adults. However, children are less easily dissuaded from pursuing their efforts to find out about us. They will snoop in desk drawers, closets, cabinets, and even try to explore the therapist's pockets or purse. They make the most intensive efforts to learn all they can about us. They will persist in endless questions about our marital status, our family, children, income, our childhood, and so on. For example, children often ask if we did the same things that they do when we were their age. One 3-year-old girl repeatedly asked, "Do you have a mommy?" (meaning a wife). Eventually she began calling my home to see who would answer the phone in hopes of satisfying her curiosity.

Telephone calls are a common problem that may raise countertransference issues. Children may call one's office on any pretext—for example, to check on appointment times that have always been the same, or to ask if they can change an appointment because they have to go play with their friends.

Children's voyeuristic impulses are sometimes so powerful that they will make extraordinary efforts to find ways to intrude on the therapist's private life in attempting to satisfy their curiosity. If the child patient calls the therapist's home and manages to reach one's children on the phone, or if the patient continually calls at night after you have gone to bed and asks, "What are you doing?," negative countertransference feelings can be stirred up. The meaning of the curiosity is obvious to us, namely, disguised sexual and primal-scene curiosity, and it must be dealt with in a therapeutic manner and analyzed or else it will persist.

As reported by Kramer and Prall (1971), Mahler pointed out that it is unwise to attempt to answer children's questions about sexual matters. "The tendency to give the child information before the defenses and underlying fantasies are worked with is quite common. Only after carefully analyzing the fantasies does one help the child to correct his mistaken ideas by supplying facts" (p. 496).

Countertransference Reactions to Resistance

Many other forms of resistive and overtly provocative behavior that children employ in therapy may give rise to negative countertransference feelings if not understood and handled properly. For example, some children bring comic books to hold in front of their faces to read, thus shutting out the therapist. Others bring their homework and insist on poring over it throughout the appointment to prevent any efforts to get at their thought life. These and other resistances must be interpreted and handled with equanimity, and the therapist must learn not to become angry and frustrated by such resistances.

Sometimes when therapists' countertransference reactions to children needing to withdraw into a book results in feelings of annoyance, they may pick up something to read themselves. This is definitely contraindicated. No matter what a child may be doing, even falling asleep, one must continually focus one's entire attention on the child throughout the session. To ignore the child and pick up a newspaper to read would serve as a severe blow to a child's narcissism. One must learn to be able to tolerate all of the children's efforts to defend themselves without permitting oneself to adopt the defense of counter withdrawal.

Countertransference Issues over Control of the Therapy

There are those therapists who may try to play God and have to be in control and show the child who is boss. This may occur when the therapist is unsure of himself or herself and tries to defend against this by insisting on being in charge at all times. This can impede the flow and progress of therapy with a child, as it may cut off avenues of access to the patient's thoughts and feelings. Flexibility is very much needed to succeed in reaching a child's inner life.

Leslie, an only child, age 7 years, was referred for rather severe school learning difficulties, stubbornness, and oppositional behavior. Careful psychological evaluation showed a high average intellectual level with no evidence of organicity or learning disabilities. The projective testing revealed unresolved oedipal problems, a close attachment to her father, and considerable hostility toward her mother.

In therapy she demonstrated her oedipal conflicts in her dollhouse play by having the mother leave town for an extended trip and placing the girl doll in bed with the father. In dealing with her school difficulties, she would frequently insist on role reversal play in which I was the "dumb kid" and she was the teacher. I would be scolded and punished and frequently shamed and made to sit in time out. She would tell me to make mistakes on my paper and then scold me for my stupidity. "How could you be so dumb!" was a frequent scathing comment.

At other times I would be the little girl and she would become the mother, and similar shaming and scolding would take place. She was doing to me what had been done to her, thus revealing a wealth of valuable insight into her family situation. If I had been too stiff or controlling to allow her to boss me around and change roles, it would not have facilitated therapeutic understanding.

The child therapist must be completely flexible and allow the child to take charge of the content of the therapy, the choice of materials, and modes of dealing with the conflictual material. One must relax and observe and participate as directed by the child. Here I depart from Anthony, who insists that he must maintain the "sessile" position in his child analytic work by not participating actively in the child's play. (See Anthony's discussion in the panel reported by Casuso [1965].) It seems to me that he must miss a wealth of valuable material by not participating in the child's role-reversal play, which I find most helpful in gaining insight into how children perceive they have been treated by the grown-ups in their lives.

COUNTERTRANSFERENCE REACTIONS TO THE CHILD'S LIBIDINAL IMPULSES

Countertransference and the Positive Transference

Countertransference reactions may arise from the positive attachment of child patients toward the therapist. For successful therapy with children a strong positive transference is essential to withstand the inevitable negative transference that will eventually emerge. However, when children evince a strong positive love claim on the therapist, there may be a tendency to seek narcissistic gratification and admiration from one's patients unless there is sufficient libidinal gratification in one's life outside the therapeutic situation. It is necessary to be comfortable with the manifestations of positive transference, but it is essential to handle them appropriately without making the patient feel either rejected or seduced.

Mahler's (1960) important caveat on handling the positive transference with children is worthy of note here. In her seminars on psychoanalytic technique she frequently emphasized that with children one should not stress the positive transference itself by saying "I see you like me," or "You are wishing that you could come and live at my house," even if there is ample evidence in the child's productions to indicate that this is true. The child's ego cannot tolerate such direct confrontations with the positive transference, which will often lead to increased

COUNTERTRANSFERENCE   263

negative transference as seen in such exclamations as "Don't think I *like* you, you old dope!" or "I don't *like* you, I *hate* you!" Instead one should wait for evidence of the ambivalence toward the therapist to evolve and then use confrontation with both sides of the ambivalent conflict, which the ego can more readily tolerate and which furthers the therapeutic process. For example, one can say with impunity, "I see that you have so many mixed feelings about this place. On the one hand, you hate to come here and are often late, but when it is time to stop, it is difficult for you to leave this place."

Mahler indicated that the child's ego can better tolerate one's using "this place" rather than "me" since this confronts the ego less directly with the positive transference. A direct confrontation of the positive transference is often defended against by increased negative transference. Thus it is imperative to watch for and enunciate *both sides* of the child's conflicts whenever they become clear. One should avoid focusing on only one side of a conflict, which does not promote therapeutic understanding.

A therapist who becomes emotionally attached to a child patient may find it difficult to foster the child's differentiation and independence. Some therapists derive so much narcissistic gratification from the child's attachment to them, once the quasi-symbiotic relationship is established in work with autistic children, that they experience difficulties recognizing when it is time to foster separation-individuation. Like some mothers of symbiotic psychotic children, they unconsciously tend to prolong the child's dependency upon them. Prall and Dealy (1965), in their discussion of countertransference problems in work with childhood psychosis, stated that "the therapist who has too much libido invested in the establishment of relationship with the child will encounter difficulties in supporting the necessary separation and the child's developing autonomy" (p. 80). This was likely to occur more often with women therapists who had no children of their own or were feeling lonely and unfulfilled.

Countertransference and the Erotic Transference

Another aspect of countertransference of which one must be aware is related to the occurrence of a positive erotic transference. This may become apparent especially with a male therapist working with female adolescent patients. The seductive nature of the transference may lead to undue countertransference reactions manifested by the therapist's response to the patient's seductive efforts, which may arouse sexual feelings. Such countertransference responses very often result in the patient responding with increased negative transference to ward off the erotic transference.

Recent studies reported in the literature regarding the frequency with which psychiatrists and other mental health workers succumb to the temptation of narcissistic gratification by becoming sexually involved with their patients attest to the presence of these countertransference problems. (See Cummings and Sobel [1985], Herman et al. [1987], Kilburg et al. [1986], Pope and Bouhoutsos [1986], and Zelen [1985].)

Mahler (1960) often emphasized that, in general, it is better for a female adolescent patient to have a woman therapist, if possible, to help avoid the need to ward off the positive erotic transference to a male therapist. Of course, one must be aware of the possibility of a positive erotic homosexual transference with a woman therapist, which may also be defended against by negative transference.

Some of the other manifestations of positive erotic transference that may lead to countertransference difficulties occur with small child patients who want the therapist to take them home to live. Others want the therapist to accompany them to the bathroom or may become overtly exhibitionistic and sexually provocative. For example, if a little girl climbs on the therapist's lap and begins to wiggle and rub her bottom on the therapist's leg, one should gently put the child down and comment to the effect that this kind of closeness is not helpful. One must avoid injuring the child's narcissism by rebuffing her attempts to show affection or to obtain erotic stimulation. However, permitting such erotic behavior to continue is countertherapeutic and should be avoided.

Similarly, a little boy may attempt to rub his penis on either a male or female therapist, and this should be dealt with in much the same way. Sometimes boys or girls who are struggling with their castration complex may suddenly pull down their pants to expose their genitals, watching closely for a reaction from the therapist. Of course, one should avoid sounding like a scolding parent or schoolteacher by telling the child to stop doing that and to pull up his or her pants! Instead one must cautiously interpret the behavior without offending the child's narcissism by saying something to the effect of "You seem to be wanting me to know that you are worried about the private parts of your body. I wonder what it is that you are worried about." As more information becomes available from the child, one may then carry the interpretations further when the specifics are known. One type of countertransference reaction I have observed with students is to be embarrassed by such sexually provocative behavior and to fail to say anything to the child, hoping that the child will stop this kind of behavior. To avoid dealing with erotic sexual behavior by avoidance is as countertherapeutic as becoming too actively involved and participating in the child's sexually seductive behavior.

With older children or adolescents, a common countertransference reaction is to get caught up in the patient's relating dirty jokes or sexually explicit details or descriptions of sexual behavior which may represent a sexual form of transference. When the patient and therapist are the same sex, this type of behavior may represent a quasi-homosexual seductive transference. One has to walk a rather narrow tightrope between permitting the patient's expression of any and all types of thoughts and feelings on the one hand, and becoming too overinvolved in the erotic material on the other.

Countertransference regarding Drive Derivatives from Oral and Anal Levels

Additional countertransference problems lie in discomfort with the drive derivatives of the earlier phases of libidinal development. The therapist's discomfort with such impulses may lead to resistance by the therapist to dealing with earlier fixations as one unconsciously deflects the child's material away from these areas of discomfort. Thus it is imperative for the successful therapist to be comfortable with all levels of psychosexual development. If one has discomfort about anality, the child's anal messiness will cause anxiety for the therapist, and the child may, during phases of positive transference, try to avoid expression of the anal impulses or, in the negative transference, may bombard the beleaguered therapist with endless messy assaults.

I am reminded of my work with 8-year-old Mark, who showed his severe anal aggression by such maneuvers as walking in mud outside my new office building and smearing mud all over the new office carpet and furniture. He would also go to the building's soda machine to buy a can of soda and then shake it violently and squirt the soda around my office and at me. One day soon after the Summer Olympics, he came into my office, approached me closely, and spit a huge mouthful of saliva into my face, shouting, "Mark Spitz!" Needless to say, I was reminded of Winnicott's (1949) admonition that the severely disturbed patient cannot deal with his own aggression unless the analyst is able to recognize and deal with his own aggression at times like these. I told Mark that his behavior made me furious and that I thought he wanted to find out what it would take to get me angry and to see if I was human like his parents, who were frequently angry with him. After this confrontation, the anal aggression gradually began to decrease.

In the work with Jami it was often necessary for me to toilet him and assist with cleaning him up for him to feel accepted by me. In addition, the manifestations of his massive oral fixation were pronounced and demanded tolerance for this regressed level of behavior as well. Just as with anal regression, the therapist's discomfort with oral or phallic manifestations may lead to therapeutic impasses when the child's conflicts center on those developmental stages.

Christ (1973) describes his concerns about his clothing during the work with a child he treated who pulled at his clothing and spit on him. It is possible to avoid a frequent source of countertransference anxiety concerning one's clothing during work with severely regressed youngsters by wearing old clothes or a smock rather than the good clothing that will be worn the rest of the day.

The child therapist must be completely comfortable with *all* of the early levels of psychosexual development in order to be able to avoid anxiety and annoyance about the child's regressive behavior. This is particularly true with psychotic and borderline children whose ego control over oral, anal, and phallic aggression and libidinal expression is often woefully inadequate.

There must also be a tolerance for the primary-process manifestations in these children. Logic and secondary-process thinking are seldom encountered with these primitive patients. Flexibility and imagination are absolute essentials for successful therapeutic work with disturbed children, and one must be prepared for *anything* that may happen.

Countertransference and Phallic Strivings

Another problem area of concern is the tendency to phallic competitiveness by the therapist. The need to play the game for the game's sake or to win at all costs often represents countertransference problems related to the therapist's childhood conflicts on the phallic level, which will lead to resistance in therapy. One should use games to gain an understanding of the child's conflicts and not respond to the child's urgings to "Hurry up and move! It's your turn!" Instead one should interpret the dynamics underlying the patient's need for the hurry. Similarly one should avoid getting swept up in the child's urgency to hurry up and play more and more games. Games can easily serve as a resistance if we allow them to, rather than using them to understand the child's inner life. Loomis's (1957) paper on checker playing is particularly helpful in this connection.

In child therapy, stereotyped board games prove less useful than more projective story games, drawing, clay modeling, and puppet or dollhouse play, which allow for free expression rather than conforming to rules of games.

THERAPIST-SPECIFIC COUNTERTRANSFERENCE REACTIONS

Countertransference Problems and Memory Failures

A therapist's inability to remember the patient's material, or certain portions of it, reflects possible areas of countertransference. When the child's productions, either verbal or behavioral, touch upon unresolved areas of conflict for the therapist, this may produce selective difficulty in recall, which should alert one to countertransference possibilities. When this phenomena is encountered in supervision, especially if it occurs frequently with one patient or at certain nodal points with a number of patients, it is imperative for the supervisor to help the therapist become aware of the problem area that is being blocked, since patients will not be able to work through difficulties in this area unless the therapist can deal meaningfully with the painful aspects of the patient's material.

Another sign of countertransference difficulties is evident when a therapist forgets, misses, or is frequently late for appointments with a certain patient. This invariably indicates that the therapist is having countertransference problems with this particular person and dreads seeing the patient.

If failure of memory continues to occur, the therapist should seek personal therapeutic help to overcome the blocks to handling conflictual material. In fact, any therapist who is experiencing countertransference difficulties should avail himself or herself of consultation with colleagues and/or personal therapeutic help in overcoming these interferences with the work.

Countertransference Problems with Acting-Out and Suicidal Patients

In regard to work with disturbed children and adolescents, in addition to the problems cited above there often arise particularly strong negative countertransference difficulties with the acting-out, self-destructive, and suicidal patient. It is especially hard for the inexperienced therapist to deal with the self-induced slow self-destruction that results from chronic drug and alcohol abuse, as well as with more acute suicidal efforts. One's therapeutic zeal and rescue fantasies are often strenuously warded off by these patients. Frustration, injured narcissism, and a sense of failure for the therapist may result. A great deal of maturity and self-confidence are required in learning to deal with these difficult patients and to enable one to handle the feelings that inevitably accompany a successful suicide attempt.

Countertransference and Exceptions to Confidentiality

If a patient reveals serious suicidal thoughts or plans, it is imperative to deal with this immediately. Such revelations are prone to arouse countertransference reactions. Even though confidentiality has been the rule, one must inform the patient that the rule must be overlooked at this point, since it is necessary for the parents to know about the suicidal trends in order to make plans to help the patient and save his or her life. It is best to arrange to meet with the patient and the parents together as soon as possible, rather than "going behind the patient's back" to inform the parents. Then appropriate plans can be made either for antidepressant medication or hospitalization, as the situation demands.

Other occasions demanding a waiver of confidentiality may occur if a youngster reveals that some dangerous behavior or situation exists. For example, one may learn that a patient has acquired a gun and plans to use it. This calls for prompt action to avoid a tragedy.

Stealing and Countertransference Reactions

Similarly, if a child repeatedly brings stolen goods to the appointments, the inexperienced therapist may experience countertransference problems and become perplexed. One must deal with this in a therapeutic manner, first by interpreting that it is clear that he or she wants the therapist to know that the stealing is going on and that help is wanted to overcome this id tendency. One must attempt to understand the origin of the symptom. However, it is usually advisable to help the child face the music and return the stolen goods to the store or other place from which it was obtained. The parents' help will usually be needed to accomplish this. Here again, it is best to have the parent join the therapy session and to help the child tell the parents what has happened and obtain their sympathetic handling of the situation, rather than their punishing the child. They should be encouraged to take the child back to the store to meet with the manager and return the stolen items. Later on in therapy it will be necessary to uncover the underlying motives of the stealing symptom.

Stealing from the therapist's office or playroom presents other countertransference problems. The therapist may become quite annoyed by a child's persistent efforts to steal things. Often children will beg to take home a special object of the therapist's such as a toy car or a doll and, when this is denied, will manage to pocket the object surreptitiously. It is essential for the therapist to pay constant attention to the child in therapy, so that one would notice such an act and deal with it promptly by indicating to the child, something to the effect of, "You have a very special attachment to that toy, and it must mean a great deal to you. We must discover together what it means to you." After attempting to analyze the taking of the object, one must still deal with the issue and not allow the child to take it home. One might say, "I really cannot allow anyone to take things home, because I know how much that toy means to you and I know how disappointed you would be to come next time and find it missing. If I let someone else take it home, you would be very angry with me. That is why I have the rule that I do not allow anyone to take things home from here."

Sometimes children will still refuse to give up the object and will become angry with the therapist. One should deal with this by interpreting the ambivalence: "I see that you like something of mine and want to keep it, while at the same time you are very angry with me. You have such mixed-up feelings, which is why we are working together here to help you get unmixed." If nothing helps the situation and the child still refuses to give up the toy, this may exacerbate negative countertransference feelings as the therapist feels powerless and inept in the face of the child's oppositional behavior. One must remain calm and firm and state that we cannot end the session until the toy is returned to its place. At this point some children may throw the treasured toy down and run out of the room, shouting that they hate the therapist and that they don't want the darn toy anyway, or that they will never come here again! It is important to go into the waiting room and talk calmly with the child before he or she leaves and to interpret, in the parent's presence, somewhat as follows: "I know how angry you are with me and that is perfectly all right. I don't mind in the least how angry you feel, because I understand why. It's because there was something that you very much wanted and I wouldn't let you have your own way. We can talk some more about this next time and try to understand more about it." Such an approach will prove helpful to a puzzled parent and will usually allow the child to calm down and leave in a less disturbed mood.

At other times, a child will simply refuse to remove the object from his or her pocket. It is imperative not to get into a wrestling match with a child by physically trying to retrieve the object. This may often evoke an eroticized-aggressive effort to obtain close bodily contact with the therapist and would be countertherapeutic.

Eventually, the child may run out to the waiting room in an effort to make a getaway with the stolen treasure. Again, it is necessary to follow the child and deal with the situation in front of the parent. This time one should attempt to get the child to tell the parent what the problem is and let the parent deal with getting the child to return the toy.

Of course such behavior represents ambivalence toward the therapist, since the object stands for the therapist whom the child really wants to keep for himself or herself but the behavior takes the form of an angry confrontation.

Countertransference and Separation Anxiety

One of the situations that causes embarrassment for some therapists is the presence of severe separation anxiety on the part of a child. In the waiting room, if a child turns his or her back on the therapist, this may hurt the inexperienced therapist's feelings and provoke negative countertransference reactions. A child's refusal to leave its mother to accompany the therapist to the playroom can stir up negative feelings accompanied by uncertainty and helplessness. The fear of having the parent see one's ineptness often causes considerable distress. Uncertainty as to whether to invite the parent into the playroom may be based on unconscious attitudes toward the parent and may include fear of having the adult see what one is doing with the child. This may well reflect unconscious unresolved childhood conflicts about being discovered by one's parents in some forbidden act.

The case of Mandy, a 3-year-old girl with severe separation anxiety, enuresis both day and night, and very oppositional behavior, may serve to illustrate the handling of separation anxiety in therapy.

Mandy's mother brought her to my office for the first evaluation interview. As soon as I entered the waiting room, the child began to fuss loudly, buried her face in her mother's lap, sobbed, and started to stamp her feet in a defiant manner. Sitting down on the floor next to her I said quietly, "Hello, Mandy, I am Dr. Bob and I am so glad to see you." The volume of the whimpering diminished to some degree and, after a few moments of patient silence, I said, "I have some toys that kids like to play with." At this point she peeked at me with one tearful eye from mother's lap.

After a further pause, I said, "I can see that you are very unhappy about being here, and I can understand that. Lots of kids feel that way the first time they come here." She relaxed a bit more, and after a while I said, "Since you like so much to be near Mommy, why don't we invite her to come in and see the toys too." With her mother's help Mandy reluctantly allowed herself to be led into the playroom. Mother sat down and Mandy immediately buried her face in mother's skirt again.

Under such circumstances, after evaluating the severity of the child's separation anxiety, it is quite permissible to have the parent accompany the child to the interview room. This offers an opportunity to observe the parent–child interaction and relationship. Most children, after they have become acquainted with the therapist and the playroom, will allow the parent to leave the room. Not Mandy! It was necessary to allow her mother to stay in the room for several visits. I suggested to the mother that she not take an active part but just watch quietly.

Sometimes it is necessary to have the parent leave in stages after the child's anxiety is somewhat diminished. This was accomplished by having mother sit near the door the next session, then in the doorway with the door wide open. Later she was able to sit farther out of the room with the door partly open. As Mandy's confidence in me increased and she began to play with some of the toys, it was possible to note the clues as to when the next step could be taken.

Because interpreting the child's fears may help allay the anxiety, I said, "It seems to me that you may be worried about Mommy not waiting for you and your being left here. Let's ask Mommy if she will be sure to wait right outside for you." After the mother reassured her that she would wait, Mandy still did not want the door shut. Eventually I said to her, "Mandy, now that you are getting a bit used to this place, I will let *you* decide when it is time to close the door to the waiting room so that we can be alone in here." Allowing the child autonomy by actively effecting the separation herself gave her enough confidence to eventually shut the door herself.

Later she wanted to go out and check on the mother's presence several times during the interviews, thus showing us that she may not have trusted the mother to wait and indicating that fear of abandonment was a crucial motivation for her behavior.

As is readily apparent, if one were to have negative countertransference reactions to a child's clinging to her mother, working through the separation anxiety would not be easily accomplished. Thus one must learn to be completely comfortable with this type of situation and relax and allow the parent to accompany the child as long as necessary.

Invitations

It frequently happens when a child is in a positive transference that the therapist will be invited to a birthday party or another special occasion such as a Bar Mitzvah party. This may arouse countertransference difficulties, and one must deal delicately with this type of situation so as not to injure the child's narcissism or offend the ego. It is usually not advisable to accept such invitations, although there may be occasional exceptions to this general rule. Instead one should inform the child that our work is done here in the therapy room, which is a very special place that allows us to deal with anything and everything without worrying about other people's reactions to what is going on. At home this would not be possible since there would be so many other people there and confidentiality would be impossible. The therapist's presence at the event might be uncomfortable for the child in view of the confidential nature of therapy and might raise conflicts in the child.

Promises

Beginning therapists, in order to win children's favor, often try to please them by trying to meet all of their demands. If a child asks for a certain new toy or game for the therapy room, it is unwise to make a promise to get it, since in therapy we should endeavor to use abstinence in order to learn children's emotional reactions and help them understand and deal with them. In addition, when such promises have been made, the therapist may fail to keep the promise, or be unable to find the desired object, and the child will be disappointed and lose faith in the therapist. It is far better not to make promises that may not be fulfilled. Instead one should hold the line and take the heat when a child becomes angry, realizing that timely limits are ego-building and are therapeutic.

I am reminded of a colleague who took a child patient in his car to go to a store to purchase something the child wanted. Unfortunately, there was an accident when the car was struck from behind, with disastrous results. It goes without saying that one should never take a child patient in one's car.

Gifts and Presents

Similarly, gifts and presents may pose countertransference problems. Many children insist on the therapist giving them birthday presents. This must also be handled delicately because giving gifts is generally not advisable. One should not attempt to buy the child's affection with gifts or favors. If one does succumb to the request, children often look crestfallen when they open the presents, which invariably will not meet their unconscious expectations. Frequently a child will ignore the gift and leave it behind in the therapy room at the end of the session to show the disappointment. Since one cannot meet a child's unmet emotional needs with concrete gifts, it is more therapeutic to avoid giving gifts and deal with the child's consequent emotional reactions and disappointments, and to help by understanding the underlying unmet needs.

The best gift that a therapist can give a child patient is a steadfast effort to be continually emotionally available, to be punctual and faithful in keeping all appointments, and by doing one's best to unravel the riddles of the child's psychopathology and to offer therapeutic understanding so that a happier life can result for the patient.

The opposite side of this coin is encountered when a child brings the therapist a gift. This is also a delicate situation since one should not, in general, accept gifts from patients. However, it may be a severe blow to a child's narcissism if one were to refuse a gift that the child had planned on his or her own. Sometimes a youngster will help mother bake cookies and bring some to the therapist. Not to accept them would be too harmful. It would be best to accept them and inquire about the baking and attempt to get at the child's feelings about bringing the gift. One could also share the cookies with the child and admire the baking.

Large gifts from patients is another issue that should be dealt with in the preparatory phase of work with the parents. Incidentally, parents may unconsciously attempt to bribe the therapist with substantial gifts with some ulterior motive in mind. Rather than accepting the gifts, the therapist should explore the underlying motivations with the parents.

Countertransference Regarding the Demands on the Therapist

There are few types of work that make more severe demands on one's time and energy than therapy with disturbed children and adults. Some therapists complain that their patients feel like "a bunch of leeches sucking them dry." Often therapists' families feel equally the stress of the demands on the dedicated therapist. Being emotionally available to so many people is problematic for some therapists. Dealing with patients' demands and still having time and energy for one's own interests and one's children is often difficult. Sometimes therapists with children the same age as their patients may resent the lack of time and energy to give to their own progeny the same degree of time, play, and empathy as is demanded in therapy of disturbed children. One must attempt to have consideration for the family, keeping in mind the emotional needs of spouse and children, in order that they do not suffer because of dedication to the work with patients.

Countertransference and Vacations

Similarly, therapists often find it quite difficult to allow themselves to take adequate vacations and time off. The demands of one's patients may lead the therapist to feel indispensable, and make it anxiety-producing to plan vacation time. The common reactions of patients who have experienced abandonment early in their lives is one of rage and resentment in response to their therapist's announcement of vacation plans. Often one must pay a penalty of increased anxiety, tension, and resentment by the patients before and after vacations.

However, it should be noted that these interruptions of therapy offer an opportunity to explore in the transference past experiences of rejection and abandonment. Much therapeutic work can surround the therapist's time off. One should not hesitate to take a reasonable amount of time off to avoid the pressures and emotional demands of working with disturbed patients.

Countertransference and the Therapist's Illness

Because therapists often feel that they are indispensable to their patients, a therapist's illness may cause strong countertransference reactions. It is a common fantasy for many therapists to think that they are indestructible, and to suddenly become ill leads to a rude awakening. Anxiety about the effect of an illness on patients is natural and must be dealt with realistically. Most patients are acutely sensitive to any changes in the therapist's appearance, posture, gait, or speech. It is virtually impossible to hide an illness from perceptive patients. Thus an attempt must be made to elicit the patient's reactions to the changes noted in the therapist. Avoidance of the issue will only lead to increased resistance by the patient and will not further the therapeutic work.

SUMMARY

This chapter represents an effort to identify many of the sources of countertransference difficulties encountered in relationship to the work with parents and the child in child analysis and in psychotherapeutic treatment of disturbed children and adolescents. Suggestions on dealing therapeutically with them are offered. Of course, the same tendencies are in operation with disturbed adult patients as well. However, they are more frequently noted and more blatant with young people whose faulty ego and superego control permits the direct expression of more raw and powerful affects and impulses than one encounters in treatment of neurotic adults. In addition, the face-to-face work with children and adolescents who are active and find it difficult to sit still makes therapeutic work with them far more difficult than work with adults, who can employ more inhibition and can sit still or use the couch and talk about their difficulties.

The therapist's personality is the most important single tool in work with children. In addition to theoretical knowledge, one must have a working acquaintance with child development, especially age-appropriate behavior and language. One must also have flexibility; infinite patience; the capacity for empathic understanding of children's communications, behavior, and painful affects; and tolerance for all of the affects encountered in work with disturbed children. The ability to tolerate the patient's anxiety, hostility, sadness, grief, or longing without experiencing anxiety, counterhostility, or despair is an absolute requirement for the successful child therapist. One must also be comfortable with regression, primary-process manifestations, and with oral, anal, and phallic-oedipal impulses.

With therapists who have countertransference difficulties, an unconscious process of self-selection tends to take place. Therapists who find it difficult to tolerate certain types of behavior attempt to avoid accepting those patients in their case load. If such a patient is inadvertently accepted, it usually does not take long for the countertransference problems to bring about a disruption of the treatment relationship and an inevitable premature termination or transfer to another therapist.

Finally, as Prall and Stennis (1964) point out, personal therapy for anyone who is to be involved in work with disturbed patients can be extremely helpful in achieving the degree of self-understanding required to avoid the types of countertransference difficulties discussed above.

It is important for therapists of all theoretical backgrounds to become aware of their own countertransference tendencies and to seek help with overcoming these pitfalls by consultation and/or personal therapy in order to become effective therapists and to avoid inflicting harm on their patients.

REFERENCES

Adler, G.(1986). Psychotherapy of the narcissistic personality disorder patient: two contrasting approaches. *American Journal of Psychiatry* 143:430–436.

Berlin, I. N. (1973). Regression as a phase in psychotherapeutic work with young schizophrenic children. In *Clinical Studies in Childhood Psychoses*, ed. S. A. Szurek and I. N. Berlin, pp. 511–521. New York: Brunner/Mazel.

Bixler, R. H. (1964). Limits are therapy. In *Child Psychotherapy*, ed. M. R. Haworth, pp. 134–147. New York: Basic Books.

Bleiberg, E. (1987). Treatment of narcissistic disorders in children. In *Basic Handbook of Child Psychiatry*, vol. 5, ed. J. D. Call, R. L. Cohen, S. I. Harrison, et al., pp. 443–449. New York: Basic Books.

Casuso, G. (1965). Report of panel on the relationship between child analysis and the theory and practice of adult psychoanalysis. *Journal of the American Psychoanalytic Association* 13:159–171.

Christ, A. E. (1973). Sexual countertransference problems with a psychotic child. In *Clinical Studies in Childhood Psychoses*, ed. S. A. Szurek and I. N. Berlin, pp. 481–497. New York: Brunner/Mazel.

Cummings, N., and Sobel, S. (1985). Malpractice insurance: update on sex claims. *Psychotherapy* 22:186–188.

Ekstein, R., Wallerstein, J., and Mandelbaum, A. (1959). Countertransference in the residential treatment of children. *Psychoanalytic Study of the Child* 14:186–218. New York: International Universities Press.

Freud, A. (1954). The widening scope of indications for psychoanalysis. In *The Writings of Anna Freud*, vol. 4, pp. 356–376. New York: International Universities press, 1968.

Freud, S. (1910). The future prospects of psycho-analytic therapy. *Standard Edition* 11:139–151.

_____ (1915). Observations on transference love. *Standard Edition* 12:159–171.

Herman, J. L., Gartrell, N., Olarte, S., et al. (1987). Psychiatrist–patient sexual contact: results of a national survey, II: psychiatrist's attitudes. *American Journal of Psychiatry* 144:164–169.

Kernberg, O., (1965). Notes on countertransference. *Journal of the American Psychoanalytic Association* 13:38–56.

_____ . (1980). *Internal World and External Reality*. New York: Jason Aronson.

Kilburg, R. R., Nathan, P. E., and Thoreson, R. W., eds. (1986). *Issues, Syndromes, and Solutions in Psychology*. Washington, DC: The American Psychological Association.

Kohut, H., (1971). *The Restoration of the Self*. New York: International Universities Press.

Kramer, S., and Prall, R. C. (1971). A child psychoanalysis training program. In *Separation-Individuation: Essays in Honor of Margaret S. Mahler*, ed. J. B. McDevitt and C. F. Settlage, pp. 486–498. New York: Basic Books.

Loomis, E. A. (1957). The use of checkers in handling resistances in child therapy and child analysis. *Journal of the American Psychoanalytic Association* 5:130–135.

Mahler, M. S. (1960). Personal communication.

_____ (1968). *On Human Symbiosis and the Vicissitudes of Individuation*. Vol. I: *Infantile Psychosis*. New York: International Universities Press.

Pope, K. S., and Bouhoutsos, J. C. (1986). *Sexual Intimacy between Therapists and Patients*. New York: Prager.

Prall, R. C. (1959). Observational research with emotionally disturbed children: session I. (Symposium, 1958.) *The American Journal of Orthopsychiatry* 29:223–249, 560–591.

_____ (1960). Training in orthopsychiatry. Introduction to panel on training in orthopsychiatry. Paper presented at the 37th Annual Meeting of the American Orthopsychiatric Association, February 25, Chicago, IL.

Prall, R. C., and Dealy, M. N. (1965). Countertransference in therapy of childhood psychosis. *Journal of the Hillside Hospital* 14:69–82, January–April.

Prall R. C., and Stennis, W. (1964). Pitfalls in psychotherapy with children. *Pennsylvania Psychiatric Quarterly* 4:3–11, Summer.

Reich, A. (1960). Further remarks on counter-transference. *International Journal of Psycho-Analysis* 41:389–395.

Szurek, S. A., and Berlin, I. N., eds. (1973). *Clinical Studies in Childhood Psychoses.* New York: Brunner/Mazel.

Winnicott, D. W. (1949). Hate in the countertransference. *Collected Papers*, pp. 194–203. London: Tavistock.

Yandell, W. (1973). Therapeutic problems related to the expression of sexual drives in psychotic children. In *Clincal Studies in Childhood Psychoses*, ed. S. A. Szurek and I. N. Berlin, pp. 498–508. New York: Brunner/Mazel.

Zelen, S. L. (1985). Sexualization of therapeutic relationships: the dual vulnerability of patient and therapist. *Psychotherapy* 22:178–185.

10

Termination

Helen R. Beiser, M.D.

Compared with the literature on adult cases, remarkably little has been written on the termination of psychotherapy with neurotic children. The early literature seems to assume that treatment will stop when the symptom for which the child was brought is no longer an issue or, in the case of child analysis, when the child has gone through the same analytic stages as would be expected in adult psychoanalysis. One of the pioneers of the early Child Guidance Clinics, Frederick Allen (1942), writes that every beginning of a child therapy has the goal of ending in mind, which is to help the child participate in making those changes necessary to assume responsibility for his or her own unique life. He also emphasizes the importance of having the child be a part of planning for the termination, requiring that the therapist be sensitive to subtle signals the child may give.

With child analysis as the focus, Anna Freud (1972) writes that between 1954 and 1957 only seventeen analyses out of forty-nine ended by mutual consent of child, parent, and therapist. In thirteen of the cases of early termination there was a geographic move of the family, in eleven the therapist finished a period of training, and in five the patient left during an adolescent stage of revolt. Although she states in 1972 that this has changed, she does not give any new figures. The reasons for the large number of unplanned terminations seem to be differences in goals between therapists and parents. Especially in psychoanalysis, reversal of early pathological personality traits, and resolution of conflicts at all developmental levels as compared with the usual parental wish to remove the presenting symptoms, probably accounts for the frequency of unplanned terminations. Another problem may develop when the therapist who wants to prevent all future psychological problems prolongs the therapy longer than is desired by the parent.

In 1980, Sandler and colleagues summarized the goals of the Hampstead Clinic founded by Anna Freud as those of restoring the child to the path of normal development, resolving the transference to the analyst, and helping the child adapt to school and home as judged by child, parents, and school. In 1965, Ekstein (1972), in a paper devoted to general problems of termination of analysis, noted that all child analysts complain of "incomplete analyses," and quoted Margaret Mahler as considering child analysis to be "intermittent." One wonders if treatment of a child ever has a clear-cut termination. Some of the differences of opinion seem related to the questions about including educational or other "therapy" techniques in a child analysis, and whether parents should be included. However, I have found the same frequency of unplanned terminations or intermittent therapy in cases where child analysis was not the treatment modality.

ISSUES IN TERMINATION

The foregoing review of a very scanty literature, as well as my own experience in a state clinic, in various social agencies, in my own private practice, and in supervision of child psychotherapy and child psychoanalysis, may help to focus on the major issues in the termination of treatment of neurotic children. First, there are many variations in what are reasonable goals or purposes for psychotherapy and/or psychoanalysis. Termination occurs when the goal is reached, but what goal? Is symptom relief enough? What about resolving various levels of developmental conflicts? Should one try to help a child adapt to parents, school, and peers, or focus on them adapting to the child? How much can a basic character or personality be changed? What is an appropriate developmental level for a given child? Can later psychological problems be prevented by early childhood therapy? Perhaps it is more important that the therapist, child, parent, and the referral source, usually a school, have some agreement about goals. I once did a preliminary study, never completed, that the most satisfactory treatment results were obtained when there was basic agreement among all of the above as to what the problems of the child were, and why therapy was being undertaken.

This leads to the next issue in termination, namely, in what way and to what extent others in the child's life have been involved in the therapy. If, as preferred by many child analysts, there has been an almost total exclusion of all others, the decision for termination is almost entirely up to the child and the analyst. Although this may sound ideal, it does not prevent a parent from suddenly withdrawing a child from treatment. At the other extreme, the therapist may have instituted contact with parents, other relatives, school, physician, and so on, all of whom become part of the decision for termination. There is a danger in such a situation of the child's input being left out, as emphasized by Allen (1942) and Sandler (1980), and leaving the child feeling totally dependent on the decisions of adults. It may be difficult for a therapist to be aware of any resentment by parents and others of the relationship of the child to the therapist, but such resentment can culminate in the sudden disruption of treatment. In such cases, no time is allowed for the child to work through what has become a very meaningful real as well as therapeutic relationship, and the time of therapy may be largely wasted. My own attitude is that some lines of communication need to be established, either by telephone or by short interviews on demand. If such lines have been established during therapy, so that parents have felt free to inform the therapist of serious events in the family, and schools have been able to inform the therapist of serious behavior that might lead to suspension, then parents are more likely to participate more constructively in the termination process.

Another major issue to be considered is whether the therapy is planned to be time limited, or allowed to go on to what can be called a "natural" termination. Therapy may be limited to a certain number of sessions, or a specific number of weeks or months. Such limits may be imposed by third-party payers, because of other financial reasons, or by the policy of a given clinic or therapist. It is probable that individual therapists with such a policy are trying to avoid the process of termination or are afraid of cases being interminable. The opposite philosophy occurs when therapists want to achieve the greatest depth, or the greatest likelihood for perfect prevention of future pathology. In my experience, these latter therapists are not limited to psychoanalysts. Termination based on the achievement of goals requires careful observation, knowledge of development stages, and special technical handling of the termination process. Time-limited therapy has its own technical demands and advantages. The goals must be set much more sharply and must be constantly reviewed. This may avoid some of the resistances often seen in long-term, open-ended therapy. Confusion over goals can be clarified, and direct suggestions made to persons in the child's environment for changes that in turn would lead to the desired changes in the child. My own personal experience with time-limited therapy has been largely with college students who have only their summer vacation to work on a problem. Some of them have returned later for further therapy that would allow for a natural termination.

PROCESS IN NATURAL OR LONG-TERM THERAPY TERMINATION

Setting the Time

I will limit the present discussion to the termination of treatment with neurotic children, with the understanding that children with severe developmental disabilities or character disorders with acting out would not be handled in the same way. When the major goals of treatment have been accomplished, it is time to begin a process of termination. How does the therapist know when this has happened? First, there is an awareness of a greater level of comfort in the child–therapist relationship along with a lack of complaints from parents and/or school. The child will give some signal that he or she is ready to stop. It is rarely very direct, especially if a very close and positive working relationship has developed between child and therapist. Depending on the age or stage of development, the child will show an interest in activities outside the therapy, different from when such interests were considered resistance earlier in treatment. The preschool child may talk about pleasurable play with peers. The school-aged child also talks about increased activities with peers, and how the therapy time interferes. A teenager may do the same, but also may miss an appointment and talk about the rival activities at the next interview. These activities may include parties, youth organizations, athletic activities, cheerleading, and so on. It is doubtful if a time clash with a favorite television program should be included. I have had teenagers bring friends to wait for them during an interview. If the therapist can accept such activities as evidence of growth and not necessarily of resistance, the possibility of termination can be brought out in the open. This allows for a review of the accomplishments in therapy, perhaps setting up other goals to be worked on, or agreeing to a termination date.

For example, a 10-year-old boy who had come because of enuresis and difficulties with peers was an interesting combination of macho masculinity and softness, as expressed by his burying his face in my fur coat hanging in the toy closet. One day he triumphantly announced that he no longer wet the bed and asked if he could stop coming so he could play more football. I told him he had certainly accomplished something very important, but he had just begun to tell me about his feelings toward his little brother, which were also important. He hung his head, said "Me and my big mouth," and agreed to continue. A little later, he put so much pressure on me to stop that I agreed to it after my return from a midwinter vacation. To our mutual surprise, he started to cry. This allowed us to continue for another 6 months to allow him to work on his feelings about being abandoned because of his demandingness, and the termination was agreed upon to coincide with the end of the school year. From later reports, he made a better late-adolescent adjustment than his brother, who had not been symptomatic enough to require treatment.

Another boy, aged 9, was in intensive treatment because of thumb-sucking and fears of going to bed. His mother was psychotic but very supportive of treatment. When he was 12, he started a pattern of chronic lateness to his sessions. When I investigated, he said 5 minutes was due to his unorganized mother, 5 minutes because of his very busy professional father, and 5 minutes because of him. Actually, he was beginning to enjoy his junior high school activities, and we agreed to stop. Two years later he returned in an anxiety state, and we resumed treatment. Throughout his high school years we worked on his fears of perhaps needing to assume responsibility for his mother and younger siblings. He learned from me that all women were not like his mother, and that he had choices that could be his alone. We terminated before he left for college. Several years later he dropped by to tell me he was moving to another part of the country to pursue his career.

If the first signal has come from the child, it is then necessary to talk with parents, and perhaps school officials, to tell them of the possibility of termination. In the process, problems might come out that the child did not mention. These can be discussed with the child and further work arranged, if necessary. For example, if it comes to light that the child has not been doing homework, he or she can be told that this will be necessary before termination can take place. The therapist must be careful not to ask the child to fit into all the demands of the environment, but such adjustment that will benefit the child in the long run can be requested.

The comfort or needs of the child and the demands of the environment can also be considered in setting the time of the termination. It is often convenient for all if termination is synchronized with school terms or family vacation plans. The latter may bring to light problems within the family, such as the patient being either the aggressor or victim of siblings. Even if therapy of an individual child is not officially "family therapy," one can still work toward better functioning of the family as a whole.

Some schools may also be brought into the termination process. The elementary school of a boy from a wealthy family with a tradition of sending its youngsters to an eastern boarding school for secondary education stated that he was too immature and poorly prepared for such at the point of graduation. His parents agreed to keep him in his local private school for the first year of high school with special emphasis on academic preparation, while I worked on his fear of growing up because of the multiple early deaths in the males in his family. Later he initiated contact with me during a school vacation and again after he finished college, to thank me and apprise me of his achievements. The last I heard, he was a law clerk to a local judge.

Sometimes the parent is not satisfied with the results of treatment, even when the child and the therapist agree that it can be stopped. I saw a very disturbed child with a phobia of insects and very poor peer relationships between the ages of 7 and 12, when she seemed to fit into her preadolescent group quite well. We stopped at that point but resumed when she began to get into the drug culture in high school. She improved again and went to a small, prestigious college from which she eventually graduated with very high grades. Her mother was very upset when she subsequently went west and took menial jobs, not utilizing her education. I saw each of them occasionally and learned from the girl that, in her view, "My mother thinks I am smarter than I am. I just memorize very well for exams." She received some therapy in her new location while I continued to help her mother accept her with her limitations. Several years later I was invited to her wedding, and her mother seemed quite pleased with her. Perhaps Mahler was right about "intermittent therapy."

Terminating with adolescents may be particularly difficult, as parents are rarely satisfied with the results. Even if they are correct in their assessment of the remaining pathology, it is best to go along with the young person unless there is some real danger in stopping. Keeping the termination a positive experience would more likely allow the patient to seek further therapy as an adult, if that becomes necessary. Although I have not had such an experience personally except with the very short, time-limited therapy of a freshman college student who returned several years later because she feared having children, others have seen patients who had previous therapy as children or adolescents. A colleague told me about a young child I had analyzed who came in young adulthood for problems of relationships. She had been such a difficult child that I believe the therapy experience greatly helped her seek therapy on her own as an adult.

Process and Content during the Termination Phase

The content of treatment interviews during the phase when termination has been agreed upon is different from the beginning and middle phases of treatment. After a varying amount of time when improvement continues or remains stable, there may be a replay of the symptoms or behavior for which treatment was initiated. This can be very disturbing for all concerned, especially if such occurs at home or at school. The therapist as well as others in the environment may wonder if the decision to terminate was correct. With some patience, however, such a replay may deepen understanding of the behavior, and it usually passes much more rapidly than it did at the beginning of treatment. After this resolution, and shortly before the actual termination date, there is opportunity to review the treatment and its accomplishments.

With preadolescent children I developed a technique of giving each child a box of his or her own to save drawings, game scores, and other productions made during the course of treatment, suitably dated. Although periodic reviews of this material may take place during the course of treatment, an unusual opportunity for review presents itself when the contents of the box are sorted chronologically a session or two before the child actually leaves. Situations in which important therapeutic gains took place can be recalled. A sequence of drawings can be particularly significant. For example, a phobic boy who had drawn many cars with rockets and other violent appendages, accompanied with appropriate violent fantasy, began to draw ordinary cars, one with a benign policeman. As we reviewed his drawings, he asked me if I remembered the day I had taken off his shoes to prevent him from kicking me in his efforts to leave the office. His affect indicated that he now perceived me as the benign policeman. Going through the box also shows the child's increasing cognitive abilities in the pattern of improving game scores. Decisions can be made as to what the therapist would like to keep as part of the case record, what the child would like to take home as a memento of the therapy, and what can be discarded. Although there may be some recurrence of old power struggles over the distribution, usually the child is pleased that the therapist values the work enough to want to keep it.

There may be ambivalence in the child, the parent, or both about stopping, especially if the therapeutic relationship has been long and very positive. The therapist may be similarly ambivalent. All may wonder if the child and/or family can get along without therapy. This is usually handled by the expression of desire for some future contact. Although the door may be left open, such contacts should not be pressed. I have found that if termination has been set for the end of the school year, a follow-up appointment can be scheduled in the fall. Most of the time, especially if the vacation has been a pleasant one, the child is distanced in his or her attachment to the therapist, and desires no further contact. As demonstrated in previous examples, if the door is left open, further necessary contacts may be sought, even years later, when new problems arise.

THE POSTTREATMENT PERIOD

There are various possibilities for handling situations after treatment has been officially terminated. As above, a common one is to have one follow-up session after an interval and determine whether the child has maintained the improvement. Some do terminate and never are heard from again. In a meaningful treatment, when therapist and family remain in the same geographic area, some further professional contact is frequent. If so it is often apparent that the child seen as the first patient was at least not the only problem. I have sometimes decided to take a parent into treatment, or referred one or both parents, either for their own problems or to advise on child-rearing issues, relating to either the original patient or other children in the family. Sometimes treatment of another child is indicated. Although some therapists will treat such a child, I have felt uncomfortable in this role, feeling that I might be betraying the original patient. I will either refer the other child to someone else or try to help both through advising the parent. Contact of this sort may last for years, as in the case of the girl whose wedding I attended.

Sometimes there is indirect contact through mutual friends. I started treatment with the phobic boy who kicked me after his mother had had a cancer operation. In treatment he worked through his feelings that his hostility had made her sick. When she died several years after his terminating treatment, I learned through mutual friends that he worked through her death better than his siblings who had had no treatment.

Another boy had a more complicated situation. When he was 5, his mother had died of a mysterious illness, which his grandmother had told him was from having another child. He showed difficult behavior when his stepmother was pregnant, and she brought him for therapy just before her second pregnancy. He was able to work through his concerns about his part, as well as that of pregnancy, in the death of his mother, and he developed a very meaningful relationship to me, even wanting to name the new baby sister after me, so that it was surprising when he and his stepmother made it impossible to continue after the birth of the baby. Several years later the parents made contact with me when he reacted severely to the death of the family dog, which father had concealed from him just as he did the death of his mother. He refused to see me at this time, so I gave the parents advice as to how to handle this, as well as some understanding of the relationship to his mother's death. I also now understood why they had stopped after his stepmother delivered a baby without any problems. To my real surprise, he made contact with me 20 years later, wanting me to see his son, who was now the same age he had been when he first saw me. The problem was not related to the death of the boy's mother, but there had been a divorce. I did very brief therapy at that time with father and son.

These examples illustrate the possibilities that exist between an ideal of treating a child so ideally well that no treatment ever need be necessary again, and keeping the door open for help when new problems arise or the old problems are reactivated. This can take place when the therapist is a private practitioner who stays put. Knowledge from a past treatment can shorten any subsequent treatment. The situation can be quite different, however, in an agency or clinic. When a former patient is heard from, there is a tendency to take that person or family back into treatment with a new therapist who may want to do a better job than was done the first time, and start the treatment process all over again, with considerable loss of efficiency.

UNPLANNED TERMINATIONS

As has been indicated, there are a great many unplanned terminations of child therapy. In order to cut down their number, the possible causes, which may be multiple, must be reviewed. I thought at first that they were more common in clinic cases, because of the generally lower socioeconomic level of the clinic population, and also because of the number of therapists in training. When I went into private practice, however, the unplanned terminations, as well as the numbers of cases who refused the recommendation for therapy, were only slightly fewer. In reaction to this, I found that I tried to give as much specific help as possible during the evaluation process, so that some change could be effected in case there was resistance to the recommendation for long-term therapy or psychoanalysis. In fact, I once was able to stop enuresis in a very intelligent 6-year-old girl, after a history-taking interview with her parents, by telling her she was old enough to go to the toilet if she had such an urge during the night. This was followed up with one more interview with her parents to support more mature expectations. However, the frustrations of having a family abruptly stop long-term therapy, especially in the midst of an improvement, are worth looking at in more detail. All parties involved may have a role in such an occurrence.

The Child

Although many children are resistant to going into therapy in the first place, some may develop resistance after a period of good therapeutic work. This may be evidence of discomfort with the issues being brought up in therapy, such as facing hostility rather than seeing themselves as victims. Another cause is a fear of intimacy, as the relationship to the therapist deepens. Some children, as part of their character structure, tend to get into power struggles with adults, including the therapist. The parent is very important in dealing with the resistance of a child, and if supportive of the treatment, can help the child–especially before adolescence–to come while working through the resistance. In the adolescent, it is more of a problem, as the parent really cannot force the child to come. Also, it is part of normal adolescent development to detach from important adults, as an intimate relationship may not be possible without the adolescent seeing it as a threat of regression. If a child of any age has been accustomed to winning in power struggles with parents, he or she will probably also win in such a struggle with a therapist.

Parents

Although parents are always involved when the resistance seems to arise primarily in the child, they may also stop treatment for other reasons. If the child shows considerable fondness for the therapist, a parent may become jealous and feel threatened or left out. He or she may feel possessive and resent the therapist who is able to obtain the child's positive regard. I expected this from the psychotic mother of a thumb-sucking boy, but her wishes to help him were stronger than her wishes to possess him. He said to me once when she called to give him a message, "You and my mother are so different, I don't understand why she likes you."

In another situation a parent may resent the attention the patient is getting from the therapist (as well as the cost in time and money) and want it for himself or herself. Such feelings are rarely expressed openly because of shame over dependent longings, and therefore are communicated by not letting the child have the therapy. After I found a 6-year-old girl taking candy from the therapy room and giving it to her mother, I arranged for a therapist for the mother. Such disruptions often occur after there has been symptomatic improvement and interfere with the gradual working through of the child's attachment to the therapist in the final phase of treatment. Some of the frustration for the therapist and damage to the child can be avoided if the feelings of the parent are explored and considered when therapy is first recommended for a child. Similarly, parents' expectations of treatment should be explored, and if these are markedly different from those of the therapist, some correction need be made. Sometimes a parent's expectation from treatment is to assure the child's happiness, which is quite unrealistic. Sometimes each parent has different expectations. If the father wants an aggressive macho boy, and the mother wants a well-behaved little gentleman, the therapist may be caught in the middle. Divorced fathers who are ordered by the court to pay for necessary treatment may stop abruptly if they see the therapist as mother's ally and their enemy. I struggled with a father who put hockey practice ahead of the therapy, in spite of the mother's desire to continue treatment. Similarly, a therapist may have a different idea of an appropriate level of development than does either parent.

The Therapist

Sometimes a therapist inadvertently causes the disruption of treatment by using techniques that are too uncomfortable for a child or family to tolerate. Rapid confrontation of a child's or parent's behavior may produce disruption of the treatment. Also, the early interpretation of what the therapist considers repressed feelings that are unacceptable to the child may make further treatment impossible. For example, the 13-year-old daughter of a woman who had been divorced twice and who had a very close relationship to this only child totally denied any hostile feelings toward her mother. She had left a previous therapist who told her she must be angry with her mother and should express it. It took her 2 more years to deal with this hostility. I once frightened off a prospective treatment case by telling the mother that the phobias of children are often related to phobias in a parent, and inviting her to tell me what she was afraid of.

A different problem is when some therapists, in their desire to achieve a positive therapeutic alliance with a child, may be seen as seductive by the child or the parent. In these days of frequent accusa-

tions of sexual abuse, a hug or any physical touching may be misinter-
preted. When a child is seductive, care must be taken not to respond in
ways that might lead to sexual arousal. There is a particular danger if the
therapist perceives that a parent is neglectful or cold. As well as physical
affection, gift giving, if excessive, or extratherapeutic contacts may be
seen as seductive or a threat to the child–parent relationship. The same
care needs to be exercised if a parent is seductive.

Overambition on the part of a therapist may also cause an earlier-
than-planned termination. Many therapists, especially those with
strong psychoanalytic leanings, want to continue, to explore the theoretical earliest stages of development. They may provide nursing bottles
to relive the oral stage, encourage messing to traverse the anal stage,
and sexually explicit dolls to help the child express oedipal feelings.
They feel that symptom relief will not hold up unless all stages of
development with their specific conflicts have been thoroughly analyzed. Such regressive play may frighten the child or parents unless the
therapist's goal has been agreed to at the beginning of the therapy. If
therapy is broken off prematurely, the resultant inability to resolve the
real relationship between child and therapist may be more damaging
than possible gains from traversing early stages of development.

Some families will terminate treatment with trainees or inexperienced
therapists and may not be able to tell why, again interfering with a
termination process. On the other hand, it can be surprising how long
some families will stay with an inexperienced therapist, forgiving them
for a degree of clumsiness because of their strong investment in the
welfare of the child.

Other Factors

A variety of other factors may produce an unplanned termination. A
school may stop giving permission for a child to miss classes after the
presenting symptom disappears. In those cases in which the symptom
has never appeared in school, such as enuresis or night fears, schools
may be reluctant to allow early dismissal for any length of time. I once
encountered a school that allowed time off only for acute illnesses, and
not for "therapy or piano lessons." More recently, however, schools
may be almost too tolerant of absences for therapy. Although public
humiliation of a child in therapy is not usual anymore, if other children
tease such a child it may produce such resistance that the child will insist
on terminating treatment.

If not clarified in the beginning, the contract with third-party payers may not cover the length of treatment desired. The therapist needs to investigate the ability and willingness of parents to pay for the continuation of therapy. Even some affluent parents are unwilling to pay those expenses not covered by third-party payers.

When the therapist is in a training program, other factors may be involved. The supervisor may require more treatment than the family is willing to support, catching the student therapist in the middle. More likely, the student therapist wishes to do more and, in spite of help from a supervisor, cannot read the signs given by the child and family indicating they wish termination.

The training program itself may require a length or depth of treatment that is not acceptable to the family. For example, psychoanalytic training requires that a child be seen four times a week. Any resultant problems in transportation, school attendance, payment, and/or social activities might lead a family to terminate prematurely. In some programs, students are judged by their ability to have a child come regularly, or for a specified period of time, which may not fit the goals of the family.

INCREASING THE PROPORTION OF PLANNED TERMINATIONS

Positive Relationships with Adults in the Environment

Although some techniques have already been indicated in the discussion of the causes of unplanned terminations, it is advisable to elaborate on some of them. It is well to emphasize that no child comes to treatment on his own. He or she depends on others for payment for treatment, for support at times of resistance, and often for transportation. The need for confidentiality is often used as the rationale for the therapist's not communicating with parents, school authorities, doctors, or other adults in authority or with influence. In some families, grandparents are more significant than parents. Others may also be in the position of immediate caretakers. In my experience, children, with the exception of adolescents, expect the adults in their environment to communicate with each other about their problems, and generally expect that communication to be for their benefit. Those adolescents who seek help without parents, and those adolescents who are seen with the permission of parents but without the parents' being included in the evaluation process, often terminate their treatment prematurely. Including the parents early is more likely to allow a proper termination process. The content of the communication requires great care and judgment. Especially with adolescents, I always inform the child about what I am going to talk about with their parents. In general, the communication should keep the welfare of the child foremost in mind.

Special communications need to be addressed to the referral source, whether school, physician, or court. These sources not only expect some information when they refer, but also may be of assistance in keeping the child in treatment as long as is necessary. Judicious contact with them–especially with the school, even if it has not been the primary referral source–can be helpful in establishing positive relationships between families and community institutions. This can be of value to the child both during and after treatment.

Third-party payers also need to be taken into consideration. Insurance companies often request information, and if this is not given, may limit or deny payment, resulting in premature termination. I prefer not to receive payment from insurance companies directly, but encourage parents to clarify their benefits and collect from the company. The therapist's contract is with the parent or guardian, not with the third-party payer. When the parent is given more responsibility, he or she is more likely to support therapy if the length is prolonged beyond the contract. It should be noted that if the contract is with the parent, insurance companies should not be charged for missed appointments. Most third-party payers are sincerely interested in the welfare of the child patient, and a respectful response to their requests can be educational, making it easier for other coverage in this area to be possible.

The most important contact to be established and maintained, however, is with the parent or guardian. When agreement is reached for long-term therapy, they can be informed that therapy optimally needs to be continued beyond the point of symptom relief. Guidelines need to be established for contacts during the course of therapy. The therapist needs to know about major incidents in the child's life, such as a death in the family, suspension from school, and so on. If the parent's concerns need more than a brief telephone call or short interview at the time the child is brought, it may be advisable to refer the parent for therapy for himself or herself. If poor parenting techniques seem to be the major problem, a therapist must be chosen who is skilled in this area. It is particularly important to tell the parent, as well as referral sources, that termination is being contemplated. This not only informs the therapist of any problems that might still be addressed, also gets the cooperation and support of the parent during the termination phase.

Accepting the Child's Growth

In order to have a smooth termination, it is necessary to note and accept signs of the child's growth and improvement. Some therapists see the wish of the child to attend other activities only as resistance, which can undermine the improvements made and may upset the child and/or family enough to have them terminate prematurely. It certainly interferes with the final termination phase when improvements should be consolidated, and separation from the therapist should be accomplished in a positive way. The activity must be phase appropriate and positive, such as nursery school for the very young child, or some after-school activity for the latency-aged child and the adolescent. For the latter, summer camp or a part-time job may also be a positive activity that the therapy has allowed to take place.

Negotiation may be needed. There might be a family plan to move away, even back to a distant country. The timing may consider the improvement of the child, and time to help the child adjust to the move. A family struggling with a decision whether to return to their Middle Eastern country of origin delayed the decision to accommodate the treatment needs of their son. It was necessary for me as well as for the boy to know their plans, because learning baseball to improve his peer relationships would be necessary if he returned to his homeland.

Flexibility in Establishing Goals

This is similar to the above. It is hard for some therapists to accept goals of child or family that do not fit with their own value systems. For example, I once saw an older adolescent girl referred by the family physician because she wished to have breast reduction surgery. After I explained to her the problems she might encounter in nursing children, but agreed to listen to her reasons, she was able to persuade me of the reasonableness of her wish. She found her breasts were so heavy that she was in considerable physical discomfort, and she had found the teasing she had undergone during he entire adolescence about the sexual nature of her development most unpleasant. She was willing to accept the risks of surgery, and I was able to support her decision with her parents and her doctor on the basis of the psychological benefit.

Older adolescents frequently set goals for themselves that may seem unrealistic to the therapist. Attempting to force a change will produce termination, but alternatives can be suggested. College students can be warned of the improbability of being able to continue the relationship with a high school sweetheart when the young people are going to widely separated colleges. However, love has been known to survive such separations. More usually, there are students starting high school with ambitions not backed up by achievement in the necessary course work. Such situations may be particularly difficult if parents have strong needs to see the child succeed in certain ways that are either impossible or too stressful for the child. Fathers who wish a son in their own image, in a certain profession or an athletic career, may put pressure on a therapist to also move in this direction. The mother of a teenager I saw wanted her son to become the concert pianist she had not been. He managed to get into police trouble, but after a year of court-ordered therapy he made his own decision to continue his musical studies, and avoided further delinquent behavior. In his therapy we considered many alternatives, but he really was a talented musician. It can also be a surprise how, with extremely hard work, some young people can achieve their goals with less than superior abilities.

Flexibility includes settling for symptom relief, if that is all that child, parents, and school will support. The therapist's acceptance will allow the termination to be as positive as possible, and the child—or more usually, the adolescent—can be informed that he or she can seek further therapy, if necessary, as an independent adult.

EXCESSIVE PROLONGATION OF TREATMENT

So far, undue shortening of treatment has been considered. Anna Freud (1972) felt that this is far more common than undue prolongation. However, there are also situations when treatment seems to continue beyond a reasonable point. Many factors may be involved.

Undue Dependence on Therapy

The child and/or parents may become unduly dependent on the therapist or on the therapy itself. This may be particularly true if the goal of therapy has been accepted as prevention of all future problems.

Sometimes the therapy is almost like an addiction. This is not common in neurotic cases, and in some cases of a borderline or psychotic nature, lifelong supportive therapy may be necessary to avoid institutionalization. In dependent personalities with neurotic symptoms, new treatment may be sought rather than looking for strengths derived from the first treatment experience. If a different therapist is contacted, care must be taken that the first therapist is not criticized as a failure, but that strengths sought are clarified before starting on a new treatment phase. Even children can use a call for therapy to avoid going to school, or other kinds of responsibility. A special case is for the parents of a developmentally retarded child to seek psychotherapy or psychoanalysis to remove a "block" to learning. I have treated such children if they also were depressed, and then instigated termination when that problem was relieved and further therapy was unrealistic. Such families are most likely to seek further help from a new therapist, who needs to be careful not to offer help beyond the child's abilities.

Countertransference Problems in the Therapist

Although countertransference is usually seen as a negative attitude toward a patient, arising either from the provocativeness in a patient or from the therapist's own pathology, there may also be an unrealistically positive attitude toward a patient, causing reluctance in the therapist to stop seeing the child. Often there is an accompanying negative attitude toward the parent, and a wish to rescue the child from a "bad" parent. The common cause for such attitudes is an unresolved negative relationship of the therapist with his or her own parent or parents. When this is extreme, such a therapist is bound to fail as a therapist of children, given that such an important part of the job is to improve the parent–child relationship.

Another countertransference problem is a characterological perfectionism. The therapist always perceives more issues that the child should deal with before terminating. Aside from prolonging treatment, such an attitude also puts a burden on a child to make changes that may not be possible. Similarly, anxiety about the stability or solidity of improvements may make a therapist reluctant to stop therapy.

Special problems may be seen in trainee therapists. They may strive for treatment of a certain length, or for a certain type of termination. Many feel guilt at the idea they have not done enough by the end of their training period, and arrange for a transfer to another therapist. If this is another student, another set of countertransference problems may arise and further prolong treatment. I once consulted on a case with a social worker who had never seen a case terminated except by geographic move of family or worker. Before routine administrative reviews at the time of transfer were instituted at the state clinic previously mentioned, transfers often took place yearly, and parents vied with each other as to the number of therapists they had worked with. Workers also seemed to see long treatments as a status symbol, apparently as closer to the model of psychoanalysis.

It is possible that some of the abrupt terminations seen in child therapy are reactions to these or other countertransference problems, as well as to the prolonged treatments supporting the dependency of families. If countertransference problems of a serious nature are seen during the course of training, therapy for the therapist may be advisable. Trained therapists who encounter similar problems repeatedly may seek therapy on their own.

Institutional Needs

Some institutions set up a rigid pattern for the length of treatment. Although these usually have the goal of shortening treatment, some lengthen it. A child or adolescent is fitted into a program rather than a program being devised according to the needs of an individual child. I have seen this more often in inpatient than outpatient settings, with 30-day programs for drug abuse, for example. Although such programs are more often seen for borderline diagnoses or conduct disorders, they may also be encountered for neurotic depressions. The struggle over the length of treatment may interfere with the optimal participation of the patient and family in the termination process, or transfer to another type of treatment. Part of the decision for termination of inpatient treatment needs to be consideration of the reentry of the child into the school, and the impact of questions from peers.

Financial Exploitation

Unfortunately, the availability of third-party payers has produced financial exploitation both by therapists and by institutions. When a contract is a generous one, there is a tendency to use all of it. Even parents may push for that, to relieve themselves of guilt over having a disturbed child. If careful clinical criteria are not used in admission and discharge of patients, a child's lifetime benefits can easily be used up in one hospitalization. It is to be remembered that the most appropriate treatment is not necessarily the longest or the most expensive. Neurotic children are not an important part of the controversy over excessive use of the psychiatric hospital.

SUMMARY

Termination of psychotherapy with a neurotic child or adolescent is a complex process that may be either planned or unplanned. Planned termination may occur by limiting the time, or number of interviews, or "naturally," that is, when the goals of treatment have been accomplished. So-called natural terminations take place through mutual agreement among child, parent, and therapist. Enough additional time is required to allow for a review of the treatment process and resolve the real relationship between child and therapist. Unplanned premature terminations occur frequently in child therapy because of various problems in the child, his or her environment, and the therapist. Overly prolonged treatment may also be a problem, and can distort the termination process.

REFERENCES

Allen, F. H. (1942). *Psychotherapy with Children*. New York: W. W. Norton.

Ekstein, R. (1972). Working through and termination of analysis. *Journal of the American Psychoanalytic Association* 13:69–73.

Freud, A. (1972). Problems of termination in child analysis. In *Problems of Psychoanalytic Technique and Therapy, 1966–1970*, pp. 3–21. London: Hogarth.

Sandler, J., Kennedy, H., and Tyson, R. L. (1980). *The Technique of Child Psychoanalysis: Discussions with Anna Freud*. London: Hogarth.

INDEX